ALL YOUR MEDICAL QUESTIONS ANSWERED

ALL YOUR MEDICAL QUESTIONS ANSWERED

Lester L. Coleman, M.D.

GRAMERCY PUBLISHING COMPANY
NEW YORK

Library of Congress Cataloging in Publication Data

Coleman, Lester Laudy, 1907–
All your medical questions answered.

    Reprint. Originally published: Good Housekeeping all
your medical questions answered. New York, N.Y.: Good
Housekeeping Books, c1977.
    Includes index.
    1. Medicine, Popular—Miscellanea. I. Title.
RC82.C64   1982   610   81-13470
ISBN 0-517-36951-6 (Crown)   AACR2

This edition is published by Gramercy Publishing Co.
distributed by Crown Publishers, Inc.
by arrangement with Hearst Books.
h g f e d c b a
GRAMERCY EDITION 1982

To Leb

ACKNOWLEDGMENT

My gratitude and devotion to Ken Giniger, Joe D'Angelo, Kay Sullivan, Jim Fisher, Tommy Thompson, Felicia Coleman and Tom Pritchard, an admirable collection of editors, publishers, friends, a wife and a collator who converted the responsibility of writing and collecting these medical columns into an inexhaustible joy.

L.L.C.

Foreword

There is no subject more fascinating to an individual than himself and certainly no subject more important to him than the state of his health.

And because in this country there are so many men and women concerned with their well-being, the phenonomen of the medical column has come about. This is a nation of shortcuts. If one can save the time involved in going to a doctor's office or the hours spent in a hospital emergency room, so much the better. Getting the answer to one's health problems via a newspaper—that's the ticket. After all, we have columns providing advice to the lovelorn, to investors, to gardeners, to cooks, to hobbyists of all kinds, so why not a keep-well column?

I started writing "Speaking of Your Health" fifteen years ago. The first few newspapers that carried the column sent me my weekly batch of reader mail tied in string. I answered each query at great length.

Today, my column is syndicated in 450 newspapers throughout the United States and Canada, Europe and South America. The average number of letters I receive each month runs into the thousands. That little piece of string has stretched quite a bit.

But as the volume of reader mail has increased, so has my concern with those readers. I make it a point to read and reply in my columns to the vast majority of mail that crosses my desk. Obviously, when someone asks whether or not a boil should be lanced, there is a brief, specific answer that suits the situation. But then there are the readers with very special problems who look to me for help. Theirs are the questions that take considered thought and judgment and the best advice I can give.

Why do people write to me, a physician they may never see face to face, someone they may not know very much about? The truth is many people regard their own health problems as terribly special, totally confidential. They do not want to talk about them to a doctor who might also treat their relatives and neighbors. They want to be sure that whatever it is they might reveal is held in confidence. And somehow they regard the mail and a printed response as the acme of confidentiality. They feel free to ask me the most serious or the most trivial questions, things they would probably never ask their own personal physician.

Incidentally, I would like to make it clear that when I answer my readers, I make it a point to avoid describing specific symptoms in detail. I know from experience that there is no speedier way to "contract" a disease than to read about all its symptoms. You'd be amazed at the number of patients who arrive at a doctor's offices positive they have tuberculosis or a heart irregularity. Once the doctor tests them and finds absolutely nothing to substantiate their convictions, he checks up on their daily routine. Invariably, it turns out that patients are overwhelmed by the man-made advertising threats to their emotional health. Posters abound with scare statistics of every conceivable illness.

I avoid going into specific details on disease symptoms in my column. Otherwise, I might outdo the Pied Piper and start a whole march of sick citizens on the way to the hospital in Hamelin.

But for those who regard the subject of health and medicine, especially new medical advances, as all-important, I have compiled this book. Some may recognize in it their own personal and family health problems spelled out in its questions and answers. Other readers may need reinforcement to help in convincing those around them of sensible health decisions. It is for all these men and women that I have prepared this book, a book that I particularly want to supplement and reinforce the relationship between patient and doctor, and open new vistas to individuals experiencing ill health or surrounded by illness.

The book represents a distillation of the most significant, most-often-asked questions from many readers. It is my sincere hope that the advice it provides will be of help to those who identify with the questions and that my oft-repeated admonition goes not unheeded. Read, ponder, and apply my advice if you will—but nonetheless, consult your own doctor. In the final analysis, he knows you best.

Lester L. Coleman, M.D.

Contents

ALL YOUR MEDICAL QUESTIONS ANSWERED

Chapter I

The Doctor-Patient Relationship

An eighty-nine-year-old woman who has been a patient of mine for twenty years recently gave me the ultimate accolade I could hope for in the doctor-patient relationship. As she was leaving my office, she turned and said to me: "Even though you don't do anything for me, you make me feel good, so I love you."

Although her statement cannot possibly be interpreted as a testimony to my medical wizardry, it does highlight the importance of an interpersonal communication between patient and physician. The gentle influence of one person on another is fundamental to the art of healing.

The dynamic interplay between physician and patient begins at the moment of initial contact. From then on, the communication process either develops or, by decay, rapidly deteriorates to eventual destruction. Of course, the third possibility exists that the relationship may remain static and without vitality.

The two dominant forces in the equation of a doctor-patient relationship must recognize their own interacting responsibilities to preserve adequate and valuable communication.

Even the basis for correct diagnosis and treatment must be closely allied to the adequacy of this relationship as it crystallizes during early visits. When patients present themselves for consultation, often their emotions are in a state of disarray. They may be fearful, untrusting, defensive, confused, even hostile.

Responses like these may result from the accumulation of anxieties, and the force with which they are liberated may produce a counter reaction on the part of the physician. Such a response does an injustice to the rapport that should be established early in the relationship.

It is virtually impossible to explain why some patients can reveal their innermost thoughts to one doctor and not to another. To attempt to explain it is to explain the vagaries and subtleties of society at large.

Distortion of communication is probably the single factor that interferes with the growth and expansion of the doctor-patient relationship.

It is estimated that one-third of all patients who present themselves to a physician have no somatic or physical disease to account for their complaints, illnesses or incapacities. Still another third have symptoms which are in part dependent on emotional factors. This group includes those with body disease in which a psychological factor materially adds to the disability and the prolongation of the illness. The last third are those with predominant body disease which may or may not have an overtone of psychological disturbance.

The common denominator of all disease is that fear plays a role in almost every medical or surgical condition brought to the attention of a physician. Both physician and patient must analyze the situation. Together, they can become beneficiaries of widened horizons of understanding if they strive to accept one another's viewpoints.

Many and varied factors fashion the architecture of the doctor-patient relationship—solidify it, alter it, and occasionally, destroy it. Each aspect of the relationship must be carefully nurtured since it contributes to an affiliation that is as fragile at times as it is solid.

The prized possession shared by doctors and patients is mutual respect. Let there be a breakdown of communications on either side and that respect can be endangered. It is an arduous task for a physician to consistently empathize with the physical, emotional and often psychosocial needs of all his patients. And it is difficult for a paitent to believe or even conceive of the possibility that the doctor too can have all the frailities of being human. When a relationship can survive the pressure of such stresses it is a testimonial to both patient and doctor. Such a relationship could not possibly flourish without a solid foundation of confidence, trust and perhaps even—as my eighty-nine-year-old patient suggested—love.

Since the format of this book is a question-and-answer one, I have selected a few representative questions which touch on the relationship between doctor and patient. The questions clearly indicate the uncertainty, even animosity, with which some patients regard their medical advisors. I trust that my answers in each instance will provide a better understanding of the doctor's role and how together doctor and patient can achieve a better understanding if they listen carefully, one to the other.

What is meant by "doctor-induced illness?" I've seen the term mentioned in medical literature.

Doctors call this iatrogenesis. It comes from the Greek, *iatros* meaning doctor and *genesis* meaning origin.

This in no way is meant to suggest that doctors purposely induce emotional fears in patients. Rather, it is meant to emphasize how sensitive patients are to the slightest gesture or facial change of the physician in whom they have implicit faith.

Recently, I was examining the larynx of a woman so fearful of cancer that she had delayed coming to be examined for months. While looking at her vocal cords, which were completely normal, I inadvertently made a soft sound through my teeth. Later, when I assured her that there were no tumors, no inflammation of the vocal chords, her first question was, "Then why did you make that sound when you were examining me?"

I was guilty of "emotional" iatrogenesis.

Here's another instance of iatrogenesis. When a doctor wants an X-ray of the chest it is to contribute to his store of information for diagnoses. If he tells the patient that he wants that X-ray of the chest in order to rule out tuberculosis, pneumonia, fracture of the rib or an enlarged heart he is burdening his patient with the fear of all these diseases. Even though none of these are later found in the X-ray, implanted in the patient's mind is the fear that they somehow might be present.

Similarly, if a doctor tells his patient that he is ordering a blood test for mononucleosis ("mono"), it imprints on the patient's mind that the disease already exists. Even though the report may be negative, that anxiety may persist long after the actual illness has disappeared.

All of us in the practice of medicine run a frenetic race against time. The pressures on us are often so great that we may lose complete awareness of the impact that a word can make on the sensitive psyche of the patient.

The patient, too, plays a role in iatrogenesis. If the patient is made anxious by an inadvertent word or facial expression, it is imperative that he specifically inquire about its meaning. Unless it is clarified, both the patient and the doctor pay a penalty.

I went to the emergency room of a hospital to be treated for a burn on my hand. It's bad enough to be treated by an intern, but they assigned someone who was not even a doctor to take care of me.

Let me immediately remind you of the obvious fallacy in your letter when you say that it is "bad enough to be treated by an intern."

An intern in a hospital is a full-fledged doctor who has earned the degree of M.D. after years of hard work and medical training. Interns are qualified to engage in private practice, but have chosen to continue advanced studies in a hospital for more thorough training. All assignments given to them by their superiors can be carried out by them with accuracy and with good judgment.

The demands of modern medicine are so great that certain routine responsibilities that are time-consuming are now being assigned to very well-trained personnel known as "paramedical" assistants. These "paramedics" do not have the M.D. degree, but have undergone rigorous training with very special supervision.

The administering of routine injections, the dressing of wounds, the preparation for surgery, and the myriad time-consuming details that would normally take up the busy time of doctors and nurses are now safely and competently handled by paramedical personnel.

Not only are emergency rooms benefitting from the paramedics, but doctors, too, in their private practices are employing them in an effort to be relieved of specific details. In this way, the doctor can better utilize his time in helping his patients. Paramedics are a valuable adjunct in modern medicine.

In one of our discussion groups much comment arose about the intimate relationship between a certain psychotherapist and his patient. Someone brought up the widely circulated story of a psychoanalyst who became sexually involved with one of his patients. How did you react to that story?

The relationship between a physician in any field and his patients is a highly complicated one. The dependency that arises is responsible for the solid interfacing between the two. Out of this often emerges a very valuable and concentrated devotion.

In psychotherapy, the forces of "transference" and "counter-transference" between doctors and their patients can become highly charged. With female patients, the intricacies are even more complicated when the therapist is a male. It is not uncommon for the patient to temporarily feel she is in love with her therapist. He represents to her the figure of authority, strength and support. This, coupled with his sensitivity to her emotional needs, makes him a formidable structure in her life.

Psychoanalysts understand this mechanism, are aware of its importance and avoid the pitfalls of such an intimate relationship. Highly trained psychotherapists are very adept at utilizing this "transference" situation for the greatest advantage to the patient.

The exploitation or violation of that faith by the therapist is a sad testimonial to the principles and ethics of psychotherapy. Fortunately, such a complication occurs rarely and must not be considered by those in psychoanalysis, or those who are contemplating psychoanalysis, as a potential threat to the value of such therapy.

My doctor refused to take a cinder out of my eye. He sent me to a specialist who took a fraction of a second to remove it. I felt annoyed when I had to pay his fee.

You really have no justification for your annoyance. In fact, your reaction should be one of gratitude to your doctor who had the good judgment to know his limitations in such a matter. The cinder may have been embedded in a highly sensitive part of the eye requiring special care.

Referring you to a specialist was entirely correct. It is a testimonial to his expert ability that it took only a "fraction of a second" to remove the cinder.

I have been asking my doctor to open me up because I have had such severe pains in my abdomen for the past ten years. He refused. Recently I had such a severe bout, that when I went to see him I was rushed to the hospital and was operated on that night. It turned out that I had a twisted cyst of the ovary. Why did I have to wait so long and suffer for so many years, when I knew that surgery would help me?

You were carefully watched over a long period of time and, up to the time of your operation, there was no suggestion that you might have a twisted ovarian cyst. You may have had a cyst which was causing no damage and did not require an operation. It was for this reason that your doctor undoubtedly kept you under close observation.

Can you imagine what would happen if a surgeon "opened up" the

5

abdomen of every patient who made his own diagnosis and requested that it be done? Few people are aware that there are many severely psychoneurotic and even psychotic patients who deliberately feign symptoms, in order to have an operation.

It seems to me that you have no right to be upset by the careful judgment of the doctor who was treating you. Surgery is not a simple physical and emotional experience that can be considered lightly. There are distinct indications and contraindications for all operations. All of these had been taken into consideration while you were being observed and later when you were rushed to the hospital for surgery. Be assured that had your ovarian cyst been twisted earlier, surgery would have been performed then.

Just ask yourself whether you would have a right to react to the dedication of your doctor as you do, if, after an operation, you had developed a complication that permanently incapacitated you. How would you then have reacted to the conservative approach, rather than to the radical one?

The harmonious relationship between doctor and patient is based on faith, respect, and recognition of sincerity of judgment. Every once in a while this relationship is threatened and almost always by insignificant attitudes that do not deserve the right to interfere with a relationship that has taken years to develop. I am impressed by your doctor's judgment.

I had a virus cold two weeks ago and had to get well for an important business meeting. I was furious because my doctor would not give me a shot of penicillin. I missed my meeting and believe this could have been avoided if I had been treated more actively.

After twenty-five years in the practice of diseases of the ear, nose and throat I have come to the definite conclusion that I do not know what a "virus" cold is. For some strange reason a virus cold seems to have greater social status than the ordinary common cold. The virus seems to flourish luxuriantly in ignorance. Patients use the virus as a social distinction especially when it is a jet-propelled "two hour" virus.

A physician's decision to use or not to use an antibiotic is a very discriminating one. When an antibiotic is used it is done with mature judgment and in the belief that it is important for the cure of a disease. The importance of a business meeting is not one of the factors that determines whether or not a doctor should use penicillin.

Physicians and patients must not become involved in a competitive race against time for the cure of an illness. No acute infection or disease ever comes at the "right time." It is important for the doctor and the patient to work harmoniously for total recovery without the added problem of a race against time. Missing a business meeting must be difficult. How much more difficult might it have been had you pressurized a physician into giving you a "shot," and then found yourself severely allergic to the penicillin you demanded.

Isn't it possible for a doctor, with his vast experience, to know how long an illness will last? I never seem able to pin our doctor down to giving us any definite answer so that we can adjust our family plans.

Your complaint is a frequent one, and is based on a lack of understanding of the complexity of the diagnosis and prognosis of an illness.

The diagnosis of a disease is the science and art of identifying it by the signs and symptoms a patient shows. Many illnesses have similar signs and symptoms. Consequently, the doctor must use the process of ruling out conditions, and make what is called a "differential diagnosis" in order to pinpoint the exact illness.

The art of prognosis is to be able to predict the course of a disease and its final outcome. So many factors enter into the prognosis of an illness that it is often impossible, and frequently foolhardy, for a doctor to prophesy the duration of an illness. Some people rebound more rapidly from an injury or illness than others. The young, expectedly, recover more quickly than the elderly. The emotional state of a patient plays a vital part in the duration of and complete recovery from a disease. The course of any illness can vary in severity and, therefore, in duration. Complications, simple and complex cannot be anticipated.

You may be imposing an unfair burden on your phsycian when you expect him to give you a definite time for recovery. I am sure that your doctor, like all others, gives you a general idea of the expected duration of an illness, and varies that prognosis as recovery progresses.

A serious medical problem has just arisen in our family. We have implicit faith in our doctor but we would like to have another medical opinion. How can we do this without hurting the feelings of our doctor?

You will learn, with surprise, that your own doctor would welcome another opinion if you ask for it. You can also be certain that, if the diagnosis and the suggested treatment were not clear, the doctor would have sought a confirmatory opinion long before you wanted it.

An honest forthright approach is the mature way to handle what you consider a ticklish situation. When you tell your doctor that you need such added assurance, he will arrange a consultation with another doctor in your city or possibly in a distant one. He then can send all the available material to the consultant and spare you the need for repetition of the many tests he accumulated.

Your anxiety about "hurting" him is unnecessary.

X-rays of my spine were taken about six weeks ago. Now I have decided to change doctors. But I simply cannot get hold of the X-rays because the first doctor says he needs them for his files. I paid for the X-rays. Aren't they mine?

I believe it is universally agreed that X-ray pictures legally belong to the doctor who takes them. Even though you have paid for them, the physical possession of the X-ray plates may not be technically yours.

However, I have never known a situation in which a doctor or a hospital has refused to make such X-rays available to another doctor. X-rays have a strange way of getting lost, and sometimes medical legal confusion results. This may explain why some doctors refuse to release them to their patients.

Will you comment on a doctor being asked to give his records or to make complete copies when a patient transfers to another doctor? I made such a request and was told very definitely that there was nothing that would be of help to my present doctor. This, in spite of the fact that the first doctor had delivered my last child and made "Pap" examinations. Don't I have a right to these records?

I don't know the exact implications of your problem from a legal point of view, because your state may have specific laws about this. Such laws do vary from state to state.

I have special feelings about problems of this nature from a moral point of view. I don't feel that a patient is the fixed private property of any one doctor. Consequently, a patient has the right to make a change for whatever reason she may have.

Unfortunately, the disruption of the relationship between a patient and a doctor is often associated with some mutual displeasure. When this occurs, sometimes a doctor may be reluctant to give up his records.

My personal feeling is that such a patient has the right to have all her records transferred, after signing a release. Then, the former doctor should send those records directly to the new doctor.

I have been told that I have some kind of hernia. I follow the doctor's orders, but I don't understand the condition. I hate to bother my doctor because of my stupidity.

"Stupidity" is the last accusation with which you should be labeled. It is not unusual for patients to be confused by a description of their condition, especially when they are in a state of anxiety.

Rightful concern interferes with the proper communication between the doctor and the patient. You can be certain that your doctor would gladly repeat and clarify what he has told you.

Physicians know that unless patients clearly understand their condition they are less likely to follow the instructions and the regimen of treatment.

Do go back to your doctor and ask him to explain again the type of hernia you have and the details of its treatment.

We seem to have exhausted our patience. We find that we are going from doctor to doctor, all over the country, to find a cure for my wife's attacks of shortness of breath. Now, friends have told us about a special treatment in Europe and we are tempted to go there.

The first error you have been making is to peddle your wife's medical problem from place to place, losing the great advantage of proper direction and continuity from your own physician. When you are sick, you are understandably impatient. But this impatience can do you a great injustice.

Medical knowledge is not the private possession of any one doctor or group of doctors. When a form of medical treatment is found effective, it is reported in medical journals throughout the world, and its success is repeated everywhere.

A firm rule of wisdom is that any medical information known by one person alone, and exclusively used by him, must be suspect.

The psychological benefits are sometimes great for those who seek far-distant cures. It takes them away from the stresses within their family and from the pressures of their jobs.

When real organic disease is present, however, there is a built-in danger of running from doctor to doctor, and town to town, while valuable time is being lost—time that might well be spent in uncovering the basic cause of your wife's condition.

Unfortunately, there are many incomplete answers to medical problems. This makes the cure of your wife's condition so difficult.

All consultations with physicians in and out of your city should be made through your own doctor. The kind advice of well-meaning friends will only confuse you further.

My husband was killed in an auto accident. My three young children and I are on relief. I have been turned down by four doctors who refuse to take Medicaid cases. Is this fair?

It most certainly is not fair. In fact, I consider it to be medically immoral to refuse to see a patient who is part of the Medicaid program. This negates the remarkable social strides in America, which include the effort to bring good medical care to everyone, everywhere.

As a physician, I know that the bureaucracy of such massive social programs delays by months the payment for services given to patients. But this must not deprive anyone of the right to be treated with total dignity at a hospital or in a doctor's office.

I do know doctors who will actually treat Medicaid patients with great devotion and never even bother to send in the forms necessary for payment. The paper work becomes so time-consuming that the doctor often feels the payment will not compensate for his time and energy.

You do have recourse by calling the county or the state medical society in which you live, if you continue to be deprived of your right to good health.

Why does it seem that the relationship between doctors and patients is so much less friendly than it used to be? I've given

10

some thought to this and I wonder if patients themselves are not responsible.

There are so many factors in the equation of the doctor-patient relationship that it is almost impossible to examine and understand all of them. What impresses me in my travels around the United States is how consistently good this valuable relationship remains.

Many people recall childhood experiences with their doctors and tend to magnify that relationship in retrospect. Yet, when today's interpersonal contacts between doctors and their patients are carefully considered, it is surprising how well this mature relationship holds up.

It is true that many physicians are overworked. They do not have the time to make house calls and sit around and chat. These pleasant amenities reduce the doctor's functioning capacity and rob him of the energy he needs for the rest of his patients.

Many people believe that the "family doctor" no longer exists. This is not so. The American Academy of Family Physicians is a remarkable organization, devoting itself to the continued education and training of the family physician. They turn out "specialists" in the field of general medicine. This "specialty" ranks in importance with every other specialty in its contribution to the health of the community.

You suggest an interesting new approach. The complexities of being a patient in this frenetic world make patients more anxious and more vulnerable to the slightest variation in the doctor's attitude.

I truly believe that patients can contribute enormously in reaffirming and solidifying the relationship with their doctors. Doctors, too, need consideration, and understanding that they are pressured and made tense by the many problems they meet.

Chapter II

The Questions Everybody Asks All The Time

I remember once going for a family drive in the country and passing a meadow where cattle were grazing. As city-dwellers are prone to do, I prodded my little six-year-old daughter to stop whatever it was she was fussing with—I think she was engaged in some important task such as undoing her braids—to look out the car window at the cows. She didn't even lift her eyes. "No, thank you," she said, "I've seen a cow before." Her comment became a family password to be repeated and relished for years.

Sometimes when I encounter a question about headaches or sties or measles or gout for what might be the 2,648th time, I recall that long-ago punch line. Yes, I've heard the questions before and very often they sound exactly like ones asked the day before or the week before or the month before that. The difference lies not so much in the question as in the questioner. And basically, that is in whom I am interested, and whom I am trying to help.

It is possible to tell a great deal about a correspondent merely by the way he or she couches a query. There is the bare-bones question from the stalwart soul, "I have asthma; can it be cured?" And the walk-around-the-block question in which the timid writer fills the letter with tremendous detail, finally getting to the point in the last sentence. And the worried questioner, "If I had a cut on my hand and if it got infected, would I possibly lose my hand?"

And then there is the mail from people who apparently are hale and hearty themselves but whose friends are total wrecks. For example, "I have a friend who has warts and acne all over her face and. . ." Or "I think my neighbor should see a doctor—he has a terrible cough and high blood pressure. . ." And finally there are those bristly questions from indignant readers demanding to know things such as "Why hasn't a cure for cancer been found yet?"

Since I have been writing my column, "Speaking of Your Health," for these many years, it should be quite understandable if there's something *deja vu* about it all. But I hasten to make one point: maybe readers ask the same old questions but medicine is not standing still, so there are dozens of new answers. New treatments, new techniques, new medications are being discovered all the time and I rejoice that I am able to share this good news with my readers.

When part of the stomach is removed by surgery, does it continue to function normally?

It is remarkable how well a portion of the stomach can function when the rest of it has been removed by operation. Many brilliantly devised operations actually hook up the remaining part of the stomach to the intestines so that good digestion can continue. With moderate eating and well-controlled diet, there is virtually no disabling effect from such extensive surgery.

What happens to the body when it has a sudden chilliness or chill?

There is a distinct difference between chilliness and real chills. Chilliness may be caused by the inability of some people to adjust quickly to changes in temperature. A sudden blast of cold air may produce the chilly feeling and the "goose pimples" on the arms, which last for a few moments until the body accommodates itself to the change. It is said that some people who are "thin" skinned, fair and blond seem to be bothered by temporary chilliness. In others there may be a change in thyroid activity, or other hormone imbalance, to account for this sensation. Certainly, if it persists, a general examination might reveal the reason.

A real chill is sudden attack of shivering with an extreme sensation of cold, accompanied by chattering of the teeth and usually followed by rising body temperature. A true chill may be the result of a sudden invasion of the bloodstream by bacteria, or a parasite such as in malaria.

There is a remarkable center in the brain in the small hypothalamus which houses the temperature-regulating mechanism of the body. This can be disturbed by a wide variety of conditions and can result in a single chill or even repeated chills. A chill readily alerts the doctor to the need for intensive study.

Why are some pills taken before meals while others are taken during or after meals?

When drugs are prescribed by a doctor he knows their purpose and how best to achieve it. The instructions should be carefully followed because there is a reason why they should be taken at a particular time.

Some medicines can be irritating to the lining of the stomach, especially when it is empty. It is for this reason that these drugs are taken during meals so that they can mix with the food and not lie in contact with the lining membrane of the stomach and upper intestines.

There may be other drugs that would be more readily absorbed from an empty stomach. These therefore are given before meals for rapid and maximum effectiveness.

There is another group of drugs that may be destroyed by the stomach juices and therefore would be best taken at intervals when the juices are at a minimum.

There are many drugs which are beneficial when taken at uninterrupted intervals throughout the entire day an night. Antibiotics, for example, build up a concentration in the blood which must be maintained at a high level to destroy the bacteria that cause infection.

Follow prescribed directions carefully for the most rapid return to good health.

How can you tell if a medicine has lost its effectiveness after being in the medicine cabinet for a long time?

The shelf or cabinet life of drugs varies tremendously. If drugs are kept in the original bottle made by the pharmaceutical company, there is always an expiration date printed on the label. As for prescriptions drugs, your pharmacist is in the best position to tell you, from his records, and from his own stock, the life span of effectiveness.

It must be remembered that watery and alcoholic solutions of drugs become concentrated by evaporation as they stand on the shelf. The originally prescribed dose, therefore, would no longer be valid. It may seem wasteful, but it is safer to get rid of most of your old medicines.

What can cause fingernails to become enlarged and curve in a person who does not do hard work with his hands?

The fingernails are a valuable diagnostic aid for physicians. All sorts of changes occur in them that suggest diseases far removed from the nails themselves.

Cracking, discoloration, brittleness and deformities are seen with fungus infections, reactions to drugs, anemias, vitamin deficiencies and a host of other conditions.

There is a very strange association of marked distortion and hardening of the nails with chronic lung conditions. Chronic bronchitis, emphysema and bronchiectasis can be responsible for these changes. The nails sometimes lead the doctor to discover the early onset of these lung and chest conditions.

The association is not definitely established, but certainly inadequate exchange between the oxygen and carbon dioxide content of the blood must also be considered.

Is the value of fluoride as a preventative against dental decay still a matter of debate?

Almost every new scientific discovery has its own protagonists and antagonists. Fluoride is not different. When it was suggested that fluoride would arbitrarily be put in the water reservoirs of many cities the hue and cry was great that this would be a violation of national, international and constitutional rights.

The fact is that the advantages of fluoridation as a preventative against dental decay are now accepted by medical and dental associations. In one New York State city, the result of fluoridation has been spectacular. It is estimated that there has been a reduction of about ninety percent in the number of missing teeth in children.

The fears that fluoride in the water might be dangerous over a long period of time do not seem to have any real basis in fact. Certainly, the occasional disadvantage is more than compensated by the dental health of the community.

A complaint that fluoride might have caused some mottling of the tooth enamel did arise. So rarely does it happen that it would be in error to sacrifice the dental health of many children because of this rare occurrence.

Is it possible for hair to turn completely white after a fright?

Every physician has heard from some patient that a severe emotional upset from fright or calamity was responsible for sudden graying of the hair. Even though there is no scientific validity to this, some people cannot be budged from insisting that it is true.

A severe illness and some drugs may, perhaps, hurry the process of graying and give the impression of suddenness. The emotions can do amazing things and may perhaps affect the cells at the root of the hair that produce pigment. But even if this did occur, the whole shaft of hair itself would not suddenly lose its color.

Is body massage an acceptable form of medical treatment?

For centuries it has been known that massage can be beneficial physically and psychologically. There are four varieties of massage which include rubbing, stroking, slapping and kneading. The greatest advantage of massage is that it increases the blood circulation, relaxes muscles and increases the general tone of the body. Professional athletes are enthusiastic about massage to loosen tight or strained muscles. Patients who are confined to bed need massage to keep up the muscle tension so that the muscles will not become atrophied by disuse. Many people benefit by massage because of the general feeling of relaxation that accompanies it. In the hands of well-trained and licensed people there can be many advantages to this form of passive exercise.

A note of warning: As a form of medical therapy for patients who are ill, the choice should be made by their physicians. Too active or too strenuous massage can be harmful to the muscles and to the joints if it is performed by anyone other than those specifically trained in its use.

Why do some people tend to faint more easily than others?

The process of fainting is known technically as syncope. It is caused by a temporary sudden reduction of the flow of blood and oxygen to the brain. Hunger, drugs or a severe emotional upset may be responsible for the change in the blood flow. Even a rapid change of position can cause fainting.

The threshold for fainting varies with different people. Some react more violently to a stimulus than do others. There is no specific profile suggesting that one person will have a greater tendency to fainting than another.

17

In the morning my feet are not swollen. At the end of the day they are. Is this a sign of a circulation problem?

Yes, it is. It is obviously due to some interference with the free flow of blood to and from the feet. Some simple causes, such as varicose veins, marked overweight or unrelieved standing at work may be responsible. A complete study of the circulatory system can readily determine the exact cause. Only then can effective treatment be started.

Many people delay visiting their doctors because the swelling disappears after a good night's rest. They feel encouraged by this and tend to neglect this important sign.

Can the body have too much blood, almost the opposite of anemia?

In a condition known as polycythemia an unusual amount of blood circulates throughout the body. There is a marked increase of the red blood cells and in the hemoglobin of the blood. Occasionally this condition is seen in patients with long-standing heart and lung disorders.

There are two types of polycythemia. One, the Vera or true type, is treated by blood-letting or removing blood in just the opposite fashion from a transfusion. Radioactive phosphorus and X-ray treatments to the bone marrow also are used to reduce the overproduction of red blood cells, because bone marrow is one of the chief sources for the production of red blood cells.

Exactly what is pernicious anemia?

Pernicious anemia is a remarkable disease which has an even more remarkable history. Strangely, it seems to occur most frequently in white people past the age of fifty who live in temperate climates. When this unusual blood condition was first discovered more than one hundred years ago, it was called Addison's anemia and was fatal in almost all instances. In 1926, it was found that pernicious anemia was caused by a deficiency of an important factor in the juices of the stomach. Later it was discovered that a deficiency of Vitamin B12 is one of the most important reasons for this condition.

Today, not a single person with pernicious anemia need be an invalid if the condition is found early and treated intensively. Almost miraculously, liver, once a discarded food, was found to be effective in the control of this disorder. Vitamin B12 given at regular intervals in addition to a highly nourishing diet supplemented with iron and minerals have kept people with pernicious anemia alive and productive. There are few greater scientific achievements than the control of this once-fatal disease.

Can the size and shape of blood vessels be seen by X-ray?

Routine X-rays cannot show normal soft tissue. When there is arteriosclerosis in arteries, the calcium within them may be seen by X-ray. There are many new specialized techniques in which dyes are injected into the blood stream. These can clearly outline the vascular structure of the body.

What is meant by a biopsy?

The word biopsy comes from the Greek *bios* meaning life and *opsis* meaning vision. Biopsy, therefore, means the microscopic examination of a piece of tissue in order to study the special kinds of cells that it contains.

When any tissue is removed in a hospital from any part of the body, it is immediately sent to the laboratory for the most detailed examination. The tissue is prepared with special solutions and imbedded in paraffin. After hardening, the tissue is cut in thin slivers. Trained pathologists examine these sections under a microscope for the presence of malignant cells. If they are found the pathologist can then grade the severity of the cancer to help the surgeon and physician decide on the exact course of further treatment.

Sometimes a tiny specimen can be painlessly removed from a growth and sent to the laboratory for analysis. If the biopsy report is negative then further surgery may be unnecessary. The biopsy studies provide valuable information for the diagnosis and treatment of many conditions.

Why are cultures and smears taken from the throat and from the nose?

The lining of the healthy mouth, nose and throat is covered by a wide variety of germs, viruses and fungi. They seem to live contentedly together and, in fact, keep their respectful distances from each other. It would be surprising to many people to realize that some really active bacteria are thriving while they are at the peak of health.

When the body's resistance is lowered these bacteria break through the barrier and start to invade the underlying tissues causing inflammation and infection responsible for the state of "illness."

A smear taken from the nose, throat or pharynx is sent to the laboratory and placed in an incubator in order to allow the germs to flourish. Under a microscopic examination, the exact germ can be identified.

An additional test is then made to find the particular antibiotic or sulfa drug that will most quickly destroy that particular germ.

The smear test placed directly under a microscope can often reveal the presence of certain cells that indicate the presence of an active allergy. Malignant cells sometimes reveal themselves by this technique. Smears can, of course, be taken from all other parts of the body and are exceedingly valuable as aids in the diagnosis of disease.

How serious is bleeding from the rectum?

Without question, the most frequent cause of rectal bleeding is some form of hemorrhoids. It is surprising to physicians that despite all educational campaigns some people still delay in coming to them for fear that their rectal bleeding is "serious." It may be, but more likely it is not. The agony of fear lasts many months after the patient has been reassured that the problem is a simple one.

Also, many people delay in seeking advice thinking that surgery is always necessary. They fall prey to expensive "magical" remedies made by those who for years have exploited the frightened and the fearful. Excellent methods are available to pinpoint the reason for bleeding.

Dietary regimes, careful hygiene, sitz baths, prescribed medicated suppositories and the readjustment of bowel habits can alleviate the bleeding caused by hemorrhoids. It is only when local treatment is not effective that surgery is necessary.

What do the three degrees describing burns mean?

A first degree burn is one in which the skin becomes red, inflamed and painful. Usually, there is no break in the skin. In a second degree burn there is a more severely inflamed appearance and the skin is blistered and even broken. In a third degree burn not only is the skin involved but the underlying muscles and tissues are affected.

The extent of these burns determines the ultimate recovery from them.

I burned my hand with boiling water. I am sure that other people do the same while working in their busy kitchens. Is there any ointment or cream that is soothing?

In recent years we have learned that one of the best home remedies for a burn is to quickly immerse the burned part in ice cold water. This brings almost immediate relief and is said to actually play a role in more rapid healing. The temptation to cover the burnt part with all sorts of fatty ointments, jellies and creams is great but should be avoided. Usually a great deal of time is spent by the doctor in removing the grease. A good rule of first aid is to do less, rather than more, and to do it slowly.

What is meant by "twilight" sleep?

I don't know where this interesting term originated. I could speculate and presume that it was created because twilight is a period between positive light and complete darkness.

"Twilight" sleep therefore is a state of lowered consciousness or sedation following the combined use of morphine and scopolamine.

Before patients are taken to an operating room they are often given this to reduce their tension and to increase the safety of general anesthesia. Patients who are in the state of "twilight" sleep can respond to instructions but the experience is then almost totally forgotten.

Is there any safe way to break the habit of insomnia?

Some reasons for inability to sleep or for repeated interruptions during sleep may be the overuse of alcohol, coffee, tea and tobacco. Severe emotional tensions at work and within the family structure can be important reasons for sleeplessness. Overexcitement and overtiredness contribute to a restless sleep or to difficulty in falling asleep.

Some drugs taken for general medical conditions may act as stimulants. Pills, like the amphetamines and thyroid tablets, can, when taken too late in the day, overactivate the body and cause insomnia. Dietary indiscretion and loading the stomach full of food before going to sleep can be disturbing.

Not all people need the same amount of sleep. Occasionally the body's own reserve is such that a few hours may be all that is necessary. Unless this is realized some people punish themselves by fitfully tossing in bed and taking their insomnia as a personal insult. For them it would be much wiser to get out of bed, read, or listen to the radio and television until the feeling of sleep overcomes them.

Very often insomnia can become a habit pattern which can be broken by studying the physical and emotional reasons with your own doctor. He will tell you that in his practice there are dozens of people who insist they have not slept more than an hour a night for the past forty years. He will also tell you that none of these patients gives any evidence of exhaustion—which they should if this were true.

I find that many patients are adult enough to examine the basic reasons for their insomnia and, by rearranging their patterns of living and avoiding emotional stress, are able to break their poor sleep habits.

Would you tell me what causes one to dream? I have been dreaming frustrating dreams every night for several years.

At one time, it was so difficult to evaluate dreams that the entire field was disregarded. This left the field wide open for exploitation by those who invented their own myths and superstitions. "Dream books" were sold to the gullible, who then based their lives on the "predictions" and false interpretations of their dreams.

Today the study of dreams is occupying the attention of psychologists and psychiatrists. It began when it was noted that infants, when asleep, had rapid eye movements beneath their closed eyelids. Now there is known to be a definite relationship between REM (Rapid Eye Movements) and vivid dreams.

The basic concept of the "master of dreams," Dr. Sigmund Freud, is now being substantiated with scientific studies not previously available. In a very simplistic way, it might be said that Dr. Freud believed that dreams were the ways an individual worked out inner conflicts.

It is now accepted that some dreams represent stresses that can interfere with normal, healthy sleep and with the replenishing of the energy afforded by sound sleep. Dreams may therefore play an important role in explaining why some people can function well with five hours of sleep while others are barely mobile after ten hours of sleep.

The fact that you are frustrated by your dreams would indicate that you may need some psychological guidance. In this way, deeper levels of your consciousness may be revealed. It is surprising how simple the explanation sometimes is when discussed with an expert in the field.

It is disconcerting when I am having dinner in a restaurant to suddenly have an attack of hiccups. Is there a fast way to stop them?

Hiccups, or hiccoughs, are spasms of the diaphragm which in most cases stop without any help. Any tensions and embarrassment tend to make them worse. I would suggest that at the first sign of them you absent yourself from the table and try one of these familiar remedies: drink a glass of cold water without stopping, or chew on a hard crust of bread, or hold your breath for twenty seconds. If this doesn't do it, breathe into a paper bag holding the opening tightly over the nose and mouth. This causes a concentration of carbon dioxide in the bag and frequently relaxes the hiccups.

What causes a growling stomach? This happens to me often and it's embarrassing.

The medical term for a "growling stomach" has a nicer sound than the condition itself. The word is "borborygmus." These rumbling growls are due to a collection of gas in the large intestine. This accumulation of gas almost always begins with air that is swallowed while eating or drinking. Try to avoid eating or drinking too rapidly. Fast, energetic conversation during mealtime favors the swallowing of air. Also, emotional upsets while eating help to accumulate air. Deep sighing and forced belching are often followed by swallowing air. The air becomes locked with unabsorbed fluid and causes the growling noises.

When noisy growling persists, the cause should be sought to be sure that it is not an early sign of some form of intestinal ailment. X-ray and barium studies of the small and large intestine may reveal the cause, and then specific treatment can be recommended.

Are there any reliable ways to prevent intoxication and a hangover through the use of drugs or certain foods?

There seem to be endless myths attached to the sophistication of alcohol drinking. Every drinker has created his own "scientific" observation. Some insist that lining their stomachs with olive oil will prevent intoxication and a hangover. Others are sure orange juice in between drinks can do the same thing.

Ask any drinker and he will give you his special advice. This advice, you can be sure, will exclude the most important suggestion; that is, to drink sensibly and to know your own limitations.

Drinking is not a competitive sport. The rate with which alcohol disappears from the body depends on the individual's metabolism. How soon he sobers up varies with each person.

It must be added that there is great danger in mixing alcohol with any kind of drug.

With all the "sure fire" cures for dandruff, why does the condition remain with so many of us who are using them?

There is a vast difference between the enthusiasm of the manufacturers of dandruff cure-all and the efficiency of their product with all users. Undoubtedly, there is some benefit to some people with some products. No one preparation is the complete solution to everyone's problem.

Dandruff is really a form of skin irritation or infection known as seborrheic dermatitis. The exact cause is unknown. There are probably many different forms of this skin and scalp condition which are all thrown into the general classification of dandruff. It is for this reason that sufferers of this unpleasant, socially distasteful condition should first consult a skin doctor.

In many instances the need to replace oil or water in the scalp may be the simple solution. Skin doctors know the exact contents of many of the more helpful preparations to suggest one or more that would be beneficial for each individual case. There are many excellent soaps, detergents and sulfur shampoos which, when used under proper direction, can minimize the dandruff and attack the basic underlying skin condition.

I have lost my sense of smell in the past seven years. Will it ever return to normal?

There are so many reasons for the loss of smell that it is difficult to speculate if it will return. Long-standing allergies, chronic sinus infection, nasal polyps and overuse of nose drops can produce "anosmia," or "loss of smell."

Doctors have used small doses of cortisone in selected cases, and have been sucessful in restoring the sense of smell. An ear, nose and throat specialist can, with X-rays and other techniques, find the reason for your problem.

What causes a kidney stone?

The formation of kidney stones can be ascribed to many causes. A diet (and water) that contains a high concentration of minerals is thought to be an important factor.

Some drugs have a tendency to produce stones in the kidney and in the ureter, which is the tube that carries urine into the bladder. Most stones have as their base the mineral calcium which can readily be seen by X-ray. Another stone is composed of uric acid, associated with gout. It cannot be visualized by X-ray.

When a kidney stone is found by X-ray should it always be removed?

Doctors have for years been trying to find a method of dissolving stones that are formed in the urinary system. Only a small percentage of cases have been successful with this treatment.

Occasionally, stones have been dissolved when the urine has been changed from acid to alkaline or from alkaline to acid. This technique, however, cannot be depended on.

As for surgery, the combined judgment of the physician and the urologist is based on the size of the stone, the position of the stone and the symptoms it causes. If they feel that the stone can be passed out of the body without surgery they will, of course, advise conservative treatment.

Diabetes runs in my family. Both my mother and father are diabetics. I am fearful that I may become one. Is there any way to prevent or offset the possibility?

It is agreed that there are family patterns of diabetes. This does not necessarily mean that you inevitably will develop this condition. It is unfair to you to assume that you will be invalided and that your potential happiness is threatened by this disorder.

There are a few precautionary measures that should be taken by anyone with a family history of diabetes. Weight should be kept within normal limits for one's age and size. High sugar and immoderate diets should be avoided. The blood and urine should be examined at regular intervals so that any trace of diabetes will be detected early and treatment started immediately.

Close observation by your family physician will relieve you of anxiety and permit you to live without the constant threat of an impending illness.

I have been treated for mild diabetes for two years. The pills that I have been taking by mouth seemed to control the condition up to now. Recently, I have been told that the only way that I now can be treated is with injections of insulin. I absolutely refuse to do this and want to know if I can continue to take the pills by myself.

You are one of the favored few whose diabetes has been controlled by taking medication by mouth. Apparently, it has been effective, but in the judgment of your physician injections of insulin are now the *only* way to control your diabetic disorder.

You, of course, do not have a medical choice of drugs. You do have the right to make your own decision about whether you want to remain in good health or to invite the probable complications of diabetes that are inevitable.

You can be sure that when once your diabetes gets out of hand because of neglect or your failure to take the insulin injections, you will eventually find them to be unavoidable.

Injections certainly are not pleasant. Neither is a severe disease. Millions of people are living perfectly normal, healthy, productive lives because insulin was discovered and because it is being administered at regular intervals according to the directions of the physician.

There are few diseases that need as much care and careful scrutiny as does diabetes. You will, I am certain, follow your doctor's advice when you realize that the unpleasantness of these painless injections are more than compensated by your sustained health.

Is there any reason why a young woman with diabetes should not marry?

Young men or women with diabetes should not hesitate to marry. The single important factor, however, is that the degree of severity of the diabetes should be known to the marriage partner.

The diabetic whose condition is controlled by diet, insulin or drugs can take on the responsibilities of marriage, job, running of the home, and having children.

There may be only one restriction. When a diabetic marries another diabetic, there is more chance that the children born of such a marriage have a greater possibility of developing diabetes.

Is the formation of adhesions after an operation a family tendency and is it possible to prevent them?

Adhesions are firm bands of fibrous tissue that occur following abdominal surgery. It is not generally accepted that there is any hereditary tendency in the formation of adhesions. There is greater likelihood that infection within the abdominal cavity, peritonitis, injury and rough handling of the delicate intestinal tract are more responsible for the formation of adhesions.

Adhesions are sometimes considered to be nature's protective way of walling off an abscess within the abdomen. Sometimes they form following difficult or long operations on the gall bladder, the appendix, the large and small intestines and in the pelvis. Undoubtedly some slight adhesions occur after most complicated abdominal surgery.

Adhesions can be prevented by the gentle handling of all organs during surgery. Modern techniques avoid harsh gauze, irritating drugs and solutions. A number of excellent drugs, cortisone and enzymes are used during and after surgery to reduce the formation of adhesions.

What does a doctor mean when he refers to the surgical risk to a patient who is about to undergo an operation?

Surgical risk is a medical term which is not as terrifying as it might sound. What it means is that the doctor takes into consideration the general conditon of the patient, the heart, the lungs, the blood pressure, the blood circulation, the content of the blood and the age of the patient and compares what he finds with the severity of the operation to be performed.

All operations, no matter how slight, must be considered to have some degree of risk. Obviously, an old person with chronic heart or lung disease would be considered a greater risk than a young athelete in the full bloom of life.

Surgical risk has been markedly reduced in the past twenty-five years with the advent of antibiotics, newer anesthetics and highly refined operative techniques.

Under what circumstances it is necessary to examine the spinal fluid?

The brain and the spinal cord are surrounded by a cushion of protective fluid called cerebrospinal fluid. In normal health this fluid is manufacturered in small amounts and is absorbed so that there is a constant amount circulating around the brain and the spinal cord at all times.

Normally the fluid contains sugar, proteins, and cells in small quantities. When there is infection (meningitis) or inflammation, the cell count may rise from six to hundreds or even thousands.

A spinal tap is performed with remarkably little pain or discomfort. When disease of the brain or the spinal cord is suspected, a small amount of fluid is drawn off and sent to the laboratory for intensive study.

The spinal fluid pressure is measured as it is withdrawn. This, too, is of special importance for diagnosis.

Occasionally, a special dye is inserted in the space that houses the spinal fluid in an effort to locate the possible presence of growths or tumors.

There was a time when patients and families would react with tremendous concern when a spinal tap was suggested. Today, there is no need for this concern. It can be done quickly and without danger.

Is muscular dystrophy an inherited disease? Two members of my family, an adolescent boy and an adult, are afflicted.

Muscular dystrophies are very complex problems associated with progressive degeneration of muscles. Two distinct groups of muscular dystrophy are receiving special attention. One is the Duchenne form which affects only boys. It may start in childhood and develop in a more advanced form during early adolescence. This is distinctly attributed to some inherited recessive gene in the family. Another form known as the Landouzy-Dejerine type may affect either sex. This disease too is considered hereditary. It usually begins later in life, in adolescence or young adulthood.

There are other variations of muscular dystrophy readily diagnosed by the characteristic symptoms they show.

With a family history such as yours, it would give you great assurance if a "genetic profile" were made of the members of your family. This would indicate disturbances of the genes and the chromosomes, if any were present. Genetic counseling for people with family histories of hereditary diseases is a new science which can spare families the heartache of inherited diseases.

What is meant by the term "sympathetic nervous system?" Is this a medical term or does it relate to emotions?

Although it appears that way, the word "sympathetic" is not used in this connection as an adjective. It is for this reason that there is confusion about this term, which has real technical meaning. Actually the sympathetic nervous system and the parasympathetic nervous system are both part of a complex network of tiny nerves called the autonomic nervous system. Unlike the central nervous system, which controls the movement of muscles and joints, the autonomic nervous system is an involuntary one.

This delicate system of nerves can narrow or open blood vessels, dilate the pupils of the eyes, accelerate the heartbeat, increase the flow of saliva and perform limitless other important functions. In some instances surgery is performed on the sympathetic nervous system to relieve certain types of pain and help enlarge narrowed arteries in order to increase the flow of blood.

I know that adrenalin comes from the adrenal glands. Where are they and why are they so important?

29

The adrenal glands are two triangular-shaped organs about one and a half inches long. Each is closely attached to the upper part of the kidney. The adrenals are two of the most important hormone-secreting glands and play a vital role in most of the functions of the body. Adrenalin, manufactured in these glands, can raise the blood pressure, stimulate the heart, induce emotional excitement, alter general fatigue, and affect the concentration of sugar in the blood and in the tissues of the body.

The adrenal glands contain two separate parts, a cortex and a medulla. Each plays a different role in the activity of the body. The relationship between the secretions from the adrenal glands and those in the pituitary gland in the brain dominates most of our health structure.

I know that antibiotics are worthless for an ordinary cold caused by a virus. Yet our doctor prescribes antibiotics every time we have a severe cold. Our family are not big pill-takers and I wonder if the antibiotics can eventually do us harm.

Yours is a sensible inquiry. The problem you brought up does need clarification. It is true that the common cold is caused by some type of virus. It is also true that antibiotics are not usually effective against viruses.

Why then are antibiotics used? It is well established that people who have a severe cold are better candidates for added bacterial infections. Complications like pneumonia, infections of the sinuses, and infections of the ears frequently accompany the ordinary common cold. It is to prevent these complications or to treat them should they arise that doctors frequently prescribe antibiotics.

The fact that you and your family are not pill-takers does not reduce your need for them. You can be sure that no doctor promiscuously prescribes antibiotics. He recognizes that there are some allergic reactions to the antibiotics, and that some of them may produce annoying side effects.

Does one attack of influenza bring on immunity?

There may be some slight immunity for a few weeks after an attack, but this is questionable. There are so many forms of the influenza virus.

It becomes even more confusing because all kinds of colds and grippes, some caused by bacteria rather than viruses, are lumped together as the "flu." Don't bank on immunity; take sensible precautions.

Are typhoid and cholera injections necessary for all foreign travel?

Most European countries have excellent control over their water and milk supply. This is not entirely true in all Far Eastern countries nor in all tropical and sub-tropical regions.

The U. S. Health Department, the medical departments of the Armed Forces or local health officials should be consulted when traveling abroad. There are changes in policy almost yearly, and therefore advice should be sought. Sometimes, a local epidemic in a particular country may exist. This information is relayed immediately through the World Health Organization to other countries everywhere. Our health officials can then tell you if there is a special need for vaccination against typhoid, paratyphoid, yellow fever or cholera.

Recently I had jaundice after a European trip. We have been trying to find the reason for the hepatitis I developed. Is there any way to track down the cause?

The yellowish discoloration of the skin that may follow an attack of hepatitis is called jaundice. There was a time when it was virtually impossible to trace the underlying cause for this condition. Now it is possible, by a series of tests, to pinpoint the cause and rule out other possibilities.

The very first tests are made on the blood to show the kind and severity of the jaundice. These same tests are taken at repeated intervals and indicate the progression or recession of the condition which affected the liver.

Exposure to other people with infectious jaundice, a recent blood transfusion, eating oysters or clams that may have come from polluted waters, and the use of toxic drugs are intently studied. A number of drugs can cause a severe and perhaps allergic reaction which affects the liver and produces a special type of jaundice. Chronic gall bladder disease, stones in the gall bladder ducts, chronic alcoholism and cirrhosis must all be considered as a possible cause.

31

The intricacy of the tests and their delicacy frequently points to the cause of jaundice and then dictates the treatment that must be used for recovery.

What is meant by a detachment of the retina of the eye? What causes it and can it be corrected?

The retina is a thin layer of light-sensitive tissues which lines the inside of the eyeball towards its back. For a better understanding, it can be likened to the film in the back of a camera. It is firmly attached to the eye. Occasionally a severe injury to the head or to the eye may cause a rip in the retina.

The blood that seeps beneath it separates it from the wall. Other causes of detachment may be a small tumor and, in the elderly, arteriosclerosis of the blood vessel to the retina.

When the retina becomes detached there may be a sudden dark patch or veil over the eye so that vision is interfered with. The degree to which sight is affected depends, of course, on how large an area of the retina is detached. Sometimes spots in front of the eye with blurring of vision and changes of shapes of objects occur.

The diagnosis of this condition is made very exactly by the eye specialist. With special instruments every millimeter of the eye can be examined for tears or rupture of the retina.

This is indeed a serious condition which demands immediate expert treatment and surgery. The past fifteen years have brought remarkable advances in treatment.

What is the best way to remove a foreign body from the eye?

The protective lubrication of the eye guards us from the soot, dust, diesel fuel and coal dust that fly freely in the polluted air of large cities. These foreign bodies are usually washed out with the tears and rarely cause trouble.

Occasionally, a speck may lodge on the lining of the upper lid. If the upper lid is gently pulled out and drawn down to cover the lower lid, in most instances that is all that is necessary to remove it.

Sometimes it is necessary to turn back the upper lid to look for an imbedded particle. The eyelashes are gently pulled downward and the lid turned over a thin pencil or a matchstick. If the particle is seen it can be wiped off gently with moist cleaning tissue or moist cotton.

If a particle is seen on the cornea of the eye it is best left alone until removed by a physician. Sometimes it is necessary for the physician to put a single drop of anesthetic in the eye to make the removal painless.

Are there different kinds of pinkeye? Are they all contagious?

Pinkeye or conjunctivitis is a sudden active acute infection of the conjunctiva, a thin delicate membrane that lines the lids and covers the eyeball. Pinkeye is a highly contagious infection, almost always caused by the staphylococcus and other bacteria. Only occasionally is a virus responsible for this eye condition which can travel with the speed of lightning from one victim to another.

At first, the eyes begin to tear profusely, followed by an itching or burning sensation of the lids. Soon there is a yellowish or white discharge between the lids and marked redness and swelling of the upper and lower lids.

A smear or culture taken from the discharge and studied under the microscope quickly helps to identify the causative germ. A particular antibiotic that can destroy the germ and keep the infection under control can then be chosen.

Extra careful hygiene is imperative to avoid passing the infection from one person to another or to keep from reinfecting oneself. Towels must be washed separately and limited to the patient's use while active treatment is being carried on.

I have had the most intolerable itching in the ears. Sometimes I can't keep my fingers out of them because the itching is so intense. What can cause this?

Itching is in reality a form of pain. It can be so intense that it can be as difficult to withstand as the most severe pain. Anyone who has ever had itching of the ears or itching of the skin due to hives or allergy will quickly attest to that.

The likelihood is that you have a fungus infection that lies on and just beneath the skin of the outer ear. This seems to be an excellent location for the growth of the fungus. Any chronic discharge or accumulation of wax is an excellent breeding place for the fungus that sets up housekeeping in this moist, warm, dark area. When the skin becomes inflamed and irritated other bacteria invade the tissues and cause considerable painful infection.

33

The treatment for the itching is based on rigorous attack against the fungus. The ear must be cleaned under direct vision with microscopic instruments in order to avoid further injury to the tender ear tissue. The fungus grows so rapidly that the doctor must constantly keep ahead of its growth to destroy the fungus, treating the ear with many of the new cortisone and antibiotic medicines that are now available.

What causes the outer ear to become swollen, red and itchy?

Infection and allergy are the two most common causes for this condition. Many people try using their fingers, pencils and paper clips to alleviate an itchy sensation. This results in injury to the skin lining of the canal and invites infection and even abscess formation.

Eczema of the ear canal is almost always caused by some allergy. Nail polish, hair dyes, lacquers and eye makeup are some of the possible allergens. When the condition is severe it becomes complicated by infection. Antibiotics are used when infection is present.

Treatment depends entirely on the local condition as seen by the doctor. Then it becomes important to try, by elimination, to find the offending substance that causes the skin irritation.

Itching of the ears can usually be controlled with a few drops or an ointment used on the prescription of one's own doctor, who must be sure there are no perforations of the eardrums or other chronic ear conditions present. Swabbing the ear with cotton-tipped applicators can be injurious unless the tightly-packed cotton tip is loosened and made softer.

Is tuberculosis an inherited disease?

Tuberculosis is mistakenly believed to be an inherited disease because it may occur in the same family. Actually, it is not inherited. It is rather a contagious disease, and thus can be passed from one member of a family to another.

When one lives in a state of anxiety about tuberculosis as you do, every ordinary cough that you or your family may have will unnecessarily cause you greater concern than it should. Bring such coughs to the attention of your doctor early, rather than speculate fearfully.

You would gain greater assurance if your chest were X-rayed at regular intervals.

Is it safe for a girl to marry a man who has recovered from tuberculosis? Can she contract it and is there a possibility that it can again affect him?

The key answer to your question lies in the word "recovered." If he has completely recovered from active tuberculosis and has no evidence of the disease, then he presents no threat to his wife-to-be.

There are very specific tests which show the presence of the tuberculosis germ in the sputum. If there is any activity, the doctor will be the first to suggest safety precautions for both the girl and the boy.

Most states issue a marriage license only if both applicants are completely free of infectious diseases. A history of tuberculosis simply means a thorough examination and X-rays by the doctor before permission to marry is given.

Once he is cleared completely, the chances are almost none that a wife may contract the disease from him. All people, however, who have had tuberculosis should be under surveillance by a physician for the rest of their lives. These examinations at six-month or yearly intervals may never again show evidence of the disease but they are a great investment in the health of a married couple and their family.

Can you tell me what "walking pneumonia" is?

There is no guesswork about pneumonia. The physical examination of the chest reveals pneumonia when it is present. Later, X-ray study is used to substantiate the diagnosis. Many patients, in telling their history to a doctor, will say "I once almost had pneumonia." This has no validity. One either has had it or has not had it. There is no "almost pneumonia" as there is no "walking pneumonia."

Is pleurisy similar to pneumonia or tuberculosis of the lungs?

Pleurisy is an infection or inflammation of the pleura, a fine membrane that covers the outside of the lungs. Another similar pleural membrane completely lines the entire chest cavity.

In health, when the lungs expand, the two layers of the pleura smoothly glide over each other. When there is an infection of the pleural lining, breathing becomes difficult because the pleura rub against each other. This is responsible for the severe stabbing, shooting pain of pleurisy.

Pleurisy is in itself not pneumonia or tuberculosis. Pleurisy may be one of the complications of these and other infections of the lungs.

Before the era of antibiotics, complications of pleurisy were frequent. Fluid accumulated between the two layers and made surgery necessary and often lifesaving. Thanks to antibiotics, the complications of pleurisy are rarely if ever seen today.

Are there different kinds of coughs? When should they be suppressed?

A cough is part of a wonderful mechanism that clears the airway, bronchial tubes and the lungs of any irritation. This reflex action protects the entire respiratory tree from foreign substances, polluted air and the accumulation of mucus.

The slightest irritant in the windpipe sends an immediate signal in a millionth of a second to the cough center in the brain. The message is immediately relayed to the muscles in the chest and an explosive cough clears the passageway of the irritant.

When a germ invades the bronchi and the lungs, inflammation sets up and becomes a source of irritation that produces a cough.

There are two basic kinds of cough. The first is a dry one which is a hacking cough and may be the result of irritation by tobacco or smoke or other pollution of the inhaled air. The second is a productive cough which brings up the accumulated mucus, sputum and pus that results from infection.

The treatment of a cough depends, of course, on attacking the underlying cause. The dry hacking cough is usually eliminated if the irritation from tobacco, pollution and industrial fumes are eliminated. Proper ventilation and increased humidity of the air will decrease the cough.

Infection is treated with antibiotics. The coughs that result from infection are encouraged rather than suppressed so that stagnant fluid will not accumulate in the lungs.

What causes the nose to suddenly run like a faucet? The fluid that comes out is thin and almost watery.

This condition is known as rhinorrhea. It is almost always caused by some substance to which a person is sensitive or allergic.

The delicate lining of the nose begins to pour out a thin, watery fluid when it is exposed to dust, pollens, fumes, or chemicals. Actually, this is a protective mechanism which washes away the irritants.

Sinus infections are less likely to cause this kind of outpouring of fluid. In cases of sinusitis, the discharge becomes thick and may be of a green or yellow color. In fact, this is a fairly good way to distinguish between an allergic response and an infection.

The fluid can be examined under the microscope and often will show cells that pinpoint an allergy or infection.

Anti-allergy drugs (antihistamines) are very effective in controlling this distressing symptom. If the condition persists or tends to become worse, the exact irritant must be found by testing the skin for special sensitivity to dusts, pollens, foods and chemicals.

Is there any advantage in using medication such as benzoin in steam inhalations?

Steam inhalations are very valuable and often used in respiratory conditions. Benzoin, aromatic herbs and flower concentrates are frequently used in the steam kettle. They may be very pleasant and give a medicinal aroma which could have some psychological effect. However, the real advantage is from the steam itself.

Can a sudden change of climate cause attacks of asthma?

Bronchial asthma is probably one of the most complex disorders of the respiratory system. It has so many forms and variations that almost any situation may set off a sudden attack.

Severe episodes of asthma are desperate ones for patients who simply cannot get air in and out of their lungs. In most instances, allergy is the offender that causes a temporary narrowing of the bronchial tubes.

Change of climate most certainly can start an attack. A new pollen in a new neighborhood, infection, smog, pollution, altitude and even a sudden drop of temperature may begin an attack. The relationship between emotional upsets and asthma is well known. To make matters even worse, a combination of any of these factors may launch an asthmatic seizure. Many patients learn from past experience the conditions they must avoid and are often successful in reducing the frequency and severity of these attacks.

How can a person with asthma cope with attacks within his home?

Few diseases are as complex and as difficult to control as asthma. It takes the greatest ingenuity on the part of the physician and the allergist and sometimes the psychiatrist to try to track down the exact cause. Sometimes an animal, a new rug, a new coat, or even house dust may be found to be the offending substance that causes an asthmatic attack.

If the environment cannot be changed by moving, then a few things can be done within the home. It should be mentioned that no one with asthma should uproot himself and his family and go to another climate without first having lived there. There can be great emotional disappointment when this drastic change is made only to find that the asthmatic attacks still occur in the new geographic location.

Within the home some attempt at dustproofing can be made. Non-allergic pillows and plastic coverings on the mattress and other furniture are sometimes effective. Woolen carpets that hold dust should be removed along with draperies and curtains.

Is it safe to wash out the sinuses?

When a sinus becomes filled with pus it must be drained, irrigated or washed out. This is exactly what happens when there is an infection anywhere else in the body. A pus pocket must be emptied.

It is entirely false to believe that once a sinus is washed out it must always be washed out. This idea is based on ignorance rather than truth. Of course, if a sinus is washed out and emptied of its infection, it does not mean that the underlying cause of the condition has been entirely removed. When pus re-forms, it must again be washed out and treated until the sinuses themselves are healthy.

Sinuses can be irrigated painlessly and then filled with antibiotic solutions to control the infection. Antibiotics taken by mouth, small amounts of nose drops and steam inhalations are an ideal combination to cure an acute sinusitis.

People sometimes fail to realize that, when the acute infection has subsided, they still should be treated for the chronic underlying sinus infection if they are eventually to be rid of this annoying condition.

How can you tell if a headache is caused by a sinus infection?

Headaches over the forehead and pains around the eyes and in the cheekbones are frequently caused by sinus infection. There are, however, many other reasons for the complaint of headache. Remember headache is a vague term frequently used indiscriminately to describe pain, discomfort, a sense of lightheadedness and even dizziness.

The sinuses are normally filled with air and are lined by a delicate membrane to protect against infection. When the sinuses become infected or when the lining becomes thickened because of allergy, air does not flow freely in and out of the sinuses. An accumulation of pus or thickening of the lining membrane with polyp formation presses outward on the sinus wall and can produce some degree of headache.

It should be remembered that there are occasional sinus infections without headache. Do not assume that because there is no headache there is no infection.

Infections of the frontal sinuses may cause a headache that is more marked in the morning and which tends to disappear towards the end of the day. Infections of the antra, on either side of the nose, may do the reverse. Actually there is no need to speculate about the presence of sinus infection. X-rays of the sinuses and the appearance of the nose can definitely help establish the diagnosis for the doctor.

Can headaches be classified as a disease?

Headache is a symptom and a complaint, but it is not in itself a disease.

It is imperative, therefore, that the cause of this symptom be tracked down before any treatment is started.

If this is not done, then the choice of drug must necessarily be a haphazard one that treats only the symptom rather than the underlying cause.

Only those burdened by persistent headaches know how their lives can be devitalized by this discomfort. Those who get an occasional mild transient headache, of course, do not necessarily need an intensive study to learn the basic cause, which is usually obvious.

Because it has been so difficult to pinpoint the reason for headaches, many people have been tagged with the diagnosis of "psychogenic" disease. With the poorly-founded diagnosis that their headaches are of psychological origin, many people are falsely considered neurotics, and dismissed as complainers.

The fact that a headache persists and defies diagnosis does not mean that the distressing symptom should be classed as neurotic in origin.

It is estimated that more than fifty percent of severe headaches can be classed as migraine, a recurring condition in those individuals who suffer from it.

In most instances, the headache is onesided and may start with strange sensations in the eyes, or with a growing sense of depression. The pain begins to mount, and within an hour's time, it almost unbearable.

It is now believed that some chemicals found in certain foods may set off a migraine headache. A chemical known as tyramine is contained in alcohol, some vegetables, coffee, tea and even in seafood. People can be studied for sensitivity to this chemical.

Another type of headache is referred to as the cluster headache, and is considered to be due to some transient change in the blood vessels to the brain. This type of headache differs from the real migraine. Unlike migraine, there is no family history, and it more frequently affects men.

How can a migraine headache be distinguished from an ordinary headache?

Migraine is a recurring headache. It lasts for as little as a half-hour or as long as a week. Between attacks there is almost complete freedom from pain.

It has never been satisfactorily explained why migraine headaches tend to become better at dusk. Tension, aggression, hostility and conflict can almost always be the trigger factor for the nausea and vomiting of a migraine headache.

Migraine attacks tend to involve only one side of the head especially at the temples. Victims of migraine are bothered by strong light and have blurring of vision, flashes of light and dark and momentary episodes of blindness.

Ordinary headache due to eye disorders and sinus disease may cause tenderness over the face, skull and sinuses.

Migraine headache is a very specific kind that needs very specific treatment. The correct diagnosis of the cause of headache must be determined by a physician before any definite form of treatment can be started.

Is it painful to have a stomach analysis? What do they look for when they pump out the fluid?

What you ask about is known as a gastric (stomach) analysis. The procedure is a painless one but undeniably somewhat uncomfortable. A thin rubber tube is passed through the nose down into the esophagus and then into the stomach. Because the tube is iced and because the throat is sprayed with a local anesthetic, it usually is not too distressing.

The purpose is to withdraw through this tube some of the stomach contents and then test them for the presence of blood, bile, digestive juices, hydrochloric acid and to obtain cells that can be studied under the microscope. The information accumulated in this way is an important contribution to the diagnosis and later treatment of stomach ailments.

What can cause a narrowing of the esophagus that prevents food from going to the stomach? Can this be repaired?

The esophagus can be narrowed by infections, injury and tumors, both benign and malignant. Accidental swallowing of lye has for years been a cause of this condition. A small pouch, or diverticulum, may interfere with food going down, but does not completely block it.

. Once the exact diagnosis is made by X-ray with barium, the treatment can be started. Sometimes the esophagus, especially in lye poisoning, can be opened and stretched with metal tubes.

When the esophagus is removed because of a cancerous condition a series of operations can now actually form another esophagus using a portion of the stomach to replace it.

Canker sores crop up in my mouth with no relationship to my diet or activity. They make me miserable.

Anyone who has had a canker sore, or aphthous ulcer of the mouth, knows how painful and unpleasant it can be. These puzzling sores remain one of the unanswered problems in medicine.

The use of yogurt and lactobacillus pills gives some people relief, and more rapid healing. Anesthetics applied to the ulcers bring temporary relief. A new form of treatment involves tetracycline, an antibiotic. About 250 milligrams in a syrupy solution is swished in the mouth for five minutes, and then swallowed. This can be repeated about five times a day. The treatment helps diminish pain and shortens the duration of the painful sores. Unless one is allergic to this antibiotic, it is worth trying.

Can the constant grinding of teeth be responsible for pain in the neck and head? I find that I have had this since a new appliance was made for my teeth.

A well-fitting appliance needs a period of adjustment. A poorly fitting one sometimes stays as an irritant until it is repaired or changed. Habit patterns of grinding the teeth during the waking hours are an easy trap to fall into with or without a new appliance.

By constantly putting pressure on the teeth, stress is referred to the jaw joint and to the muscles of the face. Later this may extend and involve the muscles of the neck. A condition known as temperomandibular joint disease occurs when the jaw joint is thrown out of its normal balance position.

I would not permit this condition to go uninterrupted for a long time because of the possibility of permanent damage to the jaw joint. The dental surgeon now has at his command many new techniques for altering the bite. This can then be corrected and relieve muscle spasm.

What causes a stone to form in one of the glands that produce saliva?

There are three sets of salivary glands which produce saliva containing substances absolutely essential to the proper beginning of the digestion of foods. Besides lubricating the mouth, saliva starts digestion, which then continues in the stomach and in the intestines.

The largest of these salivary glands, on either side of the face just in front of the ear, are the parotids which are the ones affected during an attack of mumps. Another set of glands, just under the jaw, are called the submaxillary glands and a third set, the submentals, lie in front just below the chin.

Through tiny ducts or canals, saliva pours steadily and smoothly into the mouth.

Occasionally, because of diet or drugs or infection, a tiny deposit of calcium or uric acid forms in the tiny canal and obstructs the free flow of saliva. This stone may grow until it affects the proper functioning of the entire gland. By means of X-ray and the injection of a dye into the tiny ducts, the exact position of the obstructing stone can be found for easier removal. Frequently the stone can be removed under local anesthesia.

Why do some people have to urinate so much more frequently than others?

People in good health do not usually have too great or too frequent a desire to urinate. Infections of the bladder, excess intake of fluids, drugs and nervousness are only a few of the reasons why both men and women have an urge to frequent urination.

There are some major conditions like kidney disease and the two forms of diabetes in which an unusual amount of urine is passed out of the body daily. There are also other disorders in the male and female urinary tract which may be responsible.

If the urge to urinate is no greater than four times a day and is not accompanied by burning or a feeling of incompletion, there need be no concern. If the urge is more frequent than that, it is not too difficult to find the exact cause and eliminate it.

After an operation six weeks ago, I was told that they found acetone in my urine. Is this a dangerous condition?

Finding a trace of acetone in the urine is not uncommon following surgery, especially before the patient is fully able to take adequate amounts of fluid. Sometimes the acetone is suspected by a sweetish odor to the breath during a period of fluid imbalance. This is technically known as acidosis and is readily corrected by introducing fluids by mouth or by vein.

The presence of acetone in a single specimen does not mean that there is a disorder of the kidneys or that there is an underlying disease to account for it. There is no reason to believe that your health will in any way be affected by the acetone that once was present or that it will even recur at any time in the future.

My tonsils are infected and I know that they should come out. Could diseased tonsils be responsible for neuritis of the lower back?

There was a time when there was great concentration on the concept of focal infection. The teeth, the tonsils, the sinuses, and the appendix were thought to be culprits responsible for disorders in other parts of the body. This attitude seems to be carrying less weight today than it formerly did. There is complete agreement, however, that any infection in the body should be removed. If your tonsils are diseased, they should be taken out. However, you must not be disappointed if their removal does not cure the neuritis in your lower back.

What causes a pain low in the back?

Low back pain seems to describe a very definite condition but, in reality, is a very complex and diffuse disorder that has many divisions and subdivisions.

Besides injuries caused by lifting heavy weights, too strenuous exercise, and unusual change of posture, low back pain may be caused by birth abnormalities, arthritis, bone disease, and circulatory disorders. And one must not overlook psychological causes of low back pain.

Too often, people with low back pain become their own diagnosticians. They buy the usual supporting belts, change their mattresses to firmer ones, and carry their bed boards with them wherever they go. All of these methods of self-treatment have some advantages, but, in many instances, keep the victims from seeking the advice of a physican to find the exact cause. X-ray studies and neurological tests almost always can establish the exact reason for back pain and the proper form of treatment can be started.

Everybody in my family has had lumbago. Is this an inherited condition?

Lumbago is not an inherited condition. Actually, it is a term no longer commonly used to describe aching pains around the loins and the kidney area. It is really not a disease, but rather a descriptive symptom of the painful spasms of the muscles of the lower back. A popular misconception that lumbago is related to kidney disease has no validity.

Why do people think of bursitis as a humorous condition? I have had four attacks and I can attest that it is not funny.

I agree that there is nothing funny about bursitis or any other pain.

A bursa is a soft pad of fat which lies in between most joints and serves as a lubricating device. The freedom of motion of the elbows, shoulders, knees and hips depends on the condition of the bursas.

The most frequent cause of bursitis is some kind of injury to the joint. This does not necessarily mean a blow or an accident. Lifting a heavy weight may do it.

There are many new and excellent forms of treatment for bursitis. The incapacitation is lessened by the application of cold compresses to the particular inflamed bursa. Pain-relieving drugs and large quantities of aspirin, under a doctor's supervision, can carry you through the very difficult first few days.

When necessary the bursa itself can be injected with a local anesthetic, cortisone and ACTH. A remarkable new drug, DMSO, holds tremendous promise.

What can cause pain in the heel without any other signs or symptoms of illness?

In most instances, pain the heel is a result of pounding the hard floor and pavements, especially by those unaccustomed to walking. Badly fitting shoes may be responsible. Occasionally, a bony spur can be felt or seen by X-ray examination of the foot. Tumors, bursitis, gout and arthritis can also produce a painful heel. Before any form of treatment is undertaken a complete examination by an orthopedist, a bone specialist, is imperative.

Protective foam rubber pads, heat and rest are very beneficial. Hot soaks can help reduce the discomfort. If gout or arthritis are found to be the reason for the pain in the heel, treatment must be directed to these conditions. an important piece of advice about a painful heel is that treatment should be started early rather than delayed with the thought that the pain may go away of its own accord.

Is a spur on the heel a form of arthritis? How can the pain be relieved?

Spurs are deposits of calcium in the tendons of the muscles of the heel. They can be exceedingly painful unless they are well protected by rubber sponges to avoid injury. Surgery, in well chosen cases, is very beneficial. They are not a form of arthritis.

What causes a "pins and needles" sensation in the feet and legs during the day, and muscle cramps during the night.

The cause may be an impairment of circulation of the blood through the arteries. Occasionally, nighttime cramps occur because of the position during sleep and be unrelated to circulatory problems. These cramps are painful and frightening, but they are of no great medical importance. Some physicians suggest the use of quinine to relieve the pain and frequency of nighttime cramps. In many instances, this is very effective.

The tingling sensation is known as paresthesia and, when accompanied by discoloration of the feet, is much more serious. Leg cramps that occur after walking a short distance, in addition to these tingling sensations, definitely deserve to be studied to track down the basic cause. Tobacco, especially in the young, and arteriosclerosis in the elderly, are the most common causes of such muscular cramps.

What is the difference between a contusion and an abrasion?

When the outer layers of the skin have been rubbed off without an actual break, the injury can be called an abrasion. Rubbing the skin against a wrestling mat produces the typical abrasion of the skin, with exposure of tiny blood vessels, with or without bleeding. The simple, effective remedy is cleanliness. The skin should be washed gently with a non-irritating soap and kept covered. In most instances, lots of water and soap is all that is necessary. If bleeding is excessive, pressure with dry, sterile gauze or a clean handkerchief will control it. The wound should be covered, making sure that any adhesive tape used to keep the dressing on is not in contact with the injured skin.

A contusion is an injury to the skin which is caused by a blunt, rather than a sharp, cutting object. Almost always, the skin itself is unbroken, but the injury to the underlying tissues such as muscles, blood vessels, nerves and bone, may be severe. Such an injury is almost immediately followed by swelling at the site, caused by seepage of blood into the muscles and other tissues beneath the skin. The pain that accompanies the discoloration and the swelling may be severe.

The immediate application of cold tends to reduce the swelling and to control the hemorrhage into the soft tissue. Cold applications can also diminish the intensity of the pain. A moderately tight bandage can help control the bleeding and make the patient more comfortable. Later, warm applications are used to help nature absorb the blood from the injured tissue.

Does a "simple fracture" mean that it is not a serious one?

You're under a misconception if you believe that a "simple fracture" is not a serious one. "Simple fracture" is a technical term used to describe one in which the separated fragments of bone have not broken through the skin.

A "compound fracture" is one in which the broken fragments of bone have torn through the muscles and the skin.

There is another kind known as the "green stick" fracture. The term comes from the resemblance to a new green twig of a tree which, when bent, splinters but does not break through.

Even "green stick" fractures must be carefully treated until the bone completely unites.

Is it possible to have a fracture of the ribs without severe pain after a minor injury?

Often a new or old fracture of the ribs is found in people during a routine X-ray examination of the lungs. This is explained by the fact that symptoms are caused when the lining of the chest cage, the pleura, is bruised or when the lung itself is injured by a break in one or more of the ribs.

47

Occasionally an incomplete fracture, known as a green stick fracture, causes little or no damage and remains unsuspected.

Relatively insignificant injuries, especially in the elderly, whose bones may be somewhat brittle, can cause a fracture without producing pain. A fracture may be suspected if there is pain on deep breathing or a severe longstanding cough. Every injury to the chest deserves an X-ray.

What is the present attitude toward treatment of the sprained foot? Should one try to "walk it off?"

It is a great mistake to try to self-diagnose and self-treat a foot sprain or injury. Even doctors refrain from guessing if an injury is mild, moderate or severe. Certainly you would be taking a great risk in trying to exercise a strain or a sprain of the ankle without knowing if a fracture is present.

Walking on such an injury can only invite prolonged incapacitation even if a tiny bone break or a tear in the ligament has occurred. Stay off the foot. Apply cold compresses at first to stop any inner bleeding and to keep the swelling to a minimum. Then the doctor's advice must be sought and followed. The decision to use adhesive tape, supporting stockings, or mild exercise should depend entirely on his judgment.

Chapter III

What Women Ask

When I began to assemble the questions and answers for this book I knew there would be two chapters that would outweigh all others as far as the number of questions go.

One would be the chapter on the questions that everyone asks. Obviously there is a vast area involving good health that concerns both men and women. There are multitudinous health problems shared by both sexes. And men and women are bound to ask the same questions.

The other category that I knew would make up a substantial chapter of this book would be the one devoted to women's problems. Now I am anything but a male chauvinist. I do not believe that women are more prone to illnesses or that women make more out of a sneeze or a cut than men do—as we have sometimes been led to believe over the years. None of these chauvinists have ever checked with a doctor who has watched a woman endure intense pain without a whimper and seen a man faint at the sight of a scratch.

True, hundreds of women do write to me each month—their letters flow in steady succession. But when I think of them, it is not the volume of correspondence or what is asked but how it is asked. I find in the mail from women correspondents a genuine concern with the welfare of others. More often than not, women ask questions concerning their husbands, their children, their aging parents, a suffering friend. Women, too, are surprisingly aware of medical terms and practices. They seem to know how far medical science has progressed in finding a cancer cure or what is being done about muscular dystrophy. Often they wax indignant in their letters. Why hasn't a cure been discovered for emphysema? What are the experts doing in regard to diabetes or arthritis? In fact, when I read some of this right-to-the-point mail, I find myself saying, "Bravo!" I want to know why, too.

A great many women in the world apparently are not interested in dwelling on their own minor physical upsets. They are concerned about colds and headaches and boils and mosquito bites—that's a fact. But they are just as aware of and even more concerned with the health picture on a larger scale. I tend to classify their letters as "classic" or "curious." And the "curious" part is extraordinarily satisfying.

My husband reads the medical columns in magazines and newpapers and invariably develops many of the symptoms of the diseases he reads about. How can I help him overcome his fears about illness?

I can't recall who said this but it is particularly applicable to your husband: "It's a good thing I'm a hypochondriac, otherwise I'd be awful sick."

Actually, the chronic complainer about nonexisting illnesses suffers a great deal because of his preoccupation with his own health. The hypochondriac must be considered to have a psychological illness which deserves sympathy and understanding. He may be devitalized by anxieties that keep him from being a normal, functioning human being.

The hypochondriac usually has deep-seated psychological problems that need to be uncovered by people trained in the art of listening. Sympathy from a member of the family may not relieve his fears and may even make them worse. The hypochondriac may be seeking refuge, in the excuse of illness, to avoid coming face-to-face with daily activities and to cope with the problems of living. He must be encouraged to seek psychological guidance for a better understanding of his emotional confusion and distress. When this is clarified for him, many of the symptoms may disappear.

It must be remembered that hypochondriacs do develop real diseases and have as much right to illnesses as those who are not psychologically disturbed. Only too often their illnesses may go unrecognized because of the frequency with which they "cried wolf" about a fanciful illness.

My husband works in a factory three miles from our home. During the past four years it has become increasingly more difficult for him to travel that distance because of some kind of fear. Is this a common condition and what can be done about it?

The fear of open spaces is known as agoraphobia. It comes from the Greek word *agora,* a market place, and the Latin *phobia,* meaning fear. The fact that it is a relatively rare emotional disturbance is not nearly as important as is the fact that it is destructive to your family's structure and needs immediate psychological control. You will, I am sure, recall that your husband showed other neurotic tendencies before this. Now it is imperative that you speak to your doctor and to a psychiatrist if he is to be freed of this burden of fear.

My husband has been warned that he must stop drinking any alcohol because he has cirrhosis of the liver. Why is this so dangerous?

When alcohol in any form is taken in large quantities over a long period of time it can produce changes in the delicate structure of the liver. The normal healthy tissue becomes replaced by dense, fibrous tissue which then seriously impairs the liver's function. Waste products accumulate in the blood and overwhelm the body with their toxic effects. The warning to stop drinking alcohol must not be taken lightly if your husband values his health and the happiness of his family.

My husband has cirrhosis of the liver. He is an alcoholic. Has there been any success with transplants of the liver in such cases?

Surgery on the liver was, until recently, considered impossible. Today, experimental studies indicate that the possibility of liver transplants may soon leave the area of fiction and become a reality.

Some cases of cirrhosis of the liver are being treated by a special type of vascular surgery. One of these operations is known as "the portal vein shunt." By this complex operation, pressure may be taken off the cirrhotic liver.

It is sad that cirrhosis of the liver due to chronic alcoholism is a serious condition that might have been prevented.

My husband has had a hiatus hernia since he had his gall bladder removed. Why should this happen after an operation and can it be cured?

I doubt that there is any relationship between the removal of your husband's gall bladder and his hernia. Undoubtedly this condition existed before the operation and may not have been discovered until later.

It is not unusual to try to tie up any two conditions when, in reality, they are only related by a coincidence.

A hiatus hernia is a condition in which a portion of the stomach pushes its way through an enlarged opening in the diaphragm and actually may stay in the chest cavity where the esophagus and the stomach join.

Uncomplicated hernias of this kind can be kept under control by a rigid, bland, ulcer-type diet. Frequent small meals of easily digested, nonirritating food bring relief from discomfort. A wide variety of drugs can relieve the spasm. In some instances, surgery may be necessary, but that, of course, depends on your own doctor's judgment combined with that of a surgical consultant. When the condition is kept under regular control, complications rarely occur.

What causes brittle fingernails?

Fragile splitting fingernails can be caused by inadequate diet, exposure to detergents and occasionally by metabolic disorder, especially of the thyroid gland.

Why does my doctor look at my fingernails whenever I have a general health examination?

Fingernails that break, scar, develop ridges, and discolor have a great many meanings to doctors. To most people, nails and their care are mostly of cosmetic significance.

Nails tell a story. Clubbing of the nails is strangely associated with chronic lung conditions. Brittle nails are sometimes caused by some intestinal conditions and anemias. There may also be concave or spooned nails with ridges in some medical conditions. It is remarkable how astute physicians can come to a spectacular diagnosis by the observation of the nails.

There may be some validity that high protein, gelatin, and mineral diets may strengthen the nails and it is worth a try under a doctor's supervision. Fragile, thin nails, can sometimes be supported with additional vitamins but this is rare.

I get infections around my fingernails. They are painful, and

keep me from doing my housework properly. Is there any way to avoid this?

The condition you describe is known as "paraonychia." It is an infection in the tissues surrounding the nail. The redness, the swelling, and pus formation are due to bacteria, or fungi, that enter by a break in the skin.

A hangnail, or a cut during manicuring, allows such germs to set up housekeeping and produce such tender, localized infections. These are sometimes called "felons," "whitlows" or "run-arounds." If neglected, they can extend into the deeper tissues, and may even require surgery.

In the absence of any chronic skin condition, one must seek other causes, such as minor burns, injuries, lack of protection in working in the garden, and long exposure to strong detergents and immersion in water.

Lubrication of the skin and, of course, rigid cleanliness, are good preventatives. Warm soaks are beneficial as soon as redness and swelling appear.

I have a scar from an appendectomy performed when I was a child. What would the process be to have it removed?

Scars on the abdominal wall, the face or anywhere on the body can be removed. It is rare for one to want an appendectomy scar taken out since it usually has no great cosmetic importance. As small as bikinis are, they probably can adequately cover yours and save you the trouble and expense of having it removed.

All scars can be removed by surgery or a process known as dermabrasion.

A scar removed by surgery may result in a similar scar, especially if you are prone to keloid, or thick scar formation.

Dermabrasion is a "sandpapering" method performed with a rotating burr. In many cases, this technique brings gratifying results. Your own physician, of course, can refer you to a plastic surgeon if you decide you must have this operation.

Is it safe to use hormone cream to remove excess hair on the upper lip and chin?

The promiscuous use of hormones in creams, lotions and ointments is potentially hazardous without a doctor's prescription and supervision.

Hirsutism, the technical name for excess hair, has many causes. These should be investigated before any treatment is used.

Electrolysis, when used by specially trained people, can be effective in removing unwanted hair.

What are the common causes of excess hair in young children and in adults?

Superfluous hair is technically known as hirsutism or hypertrichosis. There seems to be some familial tendency towards excess hairy growth, especially in women and children.

In most instances the excess hair is not a source of distress unless it involves the face and the arms in women.

When this is first observed it is important that the child be examined by a specialist in endocrine conditions. Sometimes a slight endocrine imbalance can be found and readily corrected before it becomes a source of psychological embarrassment. There are a number of complicated endocrine problems that are responsible for excess hair and other physical evidences of a hormone problem. In addition to correcting this, treatment is directed to cosmetic appearances.

A great number of devices are now available which remove the hair by plucking, shaving or "wax epilation." There are also chemical depilatories which must be used with a great deal of caution because they can be harsh and may irritate and damage the skin.

Bleaching with safe hair bleaches can hide the condition sufficiently to spare cosmetic discomfort. Be sure to avoid "mail order" drugs and chemicals which carry with their expensive potions a potential degree of harm.

Ever since I began to use eye makeup and eyeliner, my eyes become itchy and swell up.

As you assumed, this undoubtedly is an allergic reaction to the ingredients in your cosmetics.

Sometimes, a person may not be sensitive to one cosmetic or another, but may be sensitive to a combination of both. A good trial is to discontinue all cosmetics and see how you react. Then, slowly add one item at a time. Perhaps in this way you may be able to track down the offender.

I have seen patients with reactions such as yours whose conditions were traced to the lacquer in hair spray and nail polish. These, too, must be considered in searching for the source of your allergy.

There are a great many nonallergic cosmetics on the market. You should try them if your problem persists. During an acute phase of discomfort, antihistamine drugs are helpful.

Can you hazard a guess about what would cause burning of the eyelids? I know this is an unfair question to ask without a proper examination.

The unfairness is not to me but rather to you. I gather that you have not been checked by a doctor. In the absence of any infection or local eye condition, there is always the possibility that an allergy may be responsible for burning, itching or swelling of the eyelids.

A common offender, if allergy is the cause, is a sensitivity to nail polish. Hair sprays, hair dyes, shampoos, and eye makeup may also be responsible.

Non-allergenic cosmetics are available and should be tried if, after thorough medical examination, there is no evidence of a cause other than allergy.

What are the most common causes of swelling of the eyelids?

The usual excuses of lack of sleep or a hangover for puffy eyelids have some validity. No one knows better than the person who complains if either of these is true.

From the medical point of view, swelling of the eyelids, or edema, may be caused by some allergy. It is surprising how often the offender or the offending reason for allergic swelling of the eyes is nail polish. The shellac used in hair sprays, hair dyes, eye liners, mascara, and cosmetics may all be responsible for swelling of the lids.

Some eye drops and antibiotic ointments may be responsible. Often it is very difficult to track down the exact allergic substance. With trial and error and by eliminating one at a time, the cause may be found.

There are some diseases, such as trichinosis—which follows eating insufficiently cooked pork—that are recognized by a distinctive type of swelling in the eyelids. Occasionally, chronic lung, heart, and kidney conditions can cause persistent swelling of the eyelids. However, these reasons are far less frequent than allergic response to cosmetics and food.

What is the most common cause of swelling of the ankles?

The underlying mechanical reason for most swelling, or edema, is some interference with blood circulation. Tight garters, heart disease, chronic infections of the kidneys, severe varicose veins are a few of the reasons for this condition. The character of the swelling and its duration after a period of rest with the feet elevated, is of extreme importance to the doctor evaluating this disorder.

Just standing on one's feet at work for long periods of time may be an important cause. In the elderly, narrowing of the blood vessels because of arteriosclerosis may interfere with blood circulation and produce swelling, especially towards the end of the day.

Women who wear very tight girdles develop swelling of the legs because of interference with the return flow of blood through the veins.

What is of utmost importance is not to neglect any swelling of ankles or legs. The condition can almost always be relieved after the cause has definitely been established.

My ankles swell during the day to such a degree that I must take my shoes off. It is difficult for me to get them on again because my feet are so swollen. After a night's sleep, the swelling is gone.

Swelling, or edema, of the feet and legs is a sign of some disturbance of the circulation of the blood in those areas. In some instances varicose veins, overweight and standing on the feet all day can cause the swelling.

Not all of the causes are that simple. Chronic heart and kidney conditions can be responsible for some degree of swelling of the legs. The retention of fluids or a hormone imbalance can also cause it. The exact reason can only be found by complete study of the circulatory and lymph drainage systems. When the cause is found the treatment becomes obvious and the condition can be improved.

Too often people delay seeking the answer to such a problem because the swelling disappears in the morning and they feel encouraged by it. When any swelling recurs over a long period of time it deserves the benefit of a complete physical examination.

Is there a family tendency to varicose veins, or is it a coincidence that all the women in our family have them when they get older? Are there any new ways of treating varicose veins?

Varicose veins seem to be one of the penalties paid by man when he assumed a standing position in his evolution. Varicose veins do not occur in four-legged animals.

Veins in the legs have within them tiny intricate valves to prevent backflow of the normal stream of blood as it goes to the heart.

When these valves weaken or fail to function, the veins lose elasticity, and do not sustain the pressure of the blood. "Pooling," or stagnation, of the blood results; the veins become distended, tortuous or twisted. This is how varicose veins are produced in people whose work requires them to stand all day.

In addition to the upright position, the pull of gravity, the pressure of pregnancy, and even tight garters burden the veins. There may be some congenital weakness of the veins' walls or valves that accounts for the family tendency.

In simple cases, elastic stockings, elevation of the legs and simple exercises are beneficial. In other cases, injection of special chemicals are used for small varicosities. Modern surgery has developed many new techniques that are remarkably safe and effective when simple conservative measures have failed.

Can elastic stockings cure varicose veins?

Varicose veins are enlarged veins through which blood does not flow freely. There are tiny valves in the vein which, when ineffective, cause stagnation of blood and enlargement of the blood vessels.

The causes of varicose veins are many and the severity varies greatly. Elastic stockings give added support and may relieve the symptoms of pressure and swelling sometimes associated with this condition. These stockings are of value but should not be used as a delaying mechanism in seeking the opinion of a physician for complete evaluation of the condition.

Can varicose veins be permanently cured by injection?

Small varicose veins of the leg may not interfere with the return of the circulation of blood to the heart. Large varicose veins of the larger vessels of the legs are caused by a breakdown of tiny valves in the veins. When these large blood vessels are involved, a variety of symptoms may occur. There may be pain on standing or walking and chronic fatigue after little or no exercise or at work. For these conditions surgery is almost always the ideal form of treatment to insure the greatest chance of permanent recovery.

Small varicose veins may be annoying because of their appearance. Surgery for these smaller varicosities is almost always unnecessary.

There are now a number of ways of injecting special sclerosing solutions which close off these tiny veins and improve the appearance of the legs. This procedure is simple and safe and can be performed in a doctor's office.

What is the cause and meaning of "milk leg?" This happened to me after I gave birth to my second child.

I don't know the origin of the term "milk leg" and how it came to be used to describe a swelling of the foot, ankle or leg. Occasionally, after surgery or the delivery of a child, the deep veins of the leg may become inflamed. This is known as phlebitis. The inner lining of the veins may become irritated and form a clot that interferes with the free flow of blood.

When this happens marked swelling of the leg may occur. Recovery time depends on the size of the affected veins. The condition is usually controlled with rest, medication and supporting hose.

In addition to your arteries and veins, another system known as the lymphatics, plays a most important role in carrying nourishment in the form of lymph to various parts of the body. Blockage of this lymphatic system can cause the swelling you refer to as milk leg.

In recent years patients have been encouraged to get out of bed within twenty-four to thirty-six hours after surgery. This stimulates better circulation of the blood and has markedly reduced the number of cases of milk leg and phlebitis in post-operative patients.

**After the birth of my second child I developed a "milk leg."
Does this mean that I would be susceptible to this condition if I
decide to have more children?**

"Milk leg" is known by the rather enchanting name of "phlegmasia
alba dolens." An infection of the veins of the legs (phlebitis) or a clot in
the veins interferes with the normal circulation and results in swelling
of the legs. Milk, of course, has nothing to do with the onset of this
condition.

The only way to avoid a recurrence of a "milk leg" with subsequent
pregnancies is to seek any underlying conditions that may predispose
you to it.

**I suffer intense pain in the ear, especially in the morning. My
doctor says that my teeth are at fault. I can't understand this
since I have my teeth checked every six months.**

Your doctor probably was referring to a malocclusion of your teeth, or
an imperfect bite. This could account for changes in the jaw joint with
referred pain to the ear.

The same nerve that goes to the jaw joint goes deep down into the
outer ear canal and to the eardrum. Often no infection of the ear is
present when a patient complains of a direct pain in the ear.

I would speculate that you are one of the many people who grind their
teeth during the night and consequently put a strain on the jaw muscles. When they awake in the morning, intense pain can be referred to
the ear, to the back of the head, and even down the side of the neck.

Jaw joint changes are known as "tempero-mandibular-joint dysfunction." There are now specialists in the field of dentistry who concentrate
on jaw disorders. With special X-ray techniques, they are able to determine the exact relationship between the position of the teeth, the bite,
and the jaw joint.

**Can the esophagus be injured by drinking tea or coffee that is
too hot?**

It most certainly can. The delicate lining of the esophagus which brings food from the mouth to the stomach can be severely burned in this way. Most foods that are too hot are made safe and comfortable in the mouth before they are swallowed. It is asking too much of the protective mechanism of the mouth to make adjustments for fluid that is swallowed when too hot. The mucous membrane of the mouth can also be severely burned by taking unreasonably hot fluid.

My husband, after playing tennis, usually takes an ice-cold shower. Although he enjoys it, I wonder if it's good for him.

Many people make a fetish out of extremes of temperature in the shower, when moderation would be more beneficial. Cold showers especially after exercise may be harmful. Changes in circulation occur within twenty seconds and are equivalent to accelerating a car to forty miles an hour and then shifting it into reverse.

This sounds astonishing, yet it is a reasonable bit of information. This applies to those hardy souls who plunge into ice-cold waters to demonstrate masculinity.

Even after a good night's sleep I find myself barely able to drag myself out of bed. It is not only a sense of fatigue but an absolute inability to get moving.

The physical fatigue of running a house, doing the chores and taking care of children is an overwhelming one. I have often wondered how we men even dare complain about the "tremendous day at the office." The two morning coffee breaks followed by a "taxing" lunch and three hours of afternoon work cannot compare to the energy-expending day of the "little wife at home." I am certain that a man's trade for one day with his wife's exhausting tasks would make him forever keep silent about his fatiguing work.

Chronic fatigue is a very important symptom and must not be overlooked. It cannot be casually disregarded even if the person is in complete good health. The emotional tension of hour-by-hour solutions of the problems of the children and the preparations for being the charming wife when Pop comes home can be very exhausting.

There are many low grade infections, hormone imbalances, kidney and liver disorders and overactive thyroids which may be responsible for fatigue. Low blood pressure and low blood sugar must also be considered as possible causes of fatigue that does not abate with a moderate amount of rest.

My underarm perspiration is so profuse, even in winter, that it is ruining my life. Nothing helps. I'm at my wit's end.

Only those who have had such difficulty can appreciate the esthetic, physical and emotional problems of profuse perspiration. The discomfort of being wringing wet, even in cold weather, and the constant awareness of the disorder can truly interfere with the joys of all social pleasures.

It has long been known that the sweat glands responsible for perspiration are concentrated in a small area high in the armpit.

There is an operation that satisfactorily controls this condition, known as "hyperhydrosis." The operation is not dangerous. Surgeons specially trained in this technique can be found in major hospitals in the United States.

It may seem that an operation for the purpose of controlling perspiration is a radical procedure. Readers must understand that this operation is reserved for uncontrollable perspiration that in no way resembles the moderate perspiration that most people have and which is so easily controlled with a variety of products.

I have been using the same underarm deodorant for years. Sometimes the skin under my arm becomes fiery red and painful. What causes this?

Body odor and perspiration are not one and the same thing. Perspiration in itself is odorless. When odor develops, it is the result of the action of bacteria on the secretions from the glands just beneath the skin. For this reason bathing is important in controlling body odor.

Deodorants are chemicals meant to mask body odors. Antiperspirants are another group of chemicals whose purpose is to reduce the amount of perspiration. Both are usually incorporated in the products that are so commonly used.

Sometimes these chemicals, acting in conjunction with soap that has not been thoroughly rinsed from the underarm, may cause the type of distress you describe.

Occasionally, some people are allergic to the contents of one product and must shift to another. In your case, try to lubricate the area that is red and angry and for a short while avoid using your deodorant.

Both my father and mother had glaucoma of the eyes. I am 27 and live in dread of having the same thing. What are the early signs of glaucoma?

There is no reason why you should spend this happy period of your life anticipating a condition that may never occur. There are hardly any indications of a hereditary factor involved in glaucoma. The chances that you, too, will be afflicted with this are slight.

Early signs of glaucoma are frequently confused with similar symptoms. If I were able to say that a vague headache, or blurry vision, might be imporant, can you imagine the number of people who would be unnecessarily terrified? Symptoms are only important when they are thoroughly interpreted by the doctor during an eye examination.

Blindness from glaucoma is needless and almost always is the result of neglecting to have a simple examination that measures the pressure of fluid within the eyeball. This rapid, painless test for glaucoma is done with a tonometer and within a few seconds can give you the comfort you seek. Every eye examination must include tonometry. Modern drugs and simple surgery now preserve the sight of almost all people with glaucoma when the condition is recognized and given the advantage of early treatment.

Each morning, I wake up with extremely swollen, puffy eyes. Can eye exercises, a special diet, or special surgery cure my problem? My doctor just laughs at me.

I doubt that any doctor would offer laughter as a solution to a cosmetic problem. You have a perfect right to know what is causing your eyes to swell, and to seek a solution. Diet and exercise will do nothing to help you. Plastic surgery is used when "bags under the eyes" are a permanent fixture and do not just happen in the morning. The possibility that you may be allergic to cosmetics, nail polish, and eye makeup must be considered. Try talking to your doctor again to rule out these factors. You will find that he really has a great understanding of your needs.

I'm hoping to get contact lenses. I've read a great deal about them and I am confused whether to get soft lenses or regular hard lenses.

The decision to get soft or hard contact lenses is made in each individual case by the eye specialist who prescribes them.

There seem to be very definite advantages in the use of soft lenses. The most important one is that they can be worn for longer periods of time and with greater comfort from the first time they are used. Soft lenses cause little or no mechanical irritation, which is why they can be used for many more hours.

One of the important medical reasons for not using soft lenses is that they do not correct certain types and degrees of astigmatism as well as do the hard lenses. There are some other factors that enter into the decision.

I might add that not all people are good candidates for either type of contact lens and must, for safety and greater advantage, use eyeglasses.

Whenever I get nervous or upset with my children I get a throbbing headache. I feel that my head will burst open. Could high blood pressure do this?

Yes, indeed it could. But there need be no speculation about it because a blood pressure reading is probably the simplest and most readily accessible test.

This brings me to a message that all doctors want brought to the attention of people. High blood pressure is a dangerous condition when untreated and neglected. There was a time when hypertension (high blood pressure) could be treated only with bed rest. Today, there are excellent drugs which can keep the blood pressure well within an acceptable range and treatment can continue while patients go along with their normal activities.

Many people have a strange fascination about blood pressure numbers. These numbers (readings) are meaningful only to doctors. They compare them with the previous readings, and thus gain insight into the value of the drugs they are prescribing.

There are two blood pressure numbers, the first, or higher one, is called the systolic blood pressure. This measures the pressure in the arteries at the time that the heart pumps blood into them.

The second, or lower number, is called the diastolic. This indicates the pressure in the blood vessels in between each beat of the heart. It is for this reason that one hears reference to their blood pressure as being, for example, "120 over 80." In many instances, the lower, or diastolic, pressure is more significant than the higher one.

Numbers are always terrifying to people who do not understand their significance. One should not, therefore, compare one's own blood pressure numbers with those of another.

Health agencies are relentless in their drive to flush out of hiding people who have unrecognized high blood pressure. By bringing them out into the open and beginning intensive treatment with drugs, diet, and rest, heart disease statistics and mortality froms troke can be significantly minimized.

To reiterate: today high blood pressure in most instances is a controllable disorder. But it is only controllable if people are freed from their anxiety and seek the advice of their doctors.

I have been told by my doctor that I must avoid stress. I don't know what this means. I don't know how to do it at a busy job. I don't know how to handle it while helping to bring up a family of teenagers. How does stress adversely affect the body?

There probably are as many definitions of stress as there are people who use the term. Any unusual pressure, physical or emotional, that alters one's equilibrium is, in essence, stress. In this frenetic age, every experience, even leisure time and the inability to use it properly, can be stressful.

Just as there is a threshold for pain, so is there a threshold for stress. Some people react in degrees that are out of proportion to the pressurizing situation. Others allow stressful experiences to roll off their backs and hardly react to them.

All emotions of worry, fear, love, hate, anger, frustration, and insecurity can produce stress. Any physical exertion beyond the normal capacity of an individual can be stressful and can put pressure on the functioning of all organs of the body.

Stress can alter the entire hormone balance of the body. It can disturb the normal physiology of every organ—the liver, the spleen, the intestines, the brain, the heart, and the circulatory system. Certain types of inflammations, including rheumatoid arthritis, can be traced to unusual stress to the body and to the psyche.

Unfortunately it is impossible to direct you in the ways of avoiding stress. It takes arduous training, from childhood on, to learn the methods by which inner tranquillity can be maintained. Sometimes it takes intensive self re-evaluation and possibly psycho-direction to be able to change to patterns of living that reduce outer and inner tension. It is a great accomplishment when learned.

How many aspirin tablets can be taken in one day for arthritis? Is there any truth to the fact that too many aspirins can affect the heart?

There is no validity to the idea that aspirin has any effect on the heart. This is pure myth, and should be emphasized as such. There is not the slightest scientific or medical basis for it. In fact, some cases of rheumatic heart disease are actually treated with large doses of salicylate, the most active ingredient in aspirin.

Occasionally some people may have an allergic sensitivity to aspirin, even in small quantities. Of course, once this allergy is discovered, the drug should be avoided.

Aspirin, like any other drug, may cause toxic side effects when taken in too large a quantity. For this reason doctors carefully balance the amount of the drug they prescribe with the control of the symptoms.

Patients who have a history of stomach ulcer, or ulcerative colitis, are warned against taking aspirin, even in small quantities. Aspirin itself and combination drugs that contain aspirin should therefore be avoided by these people.

It is an established fact that aspirin may increase the bleeding tendency, and therefore is never prescribed directly after an operation.

The number of tablets that can be taken varies, of course, in all people, depending on age and weight. It is not unusual for patients to take as many as fifteen five-grain tablets of aspirin a day for some forms of arthritis.

The safety of the number of tablets should be established by your doctor.

What fruits have the most laxative effect?

Rhubarb, apples, figs, dates, prunes, raisins and oranges are all said to have mild laxative qualities.

Of course, one of the most reliable laxatives is a daily intake of six to eight glasses of water, unless there is some medical reason for limiting water.

I sincerely want to have my face lifted. My husband, to whom I have been married for thirty years, absolutely does not understand why this should be important to me. He says that he loves me as I am and sees no reason why I should do it, since I am not in a profession like the theater. Are there any dangers to the operation? How long will the benefits last?

There was a time when plastic surgery of the face seemed to be reserved only for people in the moving pictures, the theater and those who are constantly in the public eye. This is no longer so. Many people have found a new, added inner glow to their lives when, by plastic surgery, they have been given a renewed feeling of well-being.

The love your husband has for you is indeed a testimonial to the solid marriage you have enjoyed. The fact that his devotion is as great as it is should not, however, dissuade you from your decision or desire to have a "face lift."

It would do you an injustice, however, if you were to have this operation without his consent and complete understanding of the motives you have for doing it.

The "face lift" operation has been so well-refined that the results are gratifying to the patient and to the surgeon. The operation is performed under general or local anesthesia and is remarkably safe. Skilled plastic surgeons and skilled anesthesiologists have reduced the risk to a minimum. It must be understood that any operation, no matter how simple or complicated, carries with it some degree of risk. It is for this particular reason that your husband must be in complete accord with you, if you are not to undermine a happy household.

The advanced techniques of facial plastic surgery now can almost insure that the cosmetic benefits will last for as many as ten years.

How successfully can bags and wrinkles under the lower lids be removed?

Sagging of the lower lids, bagginess and wrinkling of the skin are some of the by-products of growing older. Some people may more readily show these changes than others. There are many who gracefully accept this change without an urgent feeling to do something about it.

I have never discouraged a patient from having plastic surgery to remedy this condition. I do not feel that the cosmetic repair of "bags" under the eyelids should be reserved for movie and television personalities. There is an excellent lift to one's ego when a disturbing disfigurement is removed.

Occasionally, excess skin with fatty deposit collects in the lower lids. This can be removed by plastic surgeons and bring very gratifying results.

The operation is performed under local anesthesia and is discomforting but relatively painless. The eyes are not involved in this surgery so that vision is not affected in any way except for the swelling that occurs for a few days after the operation.

The psychological benefits are great when people understand that there are limits to what can be expected of the surgery.

What is the safest and most satisfactory way to remove wrinkles of the face? Are hormone creams dangerous?

Let me answer the second part of your question by saying that expensive hormone creams are more dangerous to your pocketbook than to your body. Pure food and drug requirements have almost totally eliminated the right to include hormones in any of these cosmetic preparations.

There are some safe methods by which wrinkles can be removed. Plastic surgeons have many methods that can improve the cosmetic appearance of the face. Only such reliable people should be permitted to attempt to remove wrinkles. Unfortunately, there are a number of non-medical methods by which caustic agents are applied to the skin "to peel off the wrinkles." No one should undertake such a procedure without the definite approval of one's doctor.

Can anything be done about the stretch marks on the skin that I have had since my last baby was born?

"Stretch" marks, like the "hash" marks on the sleeve of a long service Army man, can only be considered a sign of special distinction.

Following pregnancy, *strae gravidarum* occur particularly on the skin of the abdomen, due to distention and stretching.

The marks can also occur on the thighs, the buttocks and the breasts. The cause is a slight rupture of the elastic fibers under the skin.

Unfortunately, there are no creams, hormones, or special gadgets that will completely eradicate these stretch marks. In some cases, they do tend to become less prominent with time.

It is an interesting and unexplained fact that other causes of distention of the abdomen other than pregnancy do not always produce these marks. But then, not all women carry these distinctive signs of pregnancy.

I am a schoolteacher, and after a day of work with children I am completely hoarse. My concern is the possibility of permanent damage to my vocal cords.

The vocal cords are two small muscles in the larynx, or voice box. They come together during speech, and separate when we breathe. Like all muscles, when they are overused they become fatigued.

The vocal cords, pounding against each other all day long, actually cause moderate swelling of the lining that surrounds them. The result is hoarseness.

If these muscles are not rested, the injury to the vocal cords can produce chronic changes so that eventually voice production is reduced markedly.

Hoarseness is, in your case, an occupational hazard. Many teachers, singers, preachers and salesmen must learn to modify the use of their vocal cords if chronic changes in the cords are to be avoided.

After a day's work, a good idea is to use warm steam for a few minutes. This is a very soothing treatment. In addition, it is important not to whisper, for whispering actually puts more of a strain on the vocal cords than soft or modulated speaking.

Is there a relationship between hoarseness and shortness of breath?

Hoarseness and shortness of the breath may be related under certain circumstances. There need not be, however, a tie-up between the two.

Hoarseness can be caused by anything that interferes with the vocal cords coming together. An infection, inflammation, tumor, polyp or a cancerous condition may be the underlying reason for longstanding hoarseness. Mentioning a cancerous growth is not meant in any way to frighten the reader but rather to show him that hoarseness is an important sign that demands recognition and examination.

The vocal cords, which lie in the voice box in the neck, come together when one speaks and separate when one breathes. Any interference with this delicate mechanism may cause both hoarseness and shortness of breath.

Occasionally there may be a weakness or even a paralysis of the vocal cords responsible for both hoarseness and shortness of breath. Here then is a possible relationship between the two.

In most instances the two conditions are unrelated. Their cause can readily be found.

The most common cause for sustained hoarseness is vocal abuse. People in a "speaking"profession like teachers, preachers, lecturers, singers and actors can often overuse their voices. I am always amazed how little respect these people have for their vocal cords which are so important to their profession.

Of course, the shortness of breath may be caused by a variety of conditions in the lungs and even due to heart and circulatory disturbances. Rather than build up a relationship between the two or become concerned about either, a general examination would allay anxiety about both.

Can there be any connection between temporary hoarseness and the beginning of the menstrual period?

Throat specialists have noted that the vocal cords can sometimes be temporarily swollen before menstruation. This may be related to the tendency to accumulate fluids in the body tissues during this time.

Is it common for a woman to notice definite changes of personality shortly before the menstrual period? I notice the change in my relationship with my children and my husband and even find that I don't like myself at that time. Can any special medicines spare all of us my irritability?

Shortly before the onset of the menstrual period there is a general change of the hormone balance and many physical changes occur which account for emotional stress. Many women tend to retain body fluids, become nervous, have headaches and generally are fatigued and restless.

In many primitive communities, women would relieve their unexplained personality changes by spending limitless hours in the community bakery making breads and cakes to lessen their anxieties.

But being kept busy is not the easy answer for your problems. The normal fatigue of running a household becomes worse during this time.

Mild tranquilizers taken under the supervision of a doctor tend to relieve premenstrual tensions.

I am a bundle of nerves before my menstrual period. Is this common? How can I avoid it so that my children and family can live with me?

Even in primitive times there were stories of how women got the sudden urge to bake bread during this time of the month. Polishing floors and painting walls are modern versions of the need to get rid of tensions before menstruation sets in.

Many explanations have been given for such tension, including psychological and emotional stress and hormonal imbalance. Many complicated reasons such as fluid retention may have some validity. Early childhood training about menstruation may also have some bearing on such adult behavior. The fact that this normal, healthy period in a woman's life is referred to as "the curse" or "falling off the roof" indicates a hostile or even violent reaction to it.

Your physician may prescribe "water pills" and mild tranquilizers to help carry you over these premenstrual phases. You must remember that you, too, have a right to indulge yourself occasionally with rest. There is no need to feel guilty that your family is suffering because of your emotional responses at this time.

Why do some women have severe pain during their menstrual periods? Is there any way to prevent these regular periods of severe discomfort?

Painful menstruation, or dysmenorrhea, may be caused by one of many conditions that affect the uterus and the ovaries. Physicians sometimes divide the causes into primary and secondary reasons.

The first may be due to a disorder in the growth and development of the uterus or to its unusual position.

The secondary form of painful menstruation may be due to diseases, infections and inflammation of the cervix and the uterus itself. Fibroid tumors, ovarian cysts and inflammatory changes around the ovaries may be the cause.

It is apparent, therefore, that, before this condition is treated, the exact cause must be definitely found by a complete pelvic examination.

It is unfortunate that so many women simply accept the fact that they must be miserable for a few days at the time of their menses. In most instances it is absolutely unnecessary for women to lose a few productive days of every month because they feel that this "is a woman's natural burden." It is not.

It is not enough to drug oneself into oblivion as a substitute for treating the basic reasons for the pain. Drugs, hormones and specially controlled exercises can convert these distressing days into painless ones so that normal daily activities can continue without interruption.

Is there any truth to the idea that children born to mothers past the age of forty are not as healthy as those born to younger mothers?

This is a misconception and a myth that tends to induce unnecessary fears. With normal pregnancy in a healthy woman who has no history of any significant disease, the child should be healthy and normal regardless of the mother's age.

Can a woman be pregnant and not know it?

Occasionally, the early symptoms of pregnancy may be confused with other conditions. Both patient and doctor may not know that an early pregnancy is involved.

In order to uncover early pregnancy, a new two-minute urine test is being used. At a large hospital in New York City a doctor has been routinely testing a large group of women who had medical complaints,

71

but did not have knowledge of existing pregnancy. Thirteen cases of unsuspected pregnancy were found among three hundred women.

The significance of uncovering early pregnancy in these cases is that some tests and some drugs normally used for a medical condition might possibly have an adverse effect on the unborn child.

Rapid urine tests can be easily performed in the doctor's office.

Why is it necessary for a woman to have so many examinations during pregnancy? I have an opportunity to go off on a distant trip for several months with my husband, but my doctor insists that I must have regular examinations during my pregnancy.

It is true that many pregnancies can proceed without any unusual problem or difficulty. As a matter of fact, thousands of babies are born all over the world without any medical supervision. Many of them thrive, but a great many of them and their mothers pay a heavy toll.

During routine visits, a doctor determines weight gain, does blood studies and measures the blood pressure so that any unusual complication is detected early. Only in this way does the unborn child have its greatest advantage for normal health.

The decision and responsibility for being away from your doctor are, of course, yours. In general, the safest approach to normal pregnancy is to be in constant contact with your own doctor here, or in the geographic area you plan to visit.

I am the mother of three healthy children. I am pregnant now. I would enjoy my pregnancy except that I suffer terribly with morning nausea. Is there any drug I can take to control the nausea?

Morning sickness, which sometimes extends to afternoon and evening sickness, is often associated with the first seven days to ten weeks of pregnancy. Fortunately, it seems to disappear about the twelfth week.

There are many complex factors, physical and emotional, that are responsible for the nausea of early pregnancy. The observation has been made that eating small quantities of food at very frequent intervals may reduce this unpleasant symptom. Foods relatively high in carbohydrate, taken in these small amounts six or eight times a day, may be beneficial. But even this innocuous suggestion should not be undertaken without the definite sanction of your own doctor.

In the light of the extensive unhappiness caused by a so-called "safe" drug during pregnancy, doctors everywhere are urging pregnant women to abstain from all drugs unless they have been specifically prescribed for them.

Are there any drugs that are safe to use for morning sickness in early pregnancy?

Absolutely none. I can't emphasize that enough.

Unless your doctor or obstetrician specifically suggests a drug, none should be bought over the counter or handed down to you from solicitous friends.

The accepted attitude of doctors today is that the fewer the drugs taken during pregnancy, the greater the advantage to the mother and the child for a safe pregnancy.

By eating small quantities of food and avoiding tobacco and alcohol, your morning sickness may ease. It certainly is worth a try.

I am about to have my first baby. I have been told about a stitching operation that is painful. Can you tell me what that is?

Your own physican, of course, would have relieved your anxiety about what the so-called "stitching" operation is.

At the time of birth, a clean incision is made at the opening of the vagina shortly before delivery. The purpose of this incision is to avoid a laceration or tearing of the birth canal as the baby emerges. This is known as an episotomy. It is a safe and painless procedure that is performed almost regularly with the birth of the first baby. Later pregnancies may not need this.

Is it common for a young woman to feel depressed after the birth of a healthy baby when she loves both the child and her husband very dearly?

Depression after the birth of a baby must be considered an unwelcome complication. It is no different from any physical problem that might have arisen.

With this in mind, every woman whose depression and misery is not readily controlled should be given the immediate advantage of a consultation with a psychiatrist or psychologist. The guidance they can offer may be in simply opening a new avenue leading to the relief of this unpleasant complication at a time of great potential happiness.

It might interest you to know, too, that the new baby benefits when the mother is helped to snap out of her depression. Infants often do not thrive when cared for by mothers who are overwhelmed by their own emotional problems.

Can you explain why I, as a young mother, should have developed a severe case of the blues after my baby was born? It was a happy pregnancy and a normal delivery. I just don't understand why I have crying spells.

Postpartum depression occurs with a greater ferquency than is commonly suspected. The exact reasons are not entirely known. Many normal, perfectly happy, well-adjusted women are affected this way. Pregnancy is associated with many physical changes that may temporarily affect the psychic balance.

There is no shame in having these symptoms. I emphasize this so that you will be encouraged to speak about it openly to your husband and, with his help, seek the guidance of a psychologist or psychiatrist.

Very often it takes little time to help you readjust to your normal pattern of living. You must not feel any sense of inadequacy because this so-called complication of a normal pregnancy happened to you.

Is there any medical reason why so many children seem to be born in the middle of the night? I have had four and each was born with the same frenzied rush at four in the morning.

Although I don't know the exact statistics, I would venture to say that more children are born during the day than during the night. I am certain that there is no significant reason why your night visitors arrive amidst the frenzy you speak of. After a woman has had more than one or two children, the ease of giving birth increases and the rapidity with which the final stages of labor occur tends to increase the anxiety about getting to the hospital on time.

There now is a tendency for doctors and obstetricians to control the actual time of delivery so that they, too, need not be deprived of a good wholesome night's rest.

This has all been made possible by the careful use of a hormone from the pituitary gland in the brain with which a doctor can begin active labor almost at will. The hormone used to induce labor stimulates the muscles of the uterus or womb and causes them to contract to advance the birth process. There are many advantages to use of this drug when it is employed in carefully chosen cases. I hope that day is a lovely one when your welcomed fifth first sees its light.

The advantages of mother's milk for a child are always referred to as being psychologically beneficial. Is the chemical composition of the milk itself better for the newborn child?

Milk, both mother's and cow's, is considered a nearly perfect, complete food for the nourishment and growth of the child. Rarely is it viewed, as it rightfully should be, as one of the most complex substances in the human body. Vitamins and minerals are only a few of the ingredients that give milk its importance as a total food product. Sugars, fatty acids, amino acids and proteins are only part of the vast complex of substances in milk. Biochemists have isolated dozens of other chemicals and their derivatives and they admit there are many more waiting to be uncovered.

Many hormones play an active role in the synthesis of milk. Millions of tiny cells in the breast structure are stimulated to produce the milk and carry it to its collecting point in the breast where it issues as food. This incredible system occurs in the human and in the cow with little variation. Yet there are admitted chemical advantages in the content of mother's milk over milk taken from animals when used to nourish the child.

Technically the advantages are there. Yet a mother who is unable to nurse, for any reason, should not feel guilty because she believes her child is being deprived. I must return to the greatest advantage of mother's milk by breastfeeding and re-emphasize the psychological values. These are more significant to the baby than is the greater nourishment factor of mother's milk.

Is there any danger if a pregnant woman flies at high altitudes in a pressurized airplane?

A number of studies have been attempted in an effort to find out if high altitude flying is a hazard at any stage of pregnancy. Most of the studies have been done on experimental animals and, therefore, have no real validity in humans. Yet, certain observations suggest that there is some risk because of an insufficient amount of oxygen to the unborn child at high altitudes.

One Colorado doctor suggests that women who are in the last three months of their pregnancy should not travel in unpressurized planes. If they fly below 10,000 feet, the unborn child is not affected. He further suggests than, when flying above 10,000 feet in an unpressurized plane, the mother should breathe oxygen to protect the child.

In order to avoid any confusion and to avoid anxiety in pregnant women who fly, this statement must be made once more. There is no danger to health in pressurized cabins during any stage of pregnancy.

Today, there are very few commercial planes that are not well pressurized. The problem occurs mostly in small private planes and these should be avoided during the end of pregnancy.

Before deciding on any flight during this period of pregnancy, advice from the doctor would be wise and reassuring.

I am in my eighth month of pregnancy. It may be necessary for my husband and me to fly across the country and back. Would there be any danger to the child?

Pressurized commerical planes have reduced the risk to the unborn child. Of course, the rare possibility of insufficient oxygen must be considered. Unless there is great urgency, flying during this stage of pregnancy should be avoided without explicit advice of the doctor in charge.

I have two children and will in the next few months have a third. As an active mother, I feel that I would like my hospital stay to be as short as possible so that I can get back to my children. Is this a danger to the mother or child?

During the past twenty-five years there has been an increasing tendency to shorten hospital stays. Surgeons who previously kept their patients in bed for a week after operations are now getting them up and about in twenty-four hours.

There is an excellent reason for encouraging patients to get out of bed quickly. It reduces the frequency of lung complications. However, I think there is a great psychological advantage, in addition to a physical one, for staying in a hospital for an extra few days.

Your desire to return home to your children is understandable. Yet, if you return too early, you will be bedded at home without any contribution to your family.

Childbirth and anesthesia exhaust the energy of all body organs. It is imperative, therefore, that the body and the mind be given a few extra days of concentrated rest, so that when the mother returns home she is in a better position to function as a healthy person rather than as an invalid.

Allow yourself the gift of indulgence. You'll be better off.

My fiance and I are both healthy. However, there is a family background of epilepsy. Is it safe for us to contemplate marriage?

If neither of you have epilepsy the chances are minimal that your offspring will be afflicted, even with your family history. There are so many different forms of epilepsy and so many causes that it would be unfair for you to cheat yourself of your rightful happiness by such anxiety.

Nevertheless, I would most certainly present this problem to one of the many excellent genetic counselors who specialize in these problems. The knowledge of genetics has progressed remarkably in the past ten years. With blood studies and intensive investigation of the family background, such a counselor can give you important advice and assurance.

It would be unfair to both of you if you were to pretend that this problem is not a real source of distress to you. If explained, it will not mar the joys of bringing up a family. You can be certain that the geneticist will carefully evaluate the problem and help you arrive at a clearly defined decision.

A blood examination of my pregnant daughter has just shown that the new baby will be born with an "RH factor." None of us really knows what this means and are terrified that it may be serious.

The problem of the RH factor is particularly confusing and complicated, even to those who speak of it daily. The letters RH were taken

77

from the first two letters of the rhesus monkey, which was used in the initial experiments.

Everyone has within their blood the RH factor. Most people are RH-positive. Only a few are RH-negative. If both parents are RH-positive, or if both parents are RH-negative, the newborn child will not be affected. If the mother is RH-positive and the father is RH-negative the newborn baby will still not be affected.

It is only when the mother is RH-negative and the father is RH-positive that the entire pregnancy must be carefully followed to avoid any of the possible complications that may arise. For, if the baby that is growing in the mother's womb has inherited the father's RH-positive factor, a condition of anemia and jaundice may occur at birth.

It is of interest to note that the firstborn child rarely, if ever, is an RH-problem baby. With the second or later pregnancies, a complex relationship exists between the mother, her antibodies, and those of the unborn child. This is responsible for the complications that may arise at birth—not to the mother, but to the baby.

When it is known that an RH situation is present, the doctor prepares himself and makes plans for many of the new techniques that now make it possible for such a child to survive and, in fact, quickly become completely healthy.

A special type of blood transfusion can, if necessary, be performed soon after birth. Almost all the child's blood can be replaced by new, fresh blood so that the anemia and jaundice will disappear. This remarkable method, once thought spectacular, is done now with such regularity that it is almost considered routine. Many more elaborate studies and methods are now available to give additional security that the child born with an RH factor will flourish.

Is an overdue pregnancy as significant to the newborn child as the premature completion of pregnancy?

Modern statistics of safety are remarkably encouraging in both premature and prolonged pregnancies, especially when they are under the constant supervision of a doctor. The time element in both is, of course, most important. A premature birth during the eighth month of pregnancy undoubtedly means greater safety to the child than one that occurs in the seventh month. Similarly, a post-term pregnancy of a few days or a week is hardly significant. Some women, because of a hereditary pattern, tend to have longer pregnancies than normal. The exact reason has never been definitely established.

There is always the possibility of miscalculation of dates which alters the predictability of the end of pregnancy. Physicians have their guidelines which in most instances are accurate. Any delay in giving birth should not be filled with any special anxiety, especially when there is the complete assurance by the delivering doctor.

I am two months pregnant and my doctor told me that I have veneral disease called trichomona. My husband does not have it. Will my baby be born with it? Could I have caught this disease in a hospital when I had a miscarriage six months ago?

Trichomonas vaginalis is definitely not a veneral disease. I am absolutely certain that in your anxiety your misunderstood what your physician told you. There is not a physcian in the world who would have said that you have a venereal disease since it is well known that this illness is due to a fungus or parasitic infection of the vagina.

There are many effective ways of curing this temporary, unpleasant condition with drugs used locally within the vagina. Others are taken orally.

Let me assure you that you baby will not in any way be affected by your present condition. In all likelihood you will completely cured by the time of delivery.

It is an interesting and rarely known fact that husbands may unknowingly be contaminated with the fungus and continue to reinfect their marital partners. This can be controlled by microscopic studies and smears. Please call your physician and explain your confusion so that your excellent relationship with him will not be disturbed by such obvious misunderstanding.

How long after a woman has ceased to menstruate can she become pregnant?

It is generally accepted that if a woman has had no menstrual cycle for a year after the menopause (change of life) has set in, pregnancy is hardly possible.

Cases have been reported of pregnancies in women who apparently have reached menopause. In these instances, the menstrual cycle has usually been irregular all through their lives.

Each person must be evaluated individually by her own doctor.

How often after fifty should a woman have an internal checkup by her gynecologist?

Unless there are any unusual symptoms such an examination should made once a year. The pap smear for cancer is easily performed and can give you great assurance when it is negative.

The experience of physicians has been that when cancers of the cervix of the womb are found early and treated immediately the chances of recovery are excellent.

Routine examination of the entire body is a sound investment in health. We in the practice of medicine have occasionally found that people seek such examinations too frequently because they live in constant fear of a disease that they actually do not have. A complete examination must bring with it the peace of mind and assurance you seek and need.

Can a woman who has had one ovary removed become pregnant? I am contemplating marriage and I am deeply concerned about this.

Pregnancy most certainly can occur with women who have only one ovary. You must not be hesitant to ask your doctor who will give you the added assurance you and your fiance deserve. Certainly your unnecessary concern should not deprive you of your happy decision to marry.

I have been told that my uterus is out of position. Is this common?

Women sometimes develop a condition known as prolapse of the uterus, commonly known as a falling of the womb. In women past middle age, especially those who have had a number of children, the muscles and ligaments that hold up the structure of the female organs in the pelvis become weakened and do not keep the womb and the vagina in proper position.

The symptoms that result are usually a sense of fullness and discomforting weight and occasionally interference with normal bowel movements and urination.

Modern care in the delivery of children has reduced the frequency and severity of this condition. Nevertheless, prolapse still occurs. The treatment in simple cases is the use of a pessary as a support. In difficult cases surgery is the ideal form of treatment. The results are most gratifying and almost immediately relieve the woman of the annoying symptoms. The decision must, of course, depend on the surgeon's judgment about the severity and progress of the falling womb.

For two years I have known that I have a large cyst of one ovary. Sometimes it is painful and I worry about it. When the pain disappears I again decide to do nothing about it. I know that I really worry that the removal of this cyst will prevent me from becoming pregnant and having a third child. If one ovary remains is there just as good chance of becoming pregnant?

It is generally believed that one perfectly healthy normal ovary is sufficient for pregnancy. The Fallopian tube that carries the egg into the womb must also be normal. I hope that this information will satisfy this one part of your anxiety.

There is, however, another aspect of your problem which must be separated from your desire to have another child. The fact that you have an ovarian cyst must be considered for your general health.

There are many types of ovarian cysts. Each month a small cyst forms in the ovary to house the egg which is discharged at ovulation. Almost always the cyst then disappears. Occasionally a cyst grows larger, causes pain and pressure and interferes with the normal menstrual cycle.

A special type of mucous cyst is found in young women. These may become as large as a basketball and can, by pressure, cause many odd symptoms.

Occasionally a cyst may become twisted and cause symptoms that resemble acute appendicitis with abdominal pain, nausea and disturbances of the intestines.

If your surgeon has recommended the removal of the cyst it is unwise to wait until a relatively simple operation is converted into a complicated one. It is not unusual for the surgeon to find a type of cyst which can be removed without the necessity of removing the entire ovary. Delay, in your case, is not good judgement. Follow your doctor's advice.

Surgery for fibroid tumors of my womb has been suggested. I cannot get my doctor to say definitely how extensive the operation will be. He does not know whether the total removal of the womb will be necessary. At my age of thirty-five, this causes me great concern.

Surgery that removes the womb (uterus) at any age is a source of concern. When one is in the child-bearing period, it is especially distressing if one still hopes to enlarge her family.

Fibroid tumors are benign, non-cancerous growths which grow on the surface, in the wall and on the inner lining of the womb. Their size varies from tiny ones to apple-sized and large melon-size ones. In many cases, surgeons can tell by their size and the pressure exerted by these tumors, the exact extent of the surgery. In your case, the surgeon must base his choice of operation and extent of surgery on his findings once he opens the lower abdomen. You must have complete faith that his past experience and judgment aims at your good health and the preservation of the womb whenever it is possible.

Five years ago when I first started the change of life I was told that I had a fibroid tumor of the womb about the size of a two month pregnancy. My change of life has now set in and I am not ill or uncomfortable. Will this fibroid disappear or will surgery be necessary?

A fibroid tumor of the womb or uterus is not uncommon. A large one such as the one you describe may produce in some people pressure on the bladder or on the large intestine and cause symptoms of discomfort.

Once the diagnosis of a fibroid tumor is made it should be checked at regular intervals, perhaps every six months, to note if it is getting larger or smaller.

There are many kinds of fibroids which are benign or non-cancerous. Some originate on the surface of the womb. Others in the muscle itself, and some on the inner lining. It is rare that a fibroid becomes malignant but it is wise to respect its presence and avoid neglecting it.

I have been told that I have a fibroid tumor of the womb. The doctor says he will watch it. Are there different types of tumors of the womb? Of course, I worry that it might be cancer.

The fact that your doctor wants to keep the fibroid tumor under observation should indicate to you that he is not concerned about the possibility that it might be malignant. If he were, he undoubtedly would recommend immediate surgery. Your anxiety about this is, therefore unnecessary.

A fibroid tumor is a benign, or non-cancerous, growth. Only rarely does it undergo malignant changes. Long before this happens, the tumor which has been under the doctor's observation is removed.

There are no "different types" of fibroid tumors, but they do vary in position and in the place where they originate and grow. Some are attached to the inside lining of the womb, or uterus. These may be responsible for excessive bleeding during and between the menstrual period.

Other fibroid tumors are attached to the outside of the uterus. When these are enlarged they may exert pressure on the bladder or even the rectum.

The largest number of fibroid tumors occur within the powerful muscle of the uterus itself. Here, too, pressure symptoms, chronic fatigue and low back pains may be present.

Varicose veins in the legs may result when a large fibroid tumor of the uterus compresses the blood vessels in the pelvis.

Some fibroid tumors never get any larger than they were at the time they were first discovered. Others increase in size slowly; sometimes rapidly. It is for this reason that surveillance is important.

For what reason is the entire womb removed from a young woman of thirty-five? Is it more dangerous at a young age? Must the ovaries be removed too?

Fibroid tumors are the most common reason for the removal of the womb, or hysterectomy.

Fibroid tumors themselves do not necessarily mean that such surgery must be performed. When there is severe bleeding during or between menstrual periods, or when large fibroids interfere with the bowels or passing urine, surgery may be necessary.

Occasionally an early cancerous condition is found by pap smear or by curettage. This may necessitate the removal of the uterus. The decision to remove the ovaries at the time of surgery depends on the age of the patient and on the judgment of the surgeon at the time of operation.

The decision to remove the uterus is very carefully and critically considered, because of its immense physical and emotional impact on the woman.

Other readers have asked if a hysterectomy brings on the menopause, or change of life. The ovaries and not the uterus are responsible for the female hormone activity. If one or both ovaries are left in place at the time of surgery, menopause will not occur even though the menstrual cycle will stop.

Before such important surgery patients are urged to ask their doctors to answer the many questions that will relieve their anxieties. This is wise before any operation. It spares a great deal of post-operative confusion.

I'm writing to you because I am ashamed to ask my own doctor. Where does the menstrual blood go after a hysterectomy operation? Can it cause a tumor or adhesions that later cause trouble?

There never should be any shame about the fact that you do not completely understand the way a body functions. Doctors do not expect their patients to know anatomy and physiology. They completely understand their patients' confusion. If one does not completely understand the body in health or in illness, one naturally becomes fearful.

During menstruation the inner lining of the uterus, or the womb, sheds itself about every twenty-eight days. When the uterus is removed by the operation known as a hysterectomy, there is no longer any surface from which menstrual bleeding can occur. After such surgery, artificial change of life sets in, especially when ovaries are removed at the same time.

Now that you understand there is no internal or external menstrual bleeding after a hysterectomy, you can be assured that tumors and adhesions cannot occur because of this.

I am very worried about approaching menopause. Can you help me?

Many women past the age of thirty-five live with expressed and un-expressed fears about the approach of the menopause, or change of life. Much of the unnecessary anxiety is based on the fact that false information and myths have been handed down from generation to generation about this period in a woman's life.

The word menopause is derived from the Greek *menos* meaning month and *pauein* meaning to cease. Menopause, therefore, is that period of normal change when menstruation slows down and finally ceases during middle age. The age varies with each individual woman and has been known to vary in different geographic areas. In some cases symptoms of change of life have occurred as early as thirty years of age, while in others they may not appear until past fifty.

Sudden episodes of hot flashes and unexplained perspiration, with restlessness and fatigue, are known to occur during this stage and often may alter the emotional stability of the woman. The psychological over-tones are particularly severe when women falsely believe that their at-tractiveness, sexuality, and general health will be impaired by the onset of the menopause.

The symptoms of change of life are due to a temporary imbalance or a deficiency of the hormones produced by the ovaries and other endocrine glands. Estrogen, the female hormone, is now being used extensively by a great many physicians to supplement the lagging production of this hormone period.

The decision to use this hormone, of course, depends on the physician's findings in each particular case. Since the emotions are in-timately involved with all bodily changes, it is wise for women to thoroughly discuss the problem of the menopause with their doctor to avoid the pitfalls of anxiety so frequent at the time of this change of life. It frequently comes as a surprise that many women flourish emotionally and physically when they gracefully mature into the menopause.

My mother had a very difficult time during her change of life. It was filled with severe emotional upsets that almost disrupted our entire family. Although I am only thirty-six years old and have no symptoms of menopause, I find myself looking out for possible changes.

There does not seem to be any special hereditary pattern common to all women in the same family. Therefore, I believe that you are being unduly concerned both about the onset of change of life and the possible severity of its symptoms.

It is believed that emotional makeup and personal temperament may affect the character of the menopause. Depression associated with the annoying symptoms can be alleviated by the understanding of your husband and the other members of your family.

You should discuss your anxieties and concern with your family doctor. He will tell you many doctors feel that the use of an estrogen, an important female hormone, before and during the change of life can reduce the severity of the annoying symptoms. Not all women are given these estrogen hormones but those who are chosen for it have been remarkably gratified by results.

During the menopause, the general hormone balance of the body is upset. The ovaries which produce the estrogen diminish their supply. There is a close relationship between the estrogen level in the blood and the hormone produced by the pituitary gland in the brain. When this balance is disturbed, definite changes in the body structure become apparent.

I cannot help wondering whether you, and so many other women, are afraid that the change of life means you will be less attractive physically and that it will be the end of your sexual life. This definitely is not so. As a matter of fact, many women during this period of their lives find they are past the fears of pregnancy that interfered with their total emancipation. Menopause can start a very happy time in a woman's life.

How do physicians feel about the use of hormones during a woman's change of life?

When the idea of using estrogen or female sex hormone was first introduced, there was a great deal of discussion about its value.

Positions were taken by some doctors who firmly believed in its advantages. Others were just as forcefully against its use. Today, there is greater stabilization of thought about its advantages.

However, hormones are never given indiscriminately to all people. It is for this reason that each woman who is in her pre-menopausal or menopausal phase is individually studied and evaluated before the estrogen is advised.

The general consensus is that female sex hormone is advantageous. It may reduce some of the unpleasant "flush" feelings so often associated with early change of life.

Extensive scientific studies have also shown that the absorption of calcium from the bones, known as "osteoporosis," a common condition among women of menopausal age, can be delayed by the use of estrogen hormone.

The change of life has begun for me without too much discomfort. I have consulted two doctors for their opinions about the use of hormones during this period. What are the advantages, and are there any dangers?

The question of hormone replacement during menopause has been a subject of great discussion during the past few years. There is not yet complete agreement that the estrogen hormone should be used by all patients during this period.

Reliable specialists all over America have used the estrogen hormone in thousands of women with apparent safety.

Your confusion must be the result of two divergent opinions. Perhaps you will be assured by a study in which five hundred women were given daily doses of estrogen hormone for the past nine years without any serious side effects.

Since there is only a slight suspicion, doctors who use the hormone insist that all of their patients have a complete gynecological examination with the pap test for cancer every six months.

A physician at the New York Downstate Medical Center, using the hormone extensively, has found no relationship between the use of estrogen and any kind of tumor.

Another advantage is that the tendency towards bone softening, or osteoporosis, during menopause can be slowed or stopped by the long use of the hormone.

Your gynecologist knows all these facts and can best direct you for the maximum advantage to your health.

Is there complete agreement about the use of estrogen therapy to prevent "change of life?"

Estrogen therapy does *not* prevent the onset of the menopause, or "change of life." Those who are enthusiastic about its use feel that it has many advantages for the comfort of the patient during the normal progression of menopause.

A great many gynecologists, specialists in the problems of women, have used the hormone with outstanding success. They believe that their patients do not show the processes of aging as quickly as do women who do not have the estrogen during this time.

Many scientific studies are being performed all over the country in an effort to substantiate the value and possible disadvantages of sustained doses of estrogen. The level of this hormone is kept up in patients throughout the onset and progress of the "change of life," in carefully selected cases.

There is never complete agreement about the use of this or any other prescription in all cases. The hormone is safe when taken under a doctor's direction for the time he prescribes it. If there are any unusual side effects, he will immediately stop it. Each case must be evaluated individually.

Your own physician takes into consideration your physical findings and your past background and then after a series of tests may prescribe estrogen for you. Then and only then should you take it. You should continue to be examined at regular intervals.

In your opinion is the extended use of estrogen in tablet form, during and after the change of life, harmful or dangerous?

The use of estrogen, or as it is commonly known, the female sex hormone, during and after menopause, has been extensive for the past five years. Although there is not absolute agreement by all physicians and gynecologists about its use in all cases, it has been accepted as a safe contribution to the health and well-being of women during the change of life.

You specifically ask about "the extended use of estrogen" and that intrigues me particularly. The word extended seems to carry with it the impression of long sustained use without constant supervision. This is the key to the successful and safe use of any drug. It should be used only for the time that it is prescribed. No extended time should elapse without a recheck by the physician or gynecologist who prescribes this valuable hormone.

Can cosmetics with hormones be beneficial for skin diseases? Are there any dangers to their use?

Hope springs eternal in the human breast for youthful regeneration with creams, lotions, and royal jellies that contain estrogen and other magic ingredients. I am certain that there must be some advantages to the lubricating qualities of these products. Their expense hardly justifies their advantages in many instances.

There isn't enough estrogen in these exorbitant creams to change the life of the skin of a canary. They can change the fatness of the wallet. The Food and Drug Administration has cracked down sharply against the fraudulence of "royal jellies" that were said to perform miracles of rejuvenation.

The possible dangers of estrogen hormone is exceedingly slight because of the small quantities that are used in these preparations. Nevertheless, before any such product is used it is wise to consult with one's own physician.

My husband is 41 years old. Last summer he had a complete change of personality. He became nervous and irritable. He shouts at me and the children. He cries a lot. My friends say that he is going through the male change of life. Is this possible?

The question of a male menopause is still a matter of dispute. Some physicians believe that emotional and physical changes in men that occur in middle age are due to an actual physical "change of life." Others insist that there is no validity to the concept. The reason for the confusion is that there are no distinct physiological changes in men similar to those that occur in women.

Women, at the change of life or menopause, can be given estrogen, or female sex hormone, to make up for a deficiency during this period. Testosterone, or male hormone, does not seem to produce the same positive effect when taken by men.

All body processes are different during the forties than during the twenties and thirties. But whether or not a real male menopause does occur would not affect your husband's problem and how it should be managed.

The first approach is to rule out, by thorough physical examination, the possibility of organic or bodily illness. If your doctor feels that there is a hormone deficiency, this can be replaced while psychological avenues are being explored.

You, with the help of your doctor (not your friends) can, in an understanding way, show your husband that he needs psychological guidance. He may possibly be able to express to a psychologist or a psychiatrist some of the hidden problems disturbing him. Very often free expression to a relative stranger can clarify deep conflicts. Once there is such clarification, your husband may get a better insight into his own emotions and revert to the person he really is.

Chapter IV

What Men Ask

Invariably, when I'm at a social gathering and the subject of my syndicated health column comes up, the women in the group ask about what most correspondents want to know or what was the funniest question I ever received or possibly how I answer some specific question, such as "do I recommend face-lifts." The men present say very little. But later, when a more fascinating subject than what I do is introduced and the tide of conversation veers, I know what to expect. Several of my fellow guests will make it their business to have a word with me quietly. Do I really answer all the letters I get from my readers? Do men write to me or is a newspaper column strictly the territory of nervous females? Do I preserve the anonymity of my correspondents?

While I usually manage to maintain a professional detachment in these situations, I nonetheless find it difficult to convince these doubting Thomases that just as many men as women seek advice by mail. And that I can often predict what a man will ask whereas women come up with more complicated situations and questions that require more involved replies. Men have certain basic problems—baldness, prostate trouble, hernias, smoking, arthritis—and one can pigeonhole the bulk of their queries in short order.

But women seem to be more intense in their anxiety to know the varied whys and wherefores of their particular health problems. A woman may ask a question for a friend, a distant cousin, her daughter-in-law, even project what might happen to herself five years hence. A man usually asks about what is happening to himself and happening at the moment.

Another difference in my correspondents occurs to me—very often I hear again from women who have sought my advice. They write to let me know how much my advice has helped them or allayed their concern. You do not get this kind of follow-up from men.

It is always interesting—and touching—to receive letters from men asking questions that relate to their wives' health and vice versa. Obviously they want to gain some special information that will help them make their spouses' conditions more comfortable, improved or cured. And who writes most frequently about conditions relating to their marriage partner? Surprisingly, it's the male.

Is it unusual for young men who complain of pain in the back to be suffering from arthritis?

Arthritis has no great respect for any age group but, undeniably, it occurs more frequently in older people.

Many cases of arthritis occur in young men who had chronic, nagging pain in their backs which prevented ordinary activity. Spondylitis, an inflammation of the vertebrae of the spinal column, may be responsible for persistent pain and may frequently be overlooked. One of the characteristics is that it occurs in young men, usually in their twenties. X-raying the small joints of the spine to find some of the reasons for the low back pain, the stiffness, and the tired soreness that so often incapacitates young men is necessary.

Early diagnosis and early treatment relieve the pain and prevent the progression of the disease. One of the most dramatic drugs is phenylbutazone. Another is indomethacin which, when used under the direction of a physician, is remarkably effective.

Young men with this type of spondylitis should sleep on a very firm mattress with a bedboard. Sleeping flat on the back is very helpful.

Too many of us tend to slouch in comfortable chairs, throwing our backs out of position and making the condition worse. A straight-back chair is beneficial.

It is suggested that daily exercises be used to strengthen the lower back. Specifically, breathe deeply fifteen times, three times a day. Bend your back forward and backwards ten times, at least three times a day. Lying on a hard surface with knees held straight, raise each leg ten times and do this twice daily. Even when standing, contract the muscles of the back and buttocks ten times and do this twice daily.

For years I have been bothered by sudden attacks of pain in my face, head and neck. When I am well I forget about them. Now, I have promised my wife that I will track down the cause of these

pains because I am constantly irritated and annoyed by them. How should I go about finding out the underlying reasons?

As many people do, you have neglected to seek a physician's help for the diagnosis and treatment of a long-standing illness. Almost always, such people are impatient and actually annoyed if the cause cannot be immediately pinpointed, treated and cured.

To give you a better understanding of the difficulty of diagnosis, let me outline only a few of the causes of pain in the face and neck.

The nerves of the head, jaws, face, eyes, ears and neck are a vast network that depend on each other and refer pain to distant areas. The persistent pain may come from the teeth, the bite of the teeth and the jaw joint, infections of the sinuses, tension of the muscles of the neck and jaws, allergies, drugs taken for other ailments and changes of the bone structure in the spinal column of the back and neck.

When pain is the only symptom, it becomes exceedingly difficult to track down its exact cause. But it can be done. A general physical examination is necessary to uncover far distant conditions in the liver, kidneys, circulatory system, lungs and the heart that may be responsible.

X-rays of the neck, sinuses, skull and jaw joints may reveal the cause for pain. A detailed examination of the teeth, bite and jaw joints will be an important contribution to the diagnosis that will lead to the treatment of your facial pain.

There is one special condition known as "tic douloureaux" which is an exceptionally painful one. It is characterized by sudden severe episodes of violent and excruciating pain. This condition affects one of the large nerves of the face, the trigeminal.

There are a number of other neuralgic conditions that can produce pain similar to the kind you describe.

Tic douloureux can now be treated successfully by a number of methods. Injection with hot water, alcohol and local anesthetics has been used in specific cases. There are a number of new drugs that can control these painful episodes and, in fact, reduce their occurrence to a minimum.

Finding the reason for your long-standing illness is a combined project that can only be accomplished with patience and detailed cooperation between you and your doctor.

You must not be impatient if the pain in the head and neck does not immediately respond to treatment. Diligent treatment must be continued in spite of temporary disappointment if you are eventually to be relieved of the disorder that is plaguing you.

I have had polyps removed from my nose four times and they always grow back. Can this be because they have not been taken out correctly? Now I must have them removed again and I want to find a way to get rid of them once and for all.

A polyp is a grape-like mass of watery tissue that occurs in the lining of the nose or the sinuses in people who have an allergy, infection, or both. Polyps may occur singly or, more often, in bunches, especially when the underlying condition is neglected.

Polyps become annoying when they become so large that they interfere with normal breathing through the nose. Many people do nothing about this condition until the nose is completely blocked and they can no longer breathe comfortably.

Once the polyps are removed it has been my experience that patients are so delighted to breathe freely again that they refuse to be treated for their allergy or infection. This probably is a key to your problem. It is absolutely necessary that intensive treatment for the allergy and the infection continue after surgery in order to delay or prevent the recurrence of the nasal polyps.

The side of my face sometimes suddenly becomes swollen, especially when I eat anything tart. This has happened four times. It lasts for a day and then disappears. What can cause this?

The story you describe is rather typical of some obstruction of the tiny tube which carries saliva from the parotid gland into the mouth. This gland lies in front of the ear and is the one that becomes swollen with mumps.

There are other salivary glands beneath the jaw and beneath the chin. The saliva pours into the mouth and is used in the first step for the digestion of food.

Occasionally a tiny stone, made out of calcium or uric acid, forms in the gland or in the tube. This may act as a ball valve. When you eat something tart the gland produces more saliva and may push the stone into the narrow tube and obstruct it. The saliva dams back and the result is swelling of the face.

There are now excellent techniques by which the salivary glands can be studied by special dyes and X-rays. Often the stone is found and, when necessary, it can be removed by simple surgery.

What can be done for a painful cyst at the base of the spine? It seems to come and go without any reason.

By the description this may well be a pilonidal cyst, a rather frequent condition that is due to a birth disorder. Rarely do these cysts cause trouble before entering adulthood. At that time, either by activity, injury, or infection, the cysts become infected and painful. The location is always at the base of the spine, just above the crease between the buttocks.

It is unfortunate that pilonidal cysts are rarely brought to the attention of the doctor or the surgeon before they become infected. Surgery would be far easier and the recovery more rapid if the operation were performed before rather than after an abscess is formed. Once there is an accumulation of pus the doctor has no choice but to open it and relieve the pain.

My own experience has been that once the pain has been controlled patients again forget about the existence of the cyst and do nothing about it until another abscess forms.

Surgery was once a very complicated procedure and healing took many weeks. Today when the operation is performed the wound is completely closed after the entire cyst is completely removed. Healing now occurs in a short time.

The operation is safe and should not be delayed while medicines, ointments and salves are being tried, without benefit.

My wife has been in perfect health. She is fifty-four years of age and has had three normal, healthy children who are now grown. Recently she had what we considered to be a minor illness. We were dumbfounded to learn that she has multiple sclerosis. This has been confirmed by a neurologist. Can you tell us any more about the condition and what hopes there are for its cure?

Multiple sclerosis is a strange disease and one that has occupied the attention of physicians and scientists all over the world. Despite the fact that vast information is being accumulated, the jigsaw puzzle is by no means complete and still baffles the doctor.

The cause has been attributed to infection, drugs, heavy metals and injury. All, and perhaps none, may be the real reason.

Multiple sclerosis is a neurological disease that attacks the brain and the spinal cord and the nerves that lead from them. Symptoms are so varied that they can hardly be itemized without causing a sense of concern to the people who read about them.

It has been suspected but not confirmed that there is an hereditary basis for it. Therefore it must be emphasized that members of a family in which there is a patient with this condition must not live their lives with the fear that they too will acquire it.

It takes a great diagnostic sense to suspect and identify multiple sclerosis in its early stages. Sometimes, as in the case of your wife, multiple sclerosis occurs suddenly. More commonly, the onset is slow and progressive with neurological symptoms that call a doctor's attention to its presence.

One of the most unusual and still unexplained aspects of this complicated disease is that without reason a patient suddenly seems to become well. These periods are called remissions during which the patient feels very much better and the symptoms seem to be less distressing. These remissions and a later recurrence of symptoms make doctors suspect the diagnosis.

Exciting new leads are being followed in many hospitals and universities all over the world. It is felt that soon the prevention of multiple sclerosis and the possible control of its progress may be on the horizon.

At the present time patients are treated for the symptoms they show. All efforts are made to give medical and psychological support to these patients, who manifest remarkable courage.

Massage, active and passive, is beneficial. Hydrotherapy and living in warm climates seem to offer relief. Cortisone and ACTH are two of the new possibilities for the interruption of the progress of this condition.

In addition to medical support your wife will benefit from psychological guidance and your own support and understanding.

What are the most common reasons for jaundice? My wife has had two attacks in the last four years. She recovered from both.

Jaundice is a yellowish discoloration of the skin and the lining of the eyes due to the accumulation of bile pigments in the bloodstream. The causes of jaundice are many, some more serious than others. Gall bladder stones and inflammation of the bile ducts are two. A virus infection of the liver, cirrhosis of the liver, amebic dysentery and a whole spectrum of blood diseases can also be responsible. Cancer of the pancreas and toxic reactions following blood transfusions are all part of the vast array of causes.

I deliberately mention these to illustrate how impossible it is for a layman to evaluate the reasons for jaundice. It takes a physician armed with elaborate solid studies and X-rays to pinpoint the cause of jaundice and then proceed with the treatment of its underlying cause.

My wife has been told that she will give birth to our child by Caesarean operation. Will you tell us what is involved here?

About one child in every fifty normal deliveries is born by Caesarean operation.

This method is named after Julius Caesar, who was supposedly born in this manner.

There are a number of reasons why a doctor chooses to deliver a child through an incision in the lower part of the abdominal wall. The most common is some anatomical abnormality of the pelvic bones of the mother. Only occasionally is the child so large that it cannot pass through the normal vaginal birth canal. If the surgeon believes that the life of the child or mother is threatened by a normal delivery he may suggest a Caesarean section. The decision to do this is made after very careful consideration, and usually after consultation with another doctor.

The excellent surgical techniques and the safety of anesthesia, coupled with the use of antibiotics, add great safety for the life and health of the mother and the child during such surgery.

Why should my wife, who had a perfectly normal delivery of a baby, suddenly find herself in a deep depression?

Following delivery of a child, emotional disturbances, some severe, some relatively minor, do occur. They take many forms and not all of them can really be attributed to the confinement.

Sometimes a mild neurosis may go unobserved and unrecognized until it is precipitated by some severe physical emotional experience. It must be treated early and consistently by a psychiatrist or psychologist. To take the attitude that this severe depression will disappear if left alone is unwise.

Occasionally, women who give all evidences of emotional stability may become terrified by the responsibilities of a new baby. Neuroticisms that may have been dormant are occasionally brought to the surface during this great physical and emotional event.

Six weeks after my wife had a successful operation for the removal of her uterus, she became terribly depressed. Is this a very common experience?

All surgery is, in a measure, an insult to the body and to the psyche. The uterus, or womb, has many psychologically significant involvements. This organ is a very special one that many women identify with their self-image of femininity. When that image is "removed," it is almost natural for agitation, depression, anxiety, and irritability to result. This reaction is not unlike that which a man often has when his prostate gland, his "image of masculinity," is surgically removed.

Gynecologists and surgeons are psychologically aware of the emotional upheaval in women who are having a hysterectomy. Many will spend time discussing this problem with their patients to give them added assurance and to help avoid postoperative depression. In highly tense patients, doctors may often suggest a consultation with a psychiatrist or psychologist to give added support before and after the operation.

The frequency and severity of postoperative depression are markedly relieved by the use of specially chosen hormones in addition to psychoenergizing drugs.

My wife is undergoing a change of life. She has suddenly become transformed from a calm, stable person to a highly irritable one whom I barely recognize. Is there any way that I can help her?

Yes, you can help your wife and, incidentally, help yourself by a better understanding of what happens to a woman during her menopause, or change of life.

The entire stability of the hormones balance is knocked into complete disarray. The body functions and the psychological balance are thrown out of gear. People who formally were stable and acted like the Rock of Gibraltar suddenly become tearful at the slightest provocation. Women who were able to do a gigantic amount of work find that they are exhausted after the slightest effort.

It is imperative that you discuss the entire problem both with your wife and with your doctor. It may well be that she, too, does not understand all the things that are happening to her.

She may be concerned about the sudden episodes of flushing, trembling and nervousness. She may be exhausted from the sleeplessness that may go with change of life. She may be just as confused about her own change of personality, and may hardly recognize herself as the same person at this time.

Your doctor, with his knowledge fo the psychological fears that accompany menopause, will give assurance to you both. He knows, as you may not, that women during this period are actually afraid that they are less attractive to their husbands than before. It comes as an actual surprise to them to learn that they, in reality, may become even more desirable physically during this transition period.

When the fear of pregnancy has been removed, a greater freedom may result which even enhances the sexual relationship with the husband. Women need and deserve physical, spiritual, emotional and medical support during this difficult period.

There is a great deal that you can do by surrounding your wife with the constant feeling that she is still being loved and wanted. Your kindnesses to her may have an added dividend. You may need the same kind of support from her when your male menopause occurs. It sometimes does.

Is there a male menopause?

Menopause refers to the cessation of the menses. The male climacteric (change of life), however, denotes that stage in a man's life when gonadal (testes) function diminishes, eventually resulting in complete cessation.

It's not as specific and definitive as what we see in the female, although the onset may be precipitous, occurring over three or four months. Men between the ages of 50 and 60 may develop these changes.

When the male change of life sets in, it is possible to study gonadal activity by measuring the steroid level in the blood. Occasionally, it is possible to replace hormones when they are found to be markedly deficient.

In general, there is scientific agreement that changes in body function do occur in the male, which can be classed as male change of life. Time and age are responsible for changes in gonadal function and in changes in every other organ of the body.

Do vasectomies always work? I've heard of a case where a man fathered a child after he had this operation.

Some men who have subjected themselves to vasectomy to prevent paternity have had the unpleasant surprise of learning that the procedure was ineffective.

Wives who had faith in this form of contraception found themselves pregnant despite the husband's vasectomy.

The reason for this is that the live sperm may still exist for months after the operation.

Some doctors and surgeons have been using special nitrofuran compounds at the time of surgery, to give greater assurance that the operative procedure will accomplish its contraceptive purpose.

My wife has a tendency to faint when she is upset. Can this be prevented by any drugs? What is the best way to get out of a faint?

It is undeniable that some people become faint more easily than others. One of my patients fainted at the onset of every thunderstorm. At first this sounds somewhat silly but when one understands the process of fainting, even this unusual provocation can call for sympathy rather than annoyance.

When a person faints it is due to a sudden loss of the blood that normally circulates to the brain. A sudden emotional upset, a telegram bearing a frightening message, a sudden fall of blood sugar or severe pain may cause an attack of syncope or fainting.

There are a number of physical conditions such as heart disease, lung disorders, and the hardening of the arteries to the brain which can cause fainting. Before an attack of fainting is entirely attributed to emotional causes, every avenue of study of the body must be made to be sure that a physical condition is not overlooked.

Because it is the temporary reduction in the blood flow to the brain that causes fainting, the victim should be placed flat with the head slightly lower than the rest of the body to encourage greater flow of blood to the brain. Belts, ties, bras, and tight girdles should be loosened. Under no circumstances should liquor be forced down the throat. A little patience and encouragement to the frightened fainter is all she needs for recovery.

Drugs to prevent fainting are used only after the exact physical reasons for it have been established.

———

Even in warm weather my sinuses keep me from performing a good day's work. With all the wonderful scientific advancements, can't anything be done about the cure of this national pestilence?

There are few illnesses about which there is as much misunderstanding, myths and confusion as there is about disease of the sinuses.

We all have sinuses. It is only when they are infected that we have sinusitis.

Often we are asked what function the sinuses serve other than to make us miserable. Actually, they do have a very important purpose. These cavities lighten the weight of the skull, increase our vocal resonance, and play a protective role in warming and cooling air as it is inhaled into the lungs.

The major reason why the sinuses become chronically infected is that they are so frequently neglected in the early stages. Underlying allergy of the nose undoubtedly predisposes people to infection of the sinuses. This combination of allergy and infection is responsible for nasal obstruction to breathing, nasal discharge, postnasal drip, and headache.

I believe that one of the reasons for persistent and chronic infections of the sinuses is the impatience of patients. They want a miracle cure in miracle time, and a guarantee of permanent cure.

Most patients quickly neglect to continue treatment of their sinuses as soon as they get the slightest relief from the symptoms that bring them to the doctor. This is a distinct mistake. Only by persistent treatment during the chronic phase is there a chance to completely eradicate chronic sinus infections.

With special drugs, heat, steam, and antibiotics most sinus infections can be kept in control.

Sometimes a slight operation is recommended to help clear infection.

Neglect of this advice is frequent and tends to allow the sinus disease to progress.

It is undoubtedly true that a warm, dry climate free of polluted air, smog, and pollens contribute comfort to chronic sinusitis sufferers.

The nasal septum which divides one side of the nose from the other is no longer operated on where there is a slight deviation. When this operation is chosen with great care and judgment, it is a valuable contribution to proper breathing and to the control of some types of sinus infections.

Sinusitis demands a great deal of patience by the doctor and the patient for best results.

I have been told that I am an "ulcer-type" personality, and if I don't change my habits I will surely get an ulcer. I am in a highly tense business, and at the age of forty-five I can't turn over a new leaf. What can I do?

The "ulcer-type" personality is generally a person who is energetic, tense, high-strung, competitive, and ambitious. Often he does not express his feelings and completely supresses his emotions.

This generalized description is probably responsible for the cliche that "an ulcer is not what you eat, but rather what's eating you."

Stomach ulcers and duodenal ulcers can also occur in people whose personality is the direct opposite of the one just described. They can occur in emotionally stable, well-controlled, slow-moving personalities. For this reason it is fair to prophesy that anyone can develop an ulcer.

Of course, you will benefit markedly by changing the tempo and the pressure of your daily work routine.

I have been under treatment for colitis for years. Sometimes I get better, then, after a while, it starts all over again. Is there any permanent cure?

There are a number of forms of colitis, some of which last a short while and may never come back, and others which come back at irregular intervals.

Some cases are caused by parasites and infestation with amebas which follow eating and drinking contaminated food. Mucous colitis and ulcerative colitis are the major forms of this intestinal disorder.

The hope for permanent cure is based on the exact nature of the condition, how long it has existed, the intensity with which it is treated and the recognition that the emotions play a very important role in its cause and cure.

There are few conditions in which there is as close a relationship between emotions and the onset and progress of this disease. Psychological support, therefore, in addition to medical treatment, is of untold value. The antibiotics and cortisone have helped immeasurably to control some cases of colitis.

There is a tendency for people with colitis to become careless about their diet and their medical follow-up once they seem to be getting better. This is an error. Treatment during the interval free from symptoms is perhaps more important than treatment during a flare-up.

Is there any truth that hormones can cause the regrowth of hair in severe baldness?

Hormones somehow have always had a strange, magical and mystical meaning for many people. This perhaps has induced the manufacturers of creams and lotions to suggest that hormones in their product are beneficial for baldness. There is no truth or validity to this claim.

Simple, inexpensive products cost many times their worth because a trace of hormone has been used with it.

There was a time when the male sex hormone, testosterone, was tried for male pattern baldness. Its use called forth a moderate amount of enthusiasm which unfortunately raised the hopes of the balding and left them in despair when the results were not forthcoming.

The overuse of hormones can produce some unusual side-effects and, therefore, these should never be used without the advice and follow-up of a physician.

Has the transplantation of hair been successful? How is it performed?

The technique is known as skin-punch-autografts and hundreds of such cases have been successfully reported by surgeons and dermatologists.

The "donor" area is the site of luxurious growth from which small clusters of hair are painlessly removed with specially devised skin-punch instruments. The skin and hair removed from the donor site are introduced into the bald recipient site. Anywhere from ten to forty of such "plugs" are grafted at each visit. About two or three weeks are allowed for the new site to heal before another group of grafts is implanted.

Sometimes, the recipient site may reject the autografts. Infections are rare and are easily controlled if they do happen. Intensive studies continue with the use of hormones, drugs and antibiotics to assure greater success with this type of hair regrowth technique.

Are there any new hopes on the horizon for baldness?

The type of baldness that is referred to as family pattern baldness still resists the active efforts known to hair specialists. Vitamins, hormones, outrageously expensive creams, lotions and vibratory massages may bring out an occasional quarter inch of fuzz, but in general they are ineffective.

There are types of alopecia or baldness which may be due to prolonged illness with very high fevers, ringworm infection, hormone imbalance and psychological stress. Almost always, with or without treatment except for local infections, the hair will spontaneously grow again.

The most encouraging new approach to pattern baldness has been the transplanation of hair. This is a technique of taking small tufts of hair and implanting them near the edge of the balding area. The method is painstaking but in the hands of highly specialized physicians this office procedure is said to be effective in a fair number of cases.

My car was struck from behind, and I was thrown forward. I was told by my doctor that I had a whiplash injury even though X-ray pictures do not show it. How can I convince the lawyers and insurance people that all I want is my health?

Anyone who has ever had a similar injury can attest that a whiplash injury can be very real, very painful, and long enduring. When the body is thrown forward and snaps back like a whip, muscles, tendons, blood vessels, soft tissue and bones of the spinal column can suffer. Small hemorrhages into the muscles of the neck can be responsible for persistent pain.

Unfortunately, whiplash injuries have been exploited in some instances. The result is that insurance companies look critically at this condition before they acknowledge its real presence. Yet it does people like you a great injustice for the insurers not to recognize obvious pain such as you describe. You should not be dissuaded by anyone from continuing to follow your doctor's advice until you are completely relieved.

I perspire a great deal and am embarrassed by the way the sweat pours off me not only in hot weather, but in cold weather, too.

I assume that all possible physical causes for your condition have been thoroughly studied. The disorder is known as "hyperhydrosis." A great many drugs have been tried in an effort to reduce the excessive outpouring of sweat from the sweat glands of the body. Some of these have been successful. There is, however, no consistency in all cases. A special operation known as "ganglionectomy" has been used with considerable success. Physicians and surgeons in many parts of the country can perform this operation but there is no uniform agreement that this procedure is the total answer to excessive perspiration.

When hair becomes gray at an early age does it mean that the general aging process is more rapid?

People whose hair becomes gray prematurely live as long as anyone else. Premature graying in no way indicates rapid aging, a change in health, or in longevity. Usually it is a hereditary, family characteristic.

It seems farfetched that an enlarged prostate can cause lumbargo. I have been told this and question it.

Specialists in urology recognize more and more that inflammation of the prostate may refer pain that can be confused with lumbago and sciatica.

How does one pick a reliable dandruff product that will really attack the underlying condition?

105

From a technical point of view, dandruff is considered a scaling of the outer surface of the skin. It may be associated with seborrheic dermatitis, a scaling of the skin due to some form of inflammation.

Most of the products manufactured are safe and effective. Most people try one for a reasonable period of time, and if it accomplishes its purpose, they continue with it.

Many contain keratolytics, which have a special effect on shedding the outer layer of the skin. Occasionally, these can be irritating.

The opinion of a skin specialist, or dermatologist, is important to people consistently bothered by this annoying condition. Often, the doctor may find an underlying skin condition which might be cleared with the use of a cortisone lotion, or some special shampoo.

What is the prostate gland? What does it do and when does it have to be removed?

The prostate gland is about the size of a plum and has three distinct lobes. It lies just below the urinary bladder. It is part of the chain of endocrine glands. The gland itself does not produce sperm cells but it pours out a fluid which protectively carries sperm during sexual intercourse.

The gland, like any other organ, is affected by infections, inflammations, tumors, both benign and malignant. Infections are treated as they would be in any other part of the body, with antibiotics and other drugs.

Enlargement of the prostate occurs in men as they get older. When it grows to the point that it presses on the urethra, (the small tube through which urine is eliminated from the bladder), it may cause frequency of urination day and night. As the condition progresses, the bladder may not be able to empty itself completely and some amount of urine remains within it. With progressive enlargement of the prostate, there may be some kidney complication. Or there may be a sudden obstruction of the urethra, making it impossible to urinate and necessitating urgent treatment. Enlargement of the prostate probably affects more than seventy-five percent of all men beyond the age of sixty. Not all need surgery. Sometimes gentle massage may reduce the size.

Removal of the prostate is performed in a number of different ways depending on the patient and the surgical judgment of the doctor. New techniques are now using electrocoagulation and even cryosurgery (freezing). The removal of the prostate is not a dangerous one and recovery is complete within fourteen days unless any unusual complication occurs.

The operation, called prostatectomy, contrary to most men's fears, may make them much healthier and more virile because it removes the threat to their mind and body.

Two of my friends had operations on their prostate. One had only one operation. The other had two operations. I'm curious about this because they had different surgeons.

The choice of a one-stage or a two-stage operation is not based on the surgical skill of one surgeon as against another.

There are definite reasons why the decision is made. In most instances today, the operation, known as "transurethral resection," is performed safely and almost routinely as a one-step procedure.

However, when a person is in particularly poor health and is considered a greater surgical risk, the prostate operation may be performed in two stages.

The first stage consists of making an opening into the bladder through the lower abdominal wall. Then, after a short time, when infection has been controlled and the patient is in better health, the prostate is removed through the same opening.

The ultimate result is the same regardless of the type of operation chosen by the surgeon.

I know I need a prostate operation. Some of my friends claim that the operation is better than the one where an electric needle is used. What do you think?

I think you should stay away from your friends until your prostate problem is solved by your medical friend—your doctor.

Prostate surgery depends on many factors. The age of the patient, his general physical condition, and the particular type of enlargement of the prostate gland are all meaningful to the surgeon.

His choice, therefore, is an individual one, and is a conclusion he arrives at with care and fine surgical judgment.

Some patients benefit most by a one or two stage operation where the prostate is approached by an incision low on the abdominal wall.

Others are best treated by "transurethral resection." This electrocoagulation method is probably the one you refer to. It is performed through a cystoscope and is not an "open" operation.

Let your doctor make the decision and spare yourself the anxiety of your well-meaning friends.

My friend is being treated for an acid stomach. The heartburn he tells me about is almost exactly like what happens when I drink beer. Can I take anything to avoid this unpleasant sensation?

As a physician, I really do not know what is meant by "acid stomach." I also do not know what is meant by patients who say, "I have too much acid in my body and everything I eat turns to acid."

All of us have a very important digestive juice known as hydrochloric acid in our stomach. Without it, we would be in real trouble. It is true that there are some foods, especially coffee and alcoholic beverages, that stimulate a greater production of this acid in the stomach. There may be an increase of acid after eating strawberries and anchovies in people who are allergic to them. In most people, these do not cause an increase of any importance.

This wonderful body of ours has a great mechanism for maintaining the proper balance between acid and alkali. There are two things that you can take. One is the advice of your doctor and not that of your friend. The second is your own personal advice to yourself after discovering that beer is a culprit. Stay away from it.

A friend of mine has cirrhosis of the liver. He was not always a heavy drinker of alcohol. Are there other causes for this?

The word "cirrhosis" is a descriptive one and refers to the orange-brown color of the liver when it is affected by this disorder. The liver can be damaged by other substances besides alcohol. It is a most remarkable organ and has considerable reserve power that compensates for small areas of damage. But when alcohol in large quantities over a long period of time does damage to a large part of the liver, its function diminishes. Unfortunately, this process is not always reversible, even if the alcoholism is finally controlled.

There are other reasons besides alcohol for one of the many types of cirrhosis. Some drugs, toxic chemicals, infections and untreated syphilis can affect the liver and cause the dire consequences of cirrhosis. Prevention is the key to the preservation of this vital organ of the body.

Is a needle biopsy of the liver dangerous?

Biopsy of the liver is a procedure that is safe in experienced hands. It is painless and may be of importance in verifying suspected disease of the liver. Through a needle, a small quantity of liver tissue is extracted. This is then examined carefully under the microscope. There are many other tests that establish a "profile" of the liver to provide the exact diagnosis and to direct treatment.

After a couple of beers, my stomach growls enough to make me heard at the far end of the bar. It gets lonely where I sit!

I don't like to suggest that you stop drinking beer. Perhaps you can reduce the quantity or the speed with which you drink it. That may help. The rumbling noise is due to air that is trapped in the stomach and intestines. If someone asks, "What's that noise?" your answer can be (technically), "Borborygmus." That should stop them!

What can cause a thickening of the tips of the fingers in the middle-aged man?

A condition known as clubbing of the fingers is occasionally seen in chronic lung conditions. It is an unusual relationship which does exist but has never been satisfactorily explained.

My wife says I don't hear her when she speaks to me. I can hear everybody else and I think it's her fault because she mumbles. Could her speech be changing with the years and her voice getting softer?

To pin your hearing problem on your wife's delicacy of speech is a brilliant cop-out that I cannot let you get away with.

Although you say you "hear everybody else" you probably are missing a great deal of conversation that you are not even aware of. Strangers, after all, are less likely to call this to your attention.

Many people with a mild or even a severe hearing defect stubbornly refuse to seek professional advice.

The world of silence is a lonely one, unnecessarily lived in by many who remain in self confinement because they will not admit that they cannot hear. The restoration of serviceable hearing by medical and surgical treatment and by the use of hearing aids is one of the great accomplishments of modern medicine.

A world of sound is a happier world than one of silence. There is no guesswork about a hearing deficiency. Tuning forks and audiometric tests can quickly establish for you the exact state of your hearing.

If you have a deficiency that can be benefitted by the use of the new transistorized hearing devices, the joys of hearing again are limitless.

Whenever I turn my neck I hear a clicking sound. Sometimes when I'm tired there is a shooting pain with the sound. Could this be related to a diving accident I had when I was young?

The diving accident may have been responsible, but your experience is not uncommon at your age, even without a history of an injury. Slight osteoarthritic deposits are very common in the cervical spine of the neck. Routine X-rays taken of people who have no symptoms may show these deposits in the bony vertebrae of the neck. In an effort to track down the cause of your discomfort, X-rays of the neck and skull will be helpful.

Sometimes the cartilages that house the voice box may become calcified. When they override each other, a clicking noise may result. Sitting in an upright position rather than a crouched one may be helpful if no other reason for your problem exists. You might try dry heat and an extension collar. Cradling of a telephone between the shoulder and the chin while using the hands for other purposes can also cause neck pain.

An eye doctor has told me that many of his patients who use bifocal glasses have a tendency to keep their heads in a distorted position. This occurs particularly while watching television or doing close desk work.

Strain and tension of the muscles of the neck can also be responsible for the type of pain you describe.

I have a mild form of epilepsy which is kept under control with drugs. I plan to be married this fall and my wife-to-be knows that I have the condition. Although we have never spoken about it, I know that we are both afraid that our children may inherit this condition.

If there is no long history of epilepsy on both sides of the family, the chances are negligible that your children will inherit this condition. That which stands out prominently in your letter is the fact that you have both avoided the discussion of this most important aspect of your lives. Unless you do, you are inviting hazards to a good marriage.

There now are many universities and hospitals where you can be given the advantage of genetic counseling. Here specialists are able to review your entire medical background and then assure you and spare you concern. To embark on a marriage without a clear and open study of this important problem would do you both a great injustice.

I have a growth on my wrist called a ganglion. It has grown slightly larger in the past ten years. Could it become cancerous?

These ganglions are cysts of the joints and tendons of the wrists and are usually filled with a thick gelatinous substance. They never become malignant or cancerous and rarely become infected. If there is the slightest suspicion about it, removal under local anesthesia is simple. The tissue is then examined and its negative nature frees the patient of concern.

An interesting method of "breaking" these cysts was to whack it hard with a Bible. This has no religious implication. The Bible was chosen because it is the handiest and heaviest book in the house. This Bible therapy is rarely permanently effective.

I was told that I have a hiatus hernia. Only a single X-ray was taken of my chest. Is that enough to make such a diagnosis?

A hiatus hernia is a condition in which a small portion of the stomach forces its way up into the chest cavity. Normally, the esophagus goes into the stomach through a small opening in the diaphragm. When this opening is abnormally enlarged, the stomach protrudes into the chest

111

cavity. That is why a hiatus hernia is sometimes called a "diaphragmatic" hernia.

This condition can masquerade in many different forms and can present confusing symptoms. In difficult cases, extensive X-ray studies are done. Sometimes a lighted tube, the esophagoscope is passed through the esophagus to visualize the area. You can be sure that if your doctor needed more confirmatory studies, he would have performed them.

I have been wearing a truss for a hernia for many years. I've never told anybody about it, not even a doctor. Now I have pains in my groin when I walk. Are there different kinds of hernia? Can they be dangerous?

The greatest danger of a hernia is to neglect it. Too often people do exactly what you have done and wait until a simple condition becomes a complicated one.

A hernia is simply a weakness or defect in the muscles that protect and enclose the body cavities. Besides the inguinal hernia that occurs in the groin, there are also abdominal, umbilical, incisional and esophageal hernias. Some of these hernias are found at birth (congenital). Others are acquired during adolescence and in adulthood.

The most common of all hernias is the one that you have. Groin hernias sometimes become visible after injury or excessive strain on muscles that may already be weakened.

The real concern of a neglected hernia is the possibility that a small loop of the intestine can become kinked and swollen and cannot be pushed back into the abdomen by the finger or by a truss.

People are often misled into believing that if they wear a truss long enough their hernia will disappear.

Trusses can be of benefit to the elderly or the infirm, who cannot safely be subjected to an operation.

You have now reached the point where you must be examined to know the reason for your pains. If surgery is necessary, it can be remarkably safe and successful. At operation the defective opening is closed under general anesthesia. The recovery period is short.

What danger is there in wearing a truss, rather than having surgery for a hernia?

There are many different kinds of hernia. I assume that the hernia referred to is the one that occurs in the groin in both men and women.

A hernia is a defect in the protective wall through which some organ of the body pushes and interrupts normal function. Most hernias are the result of some abnormality of development. Occasionally, a hernia may develop after injury or surgery of the abdomen.

The most frequent hernia, or rupture, occurs in the groin and may produce little or no symptoms for many years. Sometimes, as a result of overweight, straining at stool or lifting a heavy weight the opening may become larger and through it a small piece of intestine may be forced. Even in these cases, with gentle pressure the intestine can be pushed back through the hernial ring and into its proper position.

A truss does not cure a hernia, but rather it protects and keeps the intestines from becoming caught in the open ring. This is probably the single most important reason why hernias are best treated by surgery rather than by a truss.

Every once in a while, a loop of intestine may become caught in the ring and cannot be replaced. The result is that the intestine becomes strangulated and swollen and makes surgery a necessity and not a choice.

The speed of today's hernia operations and the excellence of the safe anesthetics, in addition to antibiotics, makes surgery simple and uncomplicated. Unnecessary delay because of the fear of surgery frequently makes a simple operation a very complicated one.

Is a colostomy opening into the intestine always permanent?

Let me first explain that a colostomy is an artificial opening into the large intestine through which a patient passes fecal matter instead of through the normal rectal opening.

This operation is performed as a temporary opening during some severe infections and inflammations of the large intestine.

A permanent colostomy opening is usually created when portions of the large intestine are removed because of tumors that obstruct the bowel.

There are hundreds of thousands of people who lead perfectly normal lives and are active in business and in sports with such an opening.

There are colostomy clubs all over America composed of dedicated members who are sent out to support new colostomy patients during the

113

first trying days. Patients soon learn that they are odor free and not handicapped but rather are given a new lease of life by this most successful type of operation. Specially constructed bags now make it possible for these courageous people to continue to function without any detection that such a condition exists.

When I am under severe tension or when I eat too rapidly I suddenly develop a closing of my throat and begin to gasp for breath. Can these attacks be prevented and what are the chances of choking to death?

There are two tubes leading from the mouth and the pharynx. One is the esophagus which carries food from the mouth directly to the stomach. The other is a firmer structure through which air passes down into the larynx or voice box and then into the lung.

Under most circumstances there are controlling reflexes that make it virtually impossible for food to go "down the wrong passage."

Under stress, or when eating too rapidly, some people have a tendency to inhale food or water which then hits the vocal cords and sends them into a sudden protective spasm. Air cannot go in or out and there is an oppressive sense of choking which at times becomes terrifying to the victim and to those who witness it.

These spasms tend to occur more frequently in the elderly or in people who wear dentures and are therefore less sensitive to the heat of the food. Eating rapidly with or without alcohol, talking while eating and generally being distracted may cause this contraction of the vocal cords.

When a spasm occurs breathe in and out slowly through the nose with the mouth closed. Any attempt to swallow saliva, water or food at this time will only increase the spasm or make it return if it has stopped for a few moments.

Do not worry about embarrassment. This only tends to increase the spasm. People are not annoyed by this temporary situation and are very understanding. They can be more understanding if they resist the temptation to slap you on the back, offer you a drink or generally get in the way of the normal relaxation of the spasm that will occur if you are left alone. Try to practice the technique of breathing rapidly in and out through the nose without swallowing as a preparation for the next time such a spasm occurs.

I have emphysema. I read that this condition is not reversible. Must I give up hope of any kind of cure?

Whenever I read a letter such as yours, or see a patient with emphysema, I wonder why so many people fail to heed the advice of their doctors to eliminate tobacco, the major culprit in the development of this chronic debilitating disease.

Despite the fact that emphysema is not reversible there are a great many treatments that may slow its progress when the factors responsible are eliminated. With breathing exercises and postural drainage, greater function can be brought to impaired lungs.

At the Institute for Rehabilitation Medicine in New York City, great numbers of "respiratory invalids," previously hopeless, are given a brighter outlook for living. Similar centers can be found throughout the country.

You should not be without hope, if you embark on such a program of active treatment.

Is it true that men who smoke are more likely to develop trouble with the circulation of blood to their feet?

There is one special disease that men are more prone to than women. A condition know as Buerger's Disease has the technical name of "thromboangiitis obliterans." As the name suggests, there is slow obliteration or blocking of the veins and arteries, especially in the legs and in the feet.

The disease occurs most frequently in young men about the age of thirty. Rarely is it found in women. In both, excessive smoking of cigarettes is considered a most important cause.

The onset occurs slowly and becomes full blown when the arteries become so closed that vital blood is carried in insufficient amounts to the feet. There may be swelling of the feet, attacks of phlebitis (inflammation of the veins) and spasm of the muscles of the leg after walking a few feet.

Another odd aspect of this condition is that Buerger's Disease usually occurs in those of Russian or Polish origin. Not all such people are affected, only those who are highly sensitive to tobacco in any form. Many forms of treatment are used for this condition but the single most important treatment is the total absolute abstinence from tobacco.

If cigarettes and tobacco affect the blood circulation, can they also affect the blood itself?

A study performed in Florida revealed that the blood of heavy smokers is far less able to transport oxygen to tissues and organs all over the body. Tobacco tends to narrow the blood vessels and interfere with good healthy circulation.

You recently wrote an article about a new drug for gout. Can you tell me if it is a permanent cure for this condition?

Before this excellent drug, allopurinol, was discovered, there were a number of other drugs used for gout, in conjunction with a rigid anti-gout diet.

Gout is a disturbance in the manufacture of uric acid in the body. Certain foods high in purines are responsible for an increased amount of uric acid in the blood. Pain in the joints, chronic arthritis and kidney stones are some of the complications of gout.

Before the new drug was found colchine was used in an effort to eliminate uric acid from the blood. Allopurinol approaches the problem of gout in a totally different way. It prevents the formation of uric acid and thereby does not allow the accumulation of uric acid in the blood. It interferes with the chemical reactions before uric acid is formed.

I awoke one night with excruciating pain. It was diagnosed as a kidney stone. Only later was it found that the stone was caused by gout. I wonder how it could have existed without my knowing about it.

When we speak of gout, we somehow visualize the classical picture of the self-indulgent, overweight man, sitting in his overstuffed chair with his toe swathed in bandages.

Actually, gout does not favor the rich or the self-indulgent. It can occur in every level of society.

Gout is a disturbance of the manufacture and accumulation of uric acid from certain foods. There is some hereditary tendency for this condition to occur more frequently in men than women.

Frequently, it is overlooked because the symptoms may be so meager at first. Vague pains in the joints may be overlooked as evidence of gout unless the blood is studied for abnormal amounts of uric acid.

Uric acid studies are now a part of every complete blood examination. Thus potential gout patients are flushed out of hiding long before the appearance of any symptoms.

Uric acid is produced from foods that contain a high quality of purines. Foods like liver, sardines, anchovies, kidneys, sweetbreads and gravies are high in purines.

Diet and drugs can now prevent the progress of gout when it is recognized early. Two types of drugs are used. One, probenecid, aims at increasing the amount of uric acid excreted from the body in the urine. The second, a newer drug, allopourinol, prevents the formation of uric acid, even from foods that are high in purine.

I applied for insurance and was rejected because I was found to have albumin in my urine. They said I might have kidney disease and that I was a poor risk. I am forty-one years old and have been in good health.

Most insurance companies would have referred you to your own doctor to track down the cause of albumin in your urine. Occasionally, albumin is found in a single specimen and never appears again.

Standing in one position for too long a period of time has been known to reflect itself with a trace of albumin. When albumin is constantly present in each specimen it may be due to infection, inflammation or some other urinary disorder. Normally, when blood flows through the kidneys, the protein albumin does not filter through the complex, sieve-like system, and properly remains in the blood to be used for healthy functioning of the organs.

There are many excellent tests for kidney function and for disorders in the urinary tract. Many of these disorders are remediable.

We have just moved to a cold climate. Even in the summertime, the temperature can go down to zero. We have been told that the wind can be as dangerous as the cold. Is this true?

The combination of cold and wind is recognized to be a great threat to health if proper precautions are not taken. The wind has distinct and severe cooling effects, and can damage the tips of the ears, the nose, the fingers, and the toes.

It is important for you to be aware of the wind-chill index so you can take precautions against extreme cold.

For example, on a day when the wind is blowing at twenty miles per hour and the temperature is twenty degrees Fahrenheit, the total effect on the body is the same as if the temperature were minus nine degrees Fahrenheit. This means that, from the point of view of body protection, the temperature is almost thirty degrees lower than what the thermometer reads.

Some members of my club try to outdo themselves in the steam baths. They act as if the longer they can stay in the hottest part of the baths, the better it is for their health. What do you think?

Steam and whirlpool baths are exhilarating and beneficial to the circulatory system. Nevertheless, caution should be exercised by all who use sauna baths and hydrotherapy.

I believe that, before anyone embarks on a program of intensive steam, consultation with a doctor is important. Some people, even relatively young ones, can place an unnecessary burden on their hearts and vascular systems by too intense or too long exposure. They must find their own level of comfort without pushing their level of endurance.

It is no testimonial to virility or masculinity to be competitive about how long one can stay in concentrated heat temperatures. Moderation and slow conditioning increase the value and enjoyment of these treatments.

I like to use the steam room at my club. Can excessively hot air hurt the lungs?

Although the benefits of steam are great, and although it can be soothing to the mucous lining in the entire respiratory tract, excessively hot steam can be injurious and should be avoided. This has been learned in a study of industrial workers exposed to such steam.

Moreover, it is unwise and unsafe to compete with fellow members of your club to see who can stand the highest level of steam for the longest period of time.

I am fifty-six and find that the sagging of my jowls interferes with my business image. Do you think that plastic surgery on a man is as ridiculous as some of my friends think?

For years, men in the entertainment business have had facial plastic operations. Today more and more men in other fields give themselves that extra emotional "lift" by this plastic procedure.

A good image of one's self is not limited to one sex. From the surgical point of view, the differences in the hair styles may make scars somewhat more visible in men than in women.

Before coming to a definite conclusion, discuss every aspect of the operative procedure with your surgeon so that the psychological and physical benefits will be maximal.

My father, as did his father before him, wears dental plates that were ordered by mail. I can't convince him that this is foolish and possibly dangerous.

If there is anything that should not be bought by mail it seems to me it would be dental plates, which should fit precisely. Improper bite may lead to changes in the jaw joint which can be painful and interfere with chewing and proper digestion.

One of the most important advantages of being examined by a dentist is, of course, the early recognition of diseases and tumors that might otherwise be overlooked.

Chapter V

What Parents Ask

"The joys of parents are secret, and so are their griefs and fears." So said Francis Bacon. But I would challenge his statement. I'll grant the secret joys but I cannot accept the "secret griefs and fears." Not according to the barrage of questions that spill forth from my daily mailbag. The parents I encounter aren't about to conceal their problems.

I sometimes equate parents with a certain botanical phenomenon —the sensitive plant. If a moth, a breeze, a chill shadow falls across the leaves of a sensitive plant, it reacts immediately, closing its delicate leaves in protective fashion. So with the typical parent. Let something happen to a child of theirs and they react at once. Those of my colleagues who specialize in pediatrics will certainly support me in this. Let an infant spend a sleepless night and the doctor's phone rings. Let a youngster bruise his knee in a sidewalk tumble and the phone rings. Let a small nose redden with a cold; a fingernail darken from a bruise; a small bottom blossom with reddish blotches and it's, "Help, doctor!"

I would definitely say that when it comes to their children's welfare, parents don't wait around. They are ever on the alert; they are truly concerned; they want help to solve every dilemma. And very often they write to me—perhaps to doublecheck on their own pediatrician's or doctor's advice or simply to further reassure themselves. Not so with their own problems, which are often neglected.

I am always gratified to answer questions about the health of young people. Perhaps in no other area am I so firmly and totally committed as in the parent-child one. As a parent myself, aware of the awesome role of caring for a helpless small being and guiding that little one along the bumpy road to adolescence, I can sympathize with questioning parents. I understand their anxieties. That is why I usually try to answer their mail at once and as though the child in question were my own.

Is there truth in the idea that a baby's sex can be predicted early in pregnancy?

There is now scientific proof that the sex of a child can definitely be established as early as the fifth or sixth month of pregnancy. It is done by the study of the fluid in the mother's womb. The genes that determine sex can now be seen and counted under high-powered electron microscopes.

The curiosity of humans should wait, however, because of the risk of infection both to the mother and the child.

The fact that sex can be predicted is not nearly as important as the knowledge of genetic malformations and other diseases that might be learned through this technique.

Predictability of sex in no way suggests that it can be changed. Parents will simply have to accept that which the genes have in the cards for them.

Are there a great many advantages to the breast feeding of infants?

This has been a great source of discussion for many years. Sides have been taken and many friends have been converted to intellectual enemies by the insistent beliefs in one theory or another.

From the point of view of physical health it is generally accepted that the newborn infant tolerates breast milk better than cow's milk.

It is said, too, that some protection against diseases is included in the mother's milk. In areas where pasteurization of milk is not available there is definite value in mother's milk.

Milk that is pasteurized, homogenized and supplemented with vitamins is almost as healthful and nutritive as is mother's milk.

Now that it has been shown that cold milk is as safe as warm milk for a newborn infant another nuisance of bottled milk has been removed.

By far the greatest advantage of breast feeding is the important psychological union of the mother and the baby.

Can newborn children be hurt if the soft spot on their head is touched firmly while the child is being dressed or fed?

All normal children have two "soft spots" on the top of the head when they are born. Those spots are known as fontanelles. As the child grows older, these soft spots gradually close and finally are completely covered by the permanent solid bone.

Even during the early stages, the thin covering over the brain is very firm, and serves as an excellent protection to normal handling. Parents of newborn children are understandably concerned, but they should not be afraid of injuring their child should they touch these areas.

What is the general order of the growth of teeth during early infancy and childhood?

We are confused by the terms "milk teeth" and "baby teeth."

It is difficult to believe when first you see the mouth of the newborn child that underneath those soft pink gums teeth activity is already going on.

The roots for the first teeth are setting the pattern for the permanent teeth of the adult. It is for this reason that no period of dental growth must be disregarded if healthy dentition is to be the child's heritage.

When the baby is about four or five months old, tiny baby teeth begin to appear in the middle of the lower jaw. Baby teeth are also called "milk teeth," "first teeth," or "primary teeth."

As the months go by, new teeth appear at regular intervals, and before long, the eye-teeth or "canines" make their appearance. Then the so-called "two-year molars," or back baby teeth, come out. Sometime between 2 ½ and 3 years, a normally developing child with good nutrition probably has all of his twenty baby teeth.

There was a time, not many years ago, when the general attitude toward baby teeth was to sacrifice them by removal with little provocation. Today, the attitude is to preserve baby teeth by teaching children good dental habits at a very early age.

My sixteen-month-old baby weighs thirty-four pounds. Since he has gained so much weight, I have started to get veins on my legs which sting and throb. How can I prevent more veins and get these to disappear?

I doubt that your baby's weight is responsible for the veins of your legs. Small varicose veins appear in a great many women following pregnancy. Carrying a heavy child is a burden and probably exaggerates the vein problem you have. How this is treated depends entirely on the nature and extent of the varicose veins, which can only be established by your doctor through special studies. If there are extensive and deep-vein varicosities, surgery may be the method of choice. When the condition is less severe the veins are sometimes injected, bringing relief from the tingling or throbbing sensation. The use of supporting stockings is often beneficial. May I suggest that while your veins are being treated, your child be started on a strict but nourishing diet. You both will benefit.

I seem to recall that you wrote about boric acid as a danger to young children. My mother says that she used boric acid all the time when we were young.

Your mother, like many others, did use boric acid as a powder and in solution. In fact, it was generally considered a harmless cleansing agent and was kept almost routinely in every medicine cabinet.

Almost ten years ago, it was found that boric acid dusting powder, used for diaper rashes in newborn children, was toxic, hazardous, and almost lethal.

Boric acid was once routinely used to "clean" the eyes of infants. This, too, of course, has been given up completely.

Since there are so many other medications that can safely be substituted for boric acid, it is wise to avoid using it.

Has anything further been done about manufacturing bottle caps of medicine to keep children from opening them?

Spurred by the fact that the simple household drug, aspirin, is still the leading poison endangering children under the age of five, new safety bottle tops are a legal requirement.

All bottles containing aspirin must have caps that resist the curious hands of young children. This ruling by the Federal Drug Administration will save many lives.

I am trying to break my little five-year-old girl of the habit of thumb-sucking before she goes to school. I have tried to wrap bad-tasting things on her nails. I have tried talking kindly and when this did no good I began to shame her. Nothing seems to help.

Almost always thumb-sucking offers a sense of comfort and gratification to the child when she is especially in need of greater security. This is the time that you must make her feel that she is loved and wanted rather than shamed into a defensive position which only causes more thumb-sucking.

Mittens, elbow splints and bad tasting medicines will only make your child more miserable and perhaps be responsible for neurotic patterns which will be far more difficult to erase.

Continue your kindness to her. Encouragement and understanding without embarrassment will give her support until she herself is ready to give up thumb-sucking.

With patience you can be sure that this habit will stop and that your daughter, as so many children have, will emerge from this period as a happy, healthy, young lady.

My three-year-old grandson is irritable and antagonistic. This I can overlook, knowing his mother. However, he has an old baby blanket which he will not let out of his sight. How long will this nonsense last?

Your statement, "knowing his mother," leads me to believe that you have some "irritable and antagonistic" attitude toward your own daughter. It really is unfair to base your grandson's behavior on the emotional content of his mother.

It would seem apparent that the relationship between you and your daughter needs some solution.

As for your grandchild, it is not unusual for children of this age to find security in a tattered blanket or a disreputable toy. Children have radar receptors which pick up all evidence of anxiety or hostility in the family. I wonder whether your basic antagonism toward your daughter, in a far reaching way, has reflected itself in your grandson. This may seem remote, but you should consider the possibility.

Try to re-establish a warm relationship with your own child. Be patient with your daughter and her son and when he finds the security he needs from personal relationships, you may find him discarding his security blanket and ceasing to depend upon it.

We are contemplating a divorce and want to spare our two

children, aged eight and five, as much psychological hurt as possible. Where can we go for guidance?

Despite the fact that so many so-called "amicable" divorces do occur, young children pay a great penalty. They feel, but cannot express, the physical and emotional insecurity that threatens them.

Far too often, childen become the pawns with which divorced parents express their anger and hostility. You are very wise to plan your divorce without leaving in its wake a disaster or an emotional catastrophe for the children. I suggest a consultation with your family physician who often is the bulwark of understanding for the general problem. Undoubtedly, he will refer you to a psychologist, psychiatrist or a family counseling service so that you can lay out a planned program for the children.

Only by thoughtful professional advice can the children be eased into the new situation and be given the emotional support that will sustain them through the ensuing years. The key is the constant assurance to your children that they will continue to be loved and protected by each of you. Never underestimate the child's ability to understand your explanations, if done with understanding and the direction of trained counselors.

I have a nine-year-old son who blinks his eyes and wrinkles his nose instead of just normally batting his eyes. This has continued for three months. What can I do to help him?

The condition you describe is usually classified as a habit spasm or a "tic." These movements which are habitually repeated frequently occur in children in your son's age group.

Most of these tics have emotional origins. It is always wise to first rule out any physical cause. Frequently tics spontaneously disappear, recurring sometimes during periods of emotional stress or fatigue.

Persistent tics may need the support of a psychotherapist. Often he will be able to determine the stress patterns that cause the tic. Psychotherapists can make suggestions to remedy the underlying cause for these habit spasms.

The child should never be mimicked or shamed in an effort to cure him. Undue pressure may only serve to prolong and intensify the condition. Kindness and patient understanding will be helpful to the eventual cure of your son's tic.

Our four-year-old boy becomes hysterical whenever the sky becomes cloudy and there is a threat of rain with lightning. There is no way that I can bring him out of the closet without his going into a panic.

Children are born into this world without fear. At a very early age, the fears of the parents or other members of the family are inadvertently imposed on them. Although it is sad for you to witness such terror, he obviously cannot be punished for his anxiety.

Many parents are unable to handle these situations. In most instances they only compound the problem and deeply ingrain the fears into the subconscious mind of the child. Even if your son's fear temporarily disappears, you should seek the expert opinion of a trained psychologist or psychiatrist who will be able to get to the roots of the problem and handle it effectively.

One of the children in my class constantly pretends she is going to bite anyone with whom she is angry. She hasn't done it yet but I wonder what should be done if she really does.

Most children who have this tendency do not hand out warnings; they just bite.

There are two aspects of the problem. One is to find out why her hostility and aggression is present and comes out in this form of anger.

The other is to understand the human bites, when they do occur, are almost always as dangerous as bites by animals. Wounds must be thoroughly cleaned with ordinary soap. Antibiotics should be given to prevent infection which may occur because of the germs present in saliva and the mouth. The doctor's advice, of course, should be followed as to whether tentanus antitoxin should be given to the "bitee."

The problem also deserves special consideration from the psychological point of view before the pretender carries out the threat.

What is your theory about small children between three and five years old who make up tales and insist that they are telling the truth? I do not want my children to get into the habit of telling untruths without punishing them. Will this habit disappear as they grow older?

127

It is difficult to separate the alert, vivid imagination of a child and his created stories from that which grown-ups consider lying. So vivid is the child's imaginative experience that, for him, it takes on absolute reality and truth.

When a lie is used purposefully for gainful benefit, it is imperative that the child be faced with the truth, without making him feel guilty or embarrassed. Unfortunately, there are no standard rules for handling these situations if they persist.

A devoted mother will not wait to see if this habit will pass away. Too often there are underlying problems that a young child may have and not express. A trained psychologist can learn a great deal about the child who makes up stories from psychometric tests and then can offer simple suggestions that may be of tremendous importance in the solution of this problem.

We have been told that you wrote about a drug used for the control of bed-wetting in young children. Can you tell us more about this method of curing bed-wetting? Is it safe?

Persistent bed-wetting is a complex problem that needs psychological guidance in addition to the advantageous drug treatment now available. The problem should be dealt with early to avoid embarrassment and distress for children going to school.

The drug I referred to is *imipramine*. It is sold under a different trade name. The drug works by changing the sleep patterns during the night and has been extremely successful in many cases where other methods have failed. It is a safe drug when prescribed and controlled by the physician, and certainly deserves a trial in cases of uncontrolled and persistent bed-wetting.

Two of our children are making normal progress at school and have excellent relations with their friends. Our third child, now seven, has many emotional problems and I attribute them to the fact that she was conceived while my husband was in an alcoholic state and also taking large amounts of tranquilizing drugs. Is there any validity to this idea?

I have never seen any specific statistics that relate birth abnormalities or behavior problems to the use of alcohol during conception.

That does not mean that the possibility does not exist even though the chances are remote.

We have learned by sad experience that some drugs that appear to be innocuous may be toxic to some people. The genes and chromosomes are hardy but may be affected by the use and abuse of toxic drugs. Alcohol must be classed as being toxic when taken over a long period of time in large quantities.

It is for this reason that many physicians avoid the use of drugs during pregnancy. Whether or not there is even the vaguest possibility that alcohol, at the time of conception, was responsible for your child's present state is speculative. That which is positive, however, is that irrespective of the cause, your child should be studied by psychological testing and if important clues are revealed, she should be treated without delay. A discussion with your own physician will then tell you if the specialized care of a psychologist or a psychiatrist is necesary.

How can one tell if a child is emotionally disturbed?

There is such a wide range between the normal emotional upsets of a child, and the abnormal behavior pattern, that only a well-trained physician should dare make the diagnosis of emotional disturbance in children. When I say a well-trained physician, I mean one who has had specific training in psychiatry and who is able to study and evaluate the complex behavior of the child.

For a parent to lable a child as being emotionally disturbed because his behavior is temporarily unusual, or because he is difficult to handle, is to do him a great injustice. The emotional stability of the parent, who is so intimately involved with the problems of his child, is too often affected by intense personal interest.

There is no guesswork in diagnosing emotional disturbance, just as there is no guesswork in diagnosing a heart or lung condition. A psychiatrist can readily evaluate the child's condition and his problems and suggest simple remedies that would clarify these problems for the parents. A visit to the psychiatrist is a wise investment in the emotional health of any child who seems disturbed.

Our five-year-old son has a tendency to read and write certain words backward. Almost invariably he reads "was" as "saw." Will he outgrow this?

129

ait for time to remedy this condition. The reversal of
may be but a fraction of visual problems that are not
ed correction.

_____, previously considered "slow learners," are now recog-
nized to have some form of "dyslexia." This broad term includes a
number of reading and writing disorders.

We now have many excellent ways to study muscle balance of the
eyes and errors in refraction. These, in addition to neurological and
psychological examinations, may pinpoint the exact cause of your son's
image reversal.

With proper re-education and training devices, many of these problems can be corrected. I suggest you get started at once.

**If there is any suspicion that a child may be brain-damaged are
there any special symptoms a parent can look for?**

The recognition of minimal brain damage, or dysfunction, is a very
difficult diagnosis to make, even for those specifically trained.

There is no single positive test that is absolute and unequivocal.
Every resource, medical, psychological, and educational, must be used
in the interpretation of brain damage.

Some children may show great excitation, aggressiveness, and a very
short attention span at school. Others may be hyperactive, impulsive,
unapproachable.

It must be noted how vague all these terms are and therefore how
easy it is to fall into a trap of a wrong parental diagnosis.

When unusual behavior patterns are recognized, associated with inability to keep pace with other children of the same age, every available
study must be done before labeling a child "brain-damaged."

Far too many children are unnecessarily considered damaged when,
with therapeutic drugs and psychological guidance, they can be inte-
grated into a happy world of progressive growth.

**How dangerous is it when a child is born with water on the
brain?**

The technical name for water on the brain is hydrocephalus. This is
not a common disorder in newborn children and may be caused by a
number of reasons.

The brain is surrounded by a protective layer of cerebrospinal fluid which also circulates within the brain. Sometimes there is an over-production of this fluid which makes the head grow to an unusually large size. This fluid is usually absorbed at about the same rate of speed that it is produced. Occasionally the rate of absorption may not be rapid enough and thus permits the accumulation of excess fluid.

Before any treatment for hydrocephalus is undertaken many tests are performed to pinpoint the exact cause. Only then can one of the many operations be performed to remedy the condition and to prevent the possibility of permanent brain damage. Doctors who treat newborn infants never take the "this too shall pass" attitude in handling this condition. They attack the problem immediately to give the baby the best chance at complete recovery.

Our third daughter was recognized as a Mongolian child at birth. Our other two girls are perfectly normal. We have exhausted ourselves emotionally, physically and financially in an effort to cope with this calamity. We are now faced with the difficult decision as to whether to place our child in an institution or to continue to keep her at home.

The heartbreak of having a child born with any severe physical, emotional or mental limitation can only be known to parents who experience it.

Mongolian idiocy and related disorders have been incorporated into a general classification called Downs disease. Vast research is now centering on the prevention of this strange deficiency usually noted at birth. The characteristic appearance of the face and the eyes of a child born with this condition resembles a typical Asiatic or Mongolian face. There is a broad nose and flat skull and a tendency towards slanting of the eyes.

The reason for this birth calamity is not known. What is known is that neither you nor your husband are being punished for anything you think you might have done or failed to do. Personal guilt must not play a role in the solution of this heartbreaking situation. All factors must be balanced carefully and given impartial consideration. You must first ask if your daughter will ever be able to take a place in normal society. Will your other children suffer by your decision to keep your child at home? You must also consider the fact that your child herself may be infinitely more happy in an environment where, without competition, she can be loved, taught and directed by those specially trained in this field. Your religious advisor and your doctors may help you to understand that there may be greater benefits for her away from home than in the home.

Does the brain completely recover after a severe injury to the skull? My son was unconscious after an automobile accident but seems to have recovered completely.

Injuries to the head may be very severe and yet the brain is protected by the skull and by the layers of fluid around the brain.

Brain tissue may be bruised, which is known as a contusion, or even lacerated or torn. The bleeding that is associated with such severe injuries, and the swelling of the brain that follows, are responsible for symptoms such as loss of consciousness, changes of speech, and other neurological signs.

Concussion of the brain is caused by a blow to the head which results in the loss of consciousness. This may be temporary or prolonged, depending on severity of the injury.

Even skull fractures need not result in permanent injury to the brain.

It sometimes takes a long period to fully recover physically and psychologically from such an experience. But having once recovered, there is little or no chance of any late developments that will interfere with his scholastic progress.

Our four-year-old child came home from nursery school with a fever. With it she had a sudden convulsion which lasted for about three minutes. We are terrified that our child will grow up to have epilepsy.

There are many different causes of convulsions. Epilepsy is probably the most frequent reason. It can also occur with meningitis, tetanus and many acute infectious diseases. Drugs and other toxic factors may produce a convulsion.

A convulsion is a sudden spasm of the muscles of the body followed by a temporary loss of consciousness.

The fact that your doctor was not unduly concerned means that your child's single convulsion was probably not of major importance. Frequently a child with a high fever may have a convulsion which never again appears. A convulsion does not mean that your child has been left with any brain damage. Nor does it mean that these convulsions will recur later in life.

It is most important that you do not transmit your fears and anxieties to your child everytime a cold or fever begins. There is a temptation to overprotect your child and, by doing so, you may make her believe that she is sick when she really is not.

If your physician thinks that there is the slightest reason for concern he would suggest a brain-wave test to rule out any permanent brain damage.

Are there any diseases that can be carried from a dog to a child? Our children are constantly kissing dogs.

Children should be discouraged from kissing dogs and cats and other domesticated animals. There are a number of parisitic infections in these animals that can be transmitted to humans. One parasite, the nematode, resides in animals and can be passed directly to children.

The nematode from the intestinal tract of a dog can contaminate the soil where children can ingest it. Fungus infections and molds can also be present around the lips and chins of animals.

There are other safer ways for children and adults to demonstrate affection for pets.

Our ten-year-old daughter likes to ride hoses. We are terribly concerned about the horse brain disease which we just read about. Should we keep her from riding?

It would be psychologically unwise for you to deprive your child of the pleasure of horseback riding because of a scare about equine encephalitis.

The disease, a very rare one, is caused by a virus. It is carried by mosquitoes that have built up an immunity against the insecticides used to kill them. There is no need for a generalized alarm about this condition. Federal and local health authorities keep it in check.

Our newborn baby cries whenever she hears a loud noise. Does this have any special meaning?

It is not unusual for newborn children to be startled and disturbed by loud noises. In fact, such a reaction is referred to as the "startle reflex." This is perfectly normal and has no significance in terms of future hearing. Some children may react more readily than others, of course, but the "startle reflex" is not an abnormal one.

Can loud rock music harm the ears of a child?

Fortunately, the ear has a dampening mechanism that protects us against unreasonably intense sounds, although blasting noises of any long duration can often do harm to the hearing mechanism of children and adults. I am certain that playing Bach or Mozart at high levels of intensity can do the same thing. It is not really the nature of the music but rather its intensity that injures hearing.

Are the adenoids ever removed in the four-year-old child without taking out the tonsils? We are confused by two different opinions about this.

It is my personal feeling that the removal of adenoids alone is, in most cases, a mistake. I speak only from my own experience which may vary from that of other doctors.

In some instances, in very young children of one and one-half or two years it can be considered as the method of choice. In older children it has been my experience that it later became necessary to do a second operation for the removal of the tonsils because of repeated infection of the tonsils. This turns out to be very distressing.

It means another hospital experience, another general anesthesia and all of the accompanying physical and emotional distress.

If there is confusion in this decision, the choice should be made by the doctor and not by the parents. There may be very special reasons in your particular case why your doctor insists on removing the adenoids alone.

What is the most important reason for nosebleeds in a young child? Can they be prevented and how can they be controlled?

In the absence of any blood disease or anemia the greatest cause for repeated nosebleeds is picking the nose. The most frequent bleeding spot is on the wall of the septum that divides one side of the nose from the other, just at the opening of the nose.

Crusting due to infection, allergy or extreme dryness of the room, at school and at home seems to induce children to pick at their noses.

Lubrication of the nose with a mild mineral oil, the use of steam inhalation for a few minutes before bedtime and a humidifier in the room during the winter months is beneficial.

In almost all cases of childhood nosebleeds, a large piece of dry cotton placed in the nostril with the child sitting up, and followed by pressure on the cotton, will control the nosebleed. Parents are urged not to display their anxiety which then reflects immediately on the child and disturbs him more than the bleeding. Almost always these episodes stop when the child grows older.

Our four-year-old keeps putting tiny objects in his nose. What is the safest way to remove these?

Only yesterday I removed a pussywillow bud from a five-year-old child's nose.

I have learned that when one object is removed, look immediately for another. I found two.

Any foreign body in the nose should be removed only with proper medical instruments. Too much damage can be done otherwise to the delicate lining of the nose.

For the past two winters my daughter, aged five, developed severe spells of croup. They absolutely terrify her and us. What causes croup and is there any way to avoid these attacks?

Croup is an inflammation and infection of the lining of the throat, the larynx, or windpipe, and the lungs. The disease occurs most frequently in infants and young children who have a narrow windpipe. As the child grows older, swelling of the lining of the windpipe does not as easily interfere with breathing. The disease tends to occur most frequently in late winter or early spring. Virus and streptococcus infections cause a sudden thickening of the mucous membrane and produce a thick material which interferes with breathing. Difficulty in breathing may suddenly follow an ordinary cold. High fever and a barking cough identify croup.

ıalations are probably the most soothing treatment for the
breathing and the barking cough. Physicians frequently suggest that the child be held in the mother's arms in a bathroom filled with steam until they can arrive to treat the child with other methods.

There are many excellent cold and warm vaporizers which produce a great deal of moisture. An open umbrella covered by a sheet makes an excellent steam tent.

Antibiotics are given in larger doses along with cortisone preparations in order to control the infection and to reduce the swelling of the mucous membrane in the windpipe.

Attacks of croup can very often be reduced if infected tonsils and adenoids are removed. Allergic children may benefit from the use of antihistamines during their allergic periods.

What is hyaline disease?

In this strange birth abnormality, a thin membrane lines the bronchial tubes of the lungs and interferes with the free flow of oxygen.

A special substance, fribrinolysin, has been extracted from human blood and has been used with moderate success in some cases of leukemia. Although hyaline disease and leukemia are not related, fribrinolysin has been tried experimentally on children born with hyaline disease. There was startling evidence that thousands of these desperately sick children might be saved by this new concept.

The fribrinolysin used is difficult to produce. The medication of one infant costs two thousand dollars. Manufacturers can not yet be interested in producing it other than on an experimental scale.

Here lies the true sadness of such a great scientific accomplishment. It is inconceivable that money is still the dominant factor that interferes with the benefits of such research. This is immoral if even one infant's life is threatened by the situation.

My son is six years old and has had many infections of the ear. When this happens he becomes very deaf and stays that way until the ears become normal. Now my doctor wants to open the ears and put a special tube in them. Is this an accepted form of treatment?

Let me explain why infections of the middle ear are so common in children. There is a tube, the Eustachian, which runs from the back of the nose to the middle ear.

Under normal, healthy circumstances the amount of air that goes into this tube keeps the eardrum in balance with the air that enters through the outer ear.

Large adenoids can close the Eustachian tube and cause middle ear infections. Allergy, too, can produce a blocked sensation even without infection.

When a child has repeated infections of the ears with impaired hearing resulting, removal of the tonsils and the adenoids will reduce the frequency, the severity and the duration of the ear infections. In the absence of adenoids, sinus infections may cause a similar disturbance.

Almost always the hearing loss is temporary as it is in your child's case. When the infection subsides and air once more passes into the Eustachian tube, the hearing returns to normal.

A condition occurs rather frequently that causes the accumulation of a thick gelatinous fluid with the consistency of honey in the middle ear. This is called "cerous otitis media." It means fluid in the middle ear. The normal movement of the eardrum is interfered with and is responsible for the loss of hearing.

The operation that your doctor suggests is called a myringotomy, or opening into the eardrums, to release this fluid. The operation is very safe and definitely is an accepted form of treatment.

The tube that your doctor will use is a thin polyethylene one that is inserted through the opening of the eardrum to prevent the further accumulation of the thick discharge.

The tube is frequently left in for many months without harm. When the tube has exhausted its function it is pushed out into the outer canal and easily removed.

It is obvious that the suggestion to open the ear and to insert the tube was made by an ear specialist whose advice most certainly should be followed to give your son the advantages of this operation.

Can eye problems be responsible for lack of physical coordination in a child who is just entering the first grade? The regular eye examination did not seem to show anything unusual.

Educators are learning that an intensive eye examination with highly specialized instruments must always be done in children who have learning disabilities and poor coordination. For years complex eye disturbances and neurological abnormalities were overlooked because a child appeared to have good vision during daily activity.

Clumsiness and poor coordination with games, memory defects, difficulty in reading, reversal of letters and poor concentration are only a few of the unusual characteristics of children who are suffering from eye disturbances. Dyslexia, a visual disorder of wide scope and many subdivisions, must be ruled out in all young children with developmental problems.

Is surgery necessary in all cases of crossed eyes in children?

It is estimated that more than seventy-five percent of all children with crossed eyes can be benefited, or even cured, without surgery.

Exercises and eyeglasses can be affective. Yet it is important that surgery when necessary, be performed without delay. Waiting for time to correct the condition does the child a great injustice.

My six-month-old daughter has always had tears running down her face. Is there any possibility that this will affect her vision?

Tears are formed in the lacrimal glands, two small sacs located near the outer portion of the eye. The function of tears, of course, is to keep the entire surface of the eyeball moist and to act as a cleansing mechanism for small foreign bodies that constantly enter it.

The tears run across the inside of the lower lid towards the nose. There, a tiny tube, or duct, picks up the tears and drains them into the nose. It is for this reason that an excess amount of tears, while crying, is always accompanied by nose-blowing.

The nasolacrimal duct through which the tears flow occasionally is blocked, narrowed or so curved that drainage is impaired and the overflow of tears runs onto the cheek. In a six-month-old child, the chances are great that there may be some blockage that almost always can be cured. The tear duct can be probed with very tiny metal rods and the obstruction alleviated. May I suggest that you do not "wait for this to go away by itself." Your doctor will undoubtedly direct you to an eye specialist who can easily do the necessary simple procedure.

Is there any danger in the use of contact lenses for small children?

There are a number of important medical reasons such as astigmatism, severe shortsightedness, birth defects and other abnormalities that can be greatly helped by contact lenses. Many children for whom such lenses have been prescribed, even at the age of four, have learned how to insert and remove them without help.

If there is a real medical or psychological need that can be fulfilled by contact lenses they should be considered only after discussion with your own eye specialist.

Our daughter was born with a strawberry birthmark. At what age is it safe to have it removed from her face?

The so-called strawberry birthmarks are considered to be vascular in origin—that is, they stem from a blood vessel. The exact reason why these occur is not known. They may result from some disorder of development or be related to heredity. Some reddish birthmarks get smaller and tend to disappear. Others grow as the child develops. Thus there is no single rule about the ideal time for the treatment of these birthmarks.

The doctor will keep your child under observation and will recommend one or more of the new techniques by which birthmarks can be handled. Surgery is not always necessary.

What can be done for a child's chest that has a large indentation in it?

The front part of the chest wall is called the sternum. Deformities of this bone are not unusual. Sometimes the chest bulges out with prominance and is called pigeon breast. In rare cases there may even be a total absence of the sternum. These and a funnel chest are all developmental abnormalities.

A deep funnel may be responsible for adding pressure on the lungs and even on the heart, so that both of these vital organs may be displaced from their normal position. Shortness of breath and difficulty in breathing may occur. Even slight exertion may cause fatigue if the funnel-shaped breastbone puts pressure on the lungs.

There are now excellent safe operations which can re-establish the shape of the chest, both for pigeon chest and for funnel chest. The opinion of a general or chest surgeon should be sought early to spare the patient sustained physical or emotional distress.

At what age should a crooked bone in the nose be straightened? Our twelve-year-old son hurt his nose while playing baseball a year ago. We never suspected that his nose was broken.

For many years I have suggested that injuries such as you describe should not be casually dismissed with a homemade diagnosis of the possibility of a fracture. It is surprising how often these fractures occur, are over-looked and leave a cosmetic deformity that might have been avoided.

X-ray examination of the nose and an examination by the doctor quickly establish the presence or absence of a fracture. At the time of injury repair and repositioning of the fractured bone can easily be done. Once the bones have knitted, which occurs within the first few weeks after an injury, the operation is more elaborate and difficult.

The ideal age for such an operation is an individual one. In most cases, plastic surgeons prefer to wait until about the age of sixteen. This, too, varies, especially if the nasal septum is markedly bent and interferes with breathing.

Does a firm growth on the top of the palate of a newborn child suggest trouble in later life?

This bony enlargement is called a torous or torose. It has no special significance in later life. It does not alter normal growth or affect speech. It is a peculiarity of the formation of the embryo and is not associated with any other unusual changes in the body.

Adults sometimes find that the thin delicate layer that covers this bony proturberance is easily burnt by hot tea, coffee or soup. Rarely is it ever necessary to surgically remove these growths.

What is the cause of a harelip? How soon after birth should an operation take place?

Since there is a relationship between the birth defects of harelip and cleft palate I will discuss them both, although one may occur without the other.

A harelip is a cleft or cleavage of the upper lip which sometimes may extend slightly into the opening of the nose. This is a rare birth abnormality which seems to have some semblance of a hereditary characteristic. During the average embryo's development, both sides of the lips fuse and come together normally. But sometimes there is a failure at complete fusion and a harelip results.

Surgery has developed remarkably and the new techniques are more and more successful in the excellent cosmetic repair of the lip. The operation is performed as soon as the child is thriving and in good health.

A cleft palate is a malformation during development which leaves a cleft or division in the hard and the soft palate of the mouth. There are many different types but in most instances there is an open pathway between the mouth and the back of the nose. Cleft palate, like harelip, may occur in one out of fifteen hundred births. The condition is correctable by surgery. The ideal time may be the first six months. The decision of the doctor may vary and the operation can be performed later depending on the specific and individual condition. Parents of children born with one or both defects are often severely distressed. This is understandable and they need special assurance that the condition can markedly improve with modern surgery.

Why does a child's voice change to a deeper one at puberty?

There are a number of reasons why the voice of a boy, or a girl, changes in pitch and in timbre about the time of puberty. The changes are less marked in girls, but certainly they, too, develop other voice characteristics.

The presence of added ovarian and testicular hormones plays a very definite role in these changes. In the male, there is an additional reason for changes and that is the size of the larynx, or voice box. This grows considerably through puberty and into adult life.

The gradual change from the high pitched to the masculine voice sometimes fails to occur, because of speech patterns that were established in childhood. This can, of course, become very embarrassing to a young boy whose friends comment unkindly on it.

With the help of a speech therapist, it is very often possible to lower the pitch of the voice with a few special exercises. Certainly the change will eventually occur, but, if an adolescent can be spared that embarrassment, it is very worthwhile from an emotional point of view to seek and find proper speech therapy.

141

The second of our four boys is nine years old and is developing hair under his arms and in the genital region. He is embarrassed by it, and we wonder how we can delicately handle the problem.

It is not unusual for boys before the age of ten to show such evidence of precocious puberty.

Strangely, and simply from the point of general interest, girls develop this conditon more commonly than boys. It may start even at age eight or nine.

Almost always, some kind of hormone imbalance is responsible. The readjustment soon takes place.

The cause is easily determined by definitive tests that are now available. X-rays of the joints and skull, and a general physical examination can rule out the possibility of underlying important causes for such early puberty changes.

It is most important that you follow the directions of your doctor, and even seek an opinion from a psychiatrist or psychologist as to how to handle your son's embarrassment.

One of our boys was born with an undescended testicle. Can this be corrected? If it is not, will this affect his fertility and the possibility of becoming a parent?

The developing child in the mother's womb grows in a most complicated way. The sheer wonder and magnificence of a growing embryo never fails to be exciting.

In the embryo, the testicle begins to descend from its position near the kidney and finally assumes its natural position in the scrotum. For some reason that is not completely understood, the testicle occasionally does not descend completely, and remains in the abdomen. It has been suspected that a hormone deficiency may be responsible.

There are now a number of excellent oprations which can bring the testicle down. Although paternity can be assured even with one normal functioning testicle, the operation should not be delayed, for both the physical and psychological adavantages to your growing boy.

Two of our boys were circumcised shortly after they were born. A third was not because he seemed so frail and now, at the age of eight, is having difficulty with the skin over the tip of his penis. Is there any danger in having him circumcised at this time?

Phimosis may be the condition you are describing in your eight-year-old boy. In the absence of circumcision, there sometimes occurs a tightness of the foreskin over the penis which can be distressing and painful. There certainly is not any great danger to circumcision at his age. It does mean a general anesthesia and a moderate amount of pain for a few days afterwards.

In this particular procedure, it is imperative that the child know every detail of the operation and be completely prepared for the discomfort that may ensue. It is particularly important that a child's masculinity not be threatened by any semblance of a lie. Your son should understand the exact reason for the operation, what it will accomplish, and why it is beneficial. It then will be a contribution to his physical welfare and to his psyche.

From the day my child was born she was called a colicky baby. Exactly what is colic, what causes it and what can be done about it?

The word "colic" comes from the Greek, meaning colon or large intestine. Actually, colic refers to a spasm of the intestine which is associated with pain. Colic is a temporary disorder which leaves no lasting effects as a child grows older. The sharp cramp-like pains and spasms rarely last after three to six months of age.

There are many reasons that may account for colic. An allergic reaction to the formula or too much butterfat and sugar in the formula may be responsible. Too often young infants do not have their hunger satisfied and then, while sucking on an empty bottle, swallow a great deal of air. Distention of the stomach and intestines may follow. Overfeeding as well as underfeeding are improper feeding habits which may cause colic.

The infant's doctor usually adjusts the formula and adds to the diet, constantly keeping track of any changes in colicky behavior. Drugs are used when necessary to relieve the pain.

Sometimes a small quantity of fluid is given by enema to help expel the accumulated gas. Most infants are somewhat more comfortable when lying on their abdomen with a warm, not hot, heating pad.

The best pacifier is holding the child in one's arms during crying spells. Mouth pacifiers increase the swallowed air, adding to the discomfort.

Infants, from the day they are born, are remarkably sensitive to emotional tensions and anxieties in the home. Psychological reasons for colic are accepted by all those who treat infants. It is important that a child be kept unaware of tensions, especially during the feeding time.

How can one tell if a child has an ordinary stomach ache and not an attack of appendicitis?

Even physicians and surgeons who deal with this problem every day will admit that the diagnosis of inflammation of the appendix is a most difficult one. It requires expert judgment and experience, in addition to blood studies and a careful history on the onset.

Pain in the abdomen, especially on the right side, associated with fever, nausea and vomiting, must not be considered as an ordinary stomach ache. Guesswork may turn out to be correct, but it is entirely unsafe for any mother to take this responsibility.

The first impulse of many people is to give their child a laxative or an enema when they complain of discomfort, especially if the child has not had a bowel movement that day. This is unwise and dangerous.

It is always safer to consider pains in the abdomen as being meaningful rather than a passing discomfort. A telephone call to your physician will relieve you of responsibility and allow him to make the decision about the need for further examination.

We were shocked to learn that our ten-year-old son has an ulcer of the stomach. No one ever seems to have heard of this in a child. Is it possible?

It most certainly is possible and the diagnosis is a testimonial to the keen observation and diagnostic ability of your doctor. Contrary to general opinion, young children can and do develop ulcers of the stomach and the small intestines.

True, they are not as frequent in children as they are in adults. Doctors are becoming more and more aware that an ulcer can be present with symptoms that resemble adult ulcers. Medical and psychological consultation is an excellent combination to control this condition in a child.

Can antibiotics cause discoloration of a child's teeth? Also is it possible that deafness can be the result of too much antibiotics?

The side affects of antibiotics have been reduced considerably because the drugs are given to patients with greater discrimination. Nevertheless, some side effects do occur and one of them is a discoloration of teeth in children. The offending drug thought to be responsible is in the class of tetracyclines.

This occurs so rarely that it must not mean rejection of one of the most valuable drugs for the control of severe infections. Doctors quickly discontinue antibiotics and other drugs as soon as there is the slightest suspicion of a side effect or unusual reaction.

Now about deafness. One particular antibiotic, streptomycin, has had an unfortunate selective effect on one branch of the nerve of hearing and has been responsible for cases of nerve deafness. Because of this, the drug is used only when it is the sole antibiotic that can control a severe infection.

I have had two attacks of severe reaction to penicillin. My concern is that our newborn infant might have inherited this sensitivity. Is there any way to test him before its use, should penicillin be necessary?

The chances are very slight that your child will inherit your hypersensitivity to penicillin. Yet it should be brought to the attention of the baby's doctor. Many skin tests have been devised to determine unusual sensitivity to pencillin. And fortunately there are now many excellent antibiotics as effective as penicillin that can be used for most ordinary infections.

With five children, someone is always running into trouble or having an accident. Almost always, a neighbor is sure that I should get a tetanus injection for the child. How can a mother judge the need for a tetanus shot?

The ideal way to avoid confusion is to be sure that your child is properly immunized with the tetanus vaccine that is now available. This immunity must be maintained by booster shots at regularly prescribed intervals. Only then can you be truly free of the fear and anxiety associated with injuries to your children.

This is particularly important because some rather severe reactions to tetanus antitoxin do occur, and these might be avoided with proper immunization.

In those children who are not vaccinated, the conservative judgment of the doctor must be respected. In only specific instances does the doctor give the antitoxin, and only after balancing the advantage against the possible severe allergic, or sensitivity, reaction.

There is no way that you or your neighbors can make this decision.

What are the incubation periods for the most common childhood diseases?

Mumps, German measles and chicken pox have an incubation period of fourteen to twenty-one days before symptoms begin to appear. Regular measles incubates in about eight to ten days. Whooping cough, or pertussis, takes about one week to incubate. Diphtheria takes two to five days after exposure.

It is important to know when a child has been exposed to a contagious disease. School authorities ask parents to notify them immediately so that they can relay this information to the parents of other children.

Is a mumps vaccine worthwhile? Should it be given to all children?

When, after extensive experimental studies for safety, a vaccine is released for general use to the public, it is not only worthwhile but it is imperative that it be used. Mumps is such a frequent childhood disease that its seriousness and its complications are very often overlooked. Neglect serves only to invite trouble.

Unless there is a specific reason why a child should not be vaccinated against it, a child is actually deprived of health benefits by not doing so.

One of the complications of mumps that can be avoided by vaccination is orchitis, or inflammation of the testicle. Sterility in men has been a result of such a complication of mumps. The reports about the effectiveness of the mumps vaccine are most encouraging.

One child after another in our neighborhood has been coming down with impetigo. Can you tell me something about this disease? Is it dangerous?

Impetigo, technically known as impetigo contagiosa, is a highly contagious skin condition.

It is caused by the staphylococcus or the streptococcus germ. It occurs in infants and young children and is passed from one to another in such places as camps and schools.

Immediate isolation of infected children and strict hygienic measures are the only ways to keep this infection from spreading.

It is not a dangerous condition—antibiotics can bring it under control.

One of our children has a pinworm infection. We were shocked to learn this because we have always felt that our home is immaculate.

Contrary to general knowledge, pinworm disorders occur rather frequently, even in northern climates. Pinworms, or enterobiasis, is caused by a tiny worm that deposits its eggs around the rectal opening.

The symptoms are persistent irritation and itching there. The diagnosis is made definite by finding the pinworm eggs through microscopic study of a stool specimen.

Scrupulous hygiene, coupled with new effective drugs, can completely eradicate this parasitic problem.

Your child may have picked up this condition from another child outside the home. Do not consider this as a reflection on the cleanliness of your home. It happens in the best of families. It is annoying, but curable, and leaves no aftereffects.

Is it serious if a child develops black and blue marks over the legs and arms even though he seems to be in good health?

These discolorations happen often to active children who, in play, injure themselves. Almost always, injury is the reason for these collections of blood under the skin. Small blood vessels are broken and produce these marks, technically known as ecchymoses.

If these marks are extensive and seem unrelated to real injury, the reason must be sought by the study of the blood. There are many tests that reveal deficiencies of blood coagulation and a tendency toward unusual bleeding.

There are complicated and serious blood clotting diseases like hemophilia. Our present knowledge of blood diseases and problems of blood coagulation is very extensive and can almost always identify any of the serious conditions.

What is the best way to treat a muscle bruise? One of our children is always getting a bruise of one kind or another.

The application of cold immediately after a muscle has been hurt tends to reduce the swelling. If a tiny blood vessel has been broken, the blood seeps into the fibers of the muscle and makes it tender and swollen. Cold applications will tend to stop the bleeding and minimize the discoloration.

However, after an hour or two the cold has served its function. Then, a switch to heat will lessen the pain and be helpful in absorbing the blood. The temptation to massage an injured muscle must be resisted. Vigorous massage can start the bleeding and further injure the muscle.

My son injured his knee while playing football. He has a torn cartilage and surgery has been recommended. Will this leave him with a permanent stiff knee?

A torn cartilage is probably one of the most common injuries to athletes and people doing heavy work. When the knee is suddenly twisted the cartilage can become ripped away from its attachment to the tibia, which is the larger of the two bones of the lower leg. This results in some limitation of motion of the knee, with tenderness, swelling and pain over it.

Sometimes a torn cartilage can heal itself with long periods of rest and by the use of a splint or cast. This is frequently tried but the results are usually disappointing, especially if the tear was a severe one.

Surgery, when selected, is neither difficult nor dangerous. The results are very satisfactory and cure can follow in almost all instances. Since there are two cartilages in the knee joint, one can be removed without interfering too much with movement of the knee.

The victim is not left with permanent damage or limited activity. The knee should be respected after surgery and must not be deliberately exposed to repeated injuries.

Recovery from a torn cartilage operation, with adequate rest, almost always permits resumption of physical exercise and athletics.

Every few days I notice that my eight-year-old son has some blood in his urine. Is this a dangerous condition?

When blood appears in the urine even a single time the exact cause should be sought. Certainly if it repeats itself, even after a few days absence, it is imperative that a complete examination be made of the entire urinary tract.

There are many simple, unimportant reasons for blood in the urine. There can also be more serious ones. The bleeding may be an early symptom of infection, injury or even a tumor. A general examination is usually sufficient to trace the cause. When the general physician needs a specialist's help he calls on a urologist who can pinpoint the exact cause, treat and cure it.

Is PKU disease in an infant dangerous to him when he gets older?

PKU is an inherited condition in which a new-born infant cannot properly use a special form of protein. It is inherited when both parents are carriers without themselves giving any evidence of the disease.

All new-born babies now have their urine tested for the telltale phenylpyruvic acid in the urine. When this is found, intensive treatment with special diets can prevent the progress of the PKU disease and the possibility of mental retardation.

For the early detection of this condition, many states have legal statutes that insist on routine examinations of the diapers of all new-born babies. Simple blood tests have also been devised for the early detection of PKU and these have been used with great success.

Our ten-year-old daughter has recovered from rheumatic fever with a slight heart complication. I know it may sound ridiculous,

but we are having long-range fears that our child may never be able to have children when she is married.

Ten-year-old girls become twenty-year-olds almost overnight. You are perfectly right in considering the problem now. By expressing your fears you will relieve yourself of many years of unnecessary anxiety.

A slight heart complication will undoubtedly be followed by your doctor who, I am certain, has assured you that your fears are exaggerated. Many women who have even had relatively severe heart complications after rheumatic fever have been able to bear more than one child without any difficulty at all.

Modern methods of delivery and the ease and safety of anesthesia take a great deal of the burden off the heart during the delivery process.

One of our children was born with cystic fibrosis. We have not been able to learn anything about its cause, or why it should happen in a family with no history of similar illnesses. Is it not surprising that so little is known about this terrible condition?

Cystic fibrosis has been baffling physicians for many years, although we know the symptoms and understand that this disease affects the pancreas, the lungs and the sweat glands. This odd threesome produces symptoms that appear early in infancy and threaten the lives of children unless they are treated actively and consistently.

It is known by other names such as Mucoviscidosis and is considered to be an inherited disease with some genetic background, especially if both parents have the trait. Neither need have the disease.

Cystic fibrosis was almost a calamitous condition because of the marked malnutrition, lung infections and susceptibility to heat prostration. Many children tragically succumbed, especially before the antibiotics were discovered to treat the lung complication.

Vast research projects continue all over the world in the hope that eventually this condition may be prevented and are yielding knowledge that makes it possible to control this condition and offer better chances for the survival of children stricken with this heart-breaking birth abnormality.

Our second child was born with an enlarged thymus gland. Our doctor doesn't seem to be concerned about it.

The thymus gland is a good-sized organ that lies in the upper part of the chest in front of the windpipe and the lungs. As the child grows older and approaches puberty, the thymus gland grows smaller and smaller, and finally practically disappears.

In the past, the scientific ignorance about the functions of the thymus gland tended to bypass its real importance. Today, more and more evidence points to the fact that this gland plays a very important role in the formation of antibodies to protect the infant and the growing child against infections.

In the last ten years, a great deal of information has been accumulated about the role the thymus gland plays in muscle strength. A condition known as "myasthenia gravis" can in some cases be improved by the removal of the thymus gland that persists in the adult. As for your child's problem, you should have confidence in your doctor's impression that you have no cause for concern.

Can a child born with an abnormality of the kidney develop normally into adulthood? We are concerned because our child was born with only one kidney.

I am certain that your doctor has given you complete reassurance that a child with a single, well-functioning kidney can grow to maturity and be in perfectly normal health. It is not a rare condition.

There are many other types of congenital birth defects related to the kidney. Occasionally, there may be one or more *additional* kidneys. These usually are non-functioning. Sometimes both kidneys may be on one side. Once in a while both kidneys are joined together. There are many other variations, but what is most important is to determine how well each of these kidneys is functioning. Many tests are now available to establish this and to alleviate concern.

151

Chapter VI

Teenagers Have Problems Too

Whenever I go through a new batch of mail from readers, I can pick out immediately those letters written by young people. And it isn't necessarily the handwriting or the wildly decorated paper that betrays the senders. It is the way they express their problems, the way they speak of themselves and their ambitions. They pretend to be unconcerned, almost nonchalant—in fact, they very often explain that they are only writing "on a friend's behalf." But I can sense the urgency and concern behind the seeming flipness; the anxieties born of tensions, insecurity, rebellion and confusion. Their inner conflict is not consistent with their surface "devil-may-care" attitudes. It is always my habit to give very full answers to questions but especially so to the adolescent. Or to the mother or father who takes the time to write about some pressing problem their son or daughter may have.

The adolescent is a very special human being who needs and deserves a great deal more patience and understanding than he frequently gets. He is going through a period of enormous transition. Psychological and sexual conflicts overwhelm him. Confusion and frustration are rampant. And, too often, he irritates the adults around him. Physically, he is almost reaching mature adult size. Emotionally, he is just graduating from the post-puberty phase. He may have an adult body but he also has a relatively immature set of emotions.

The teenager and the adolescent have physical, sexual and emotional drives that they have a great difficulty expressing, especially to their parents. The art of listening to them is a highly developed skill. It is for this reason that I believe now more than ever that we need doctors trained as specialists in adolescent medicine. Such doctors could establish relationships with young patients, encouraging them to express their conflicts and doubts, not to mention their very real physical complaints. Young people need to be listened to and heard out. Physicians trained·in the science of adolescent medicine could be a dominant force in narrowing the so-called generation gap which I believe is more artificial than real.

Some adolescents in a stage of volcanic emotional eruption may be enduring complex hormone changes. Some may have nothing more serious than a flare-up of surface acne or an annoying body odor. Young women write nervously about whether or not their breasts will ever grow; young men are just as upset about beards or, rather, the lack of them. Yes, the questions are simple, but the feelings behind them are intense. That's why my responses to teenage letters go on and on.

I know my question sounds silly, but only a girl who wants to wear a bikini will understand my embarrassment. My bellybutton protrudes. Would it be harmful if I had an operation to remove it?

As you know, the bellybutton is another word for the navel or umbilicus. It is a small stump that remains when the umbilical cord that attaches a newborn baby to its mother is cut and tied at the time of birth.

Sometimes a small lump, rather than a normal depression, is left. Mothers sometimes try to tape down a protruding navel, but this rarely is effective. Occasionally, a protrusion may be a small hernia which should be examined by a doctor for such a possibility. Only after this should plastic surgery be considered for the cosmetic repair you desire.

Is there any special vitamin that one takes to gain weight? I am fourteen years old and skinny.

Vitamin pills themselves do not have any calories that would help put on weight. Sometimes they do stimulate the appetite, and in this way could be responsible for gaining weight. A nourishing balanced diet that is high in calories will, of course, help you put on weight. Sometimes it is difficult for people to eat a great deal at one meal. If this is so with you, try to eat smaller meals at more frequent intervals.

I am fifteen years old and am in high school. I have a problem about my ears and feel silly about talking to my parents about it. My ears stick out so that I am embarrassed to wear my hair up.

There is no reason why you should feel silly or embarrassed by a situation which is completely reasonable. What is not understandable is your inability to discuss this matter with your parents. Parents are remarkably good listeners and are usually sympathetic to the problems of their children. I am certain that if you were to discuss the question of your ears with them they would follow the usual process of seeking an opinion through your family doctor as to how and when surgery on the ears should be performed.

Plastic surgeons have developed many excellent techniques by which the cartilage of the ears can be reduced and reshaped in order to bring the ears closer to the head. The operation is not a dangerous one. Frequently it is performed without putting the patient completely to sleep, except in the very young. The surgery is painless and within three to four days the bandages are removed. Within a week the ears are well on their way to complete healing.

I am embarrassed because my eyelashes have fallen out completely. I am a sixteen-year-old student. What can I do about it?

If there is no local infection around the eyelashes then the answer to your problem must be sought in allergic studies. Cosmetics, eye makeup and even nail polish could be the offenders. It is also known that people under severe emotional stress may sometimes lose their eyelashes. The stress of examinations, for example, may be the cause of your problem.

I am fourteen years old and have vitiligo. What causes these white spots on my skin and how can I get rid of them?

Since you know the name of the condition, the assumption is that you were examined by a physician. The exact cause of the lack of pigmentation in certain areas of the skin is not known. Vitamin deficiencies have been considered but not definitely established as a cause. Allergies to dyes and preservatives in rubber have, too, been considered as possible causes.

Sometimes the condition tends to disappear of its own accord during the late teens. The embarrassment you speak of can be avoided by the skillful application of makeup. You should discuss your condition with the doctor who originally made the diagnosis.

My job requires me to stand on my feet most of the day. Some

noticeable blood vessels are accumulating just above my knees, although I am only eighteen. Can these be removed by plastic surgery?

Understandably, at your age you are particularly conscious of your appearance and therefore want something done immediately.

Plastic surgery is not the way to treat this condition. Your own doctor will tell you that these tiny blood vessels cannot be "drained" and rarely can be removed by injections. Small varicose veins, however, are treated in selected cases by injections.

One way you might keep these blood vessels from accumulating further is to use supportive stockings while at work. Whenever possible, you might also take a short rest period and elevate your feet and legs.

Is it possible to have an allergy to cold weather? Every time my teenage daughter goes out in weather below freezing, she develops hives.

It is not uncommon for people to develop hives when exposed to extremes of heat or cold. Some believe that it is the change from one temperature to another that may be responsible. These hives have responded rather readily to concentrated use of the anti-allery, or antihistamine drugs. For real effect there must be consistent use in order to build up a concentration of antihistamines in the body.

Is there any kind of hormone or hormone cream that can be bought to help enlarge my breasts? I am seventeen years old and flat-chested.

I have seen mail order advertisements suggesting immediate results with the use of expensive creams. These are tempting to anyone in your situation. But they must be avoided because they are totally valueless. All hormones prescribed by a doctor must be carefully used under his constant supervision. Specific hormones are occasionally suggested by physicians after intensive study for hormone deficiencies.

Your answer may be in plastic surgery, which now offers gratifying results to the flat-chested woman. During the past ten years, tremendous advances have been made in this field. Soft, synthetic implants are inserted, bringing much-improve contours to the chest wall. An encouraging aspect to this kind of surgery is that it does not interfere with the functioning of the breast following pregnancy and the birth of of a child.

Our daughter is seventeen years old and has large, pendulous breasts. She refuses to socialize because she is so self-conscious. Is surgery safe at this age? We are considering it.

The age of seventeen is not too young to consider plastic repair of pendulous breasts. The results are most gratifying and can be of tremendous psychological support to young people like your daughter. Scars are minimal and the functioning of the breasts is preserved. It is of vital importance to obtain an opinion about your daughter's psychological makeup before any such operation is undertaken. This may give a clue as to whether or not having the large breasts is the only distressing factor in her life. The decision as to when to do the operation should be left to the surgeon.

Is it unusual for a girl of thirteen to have a marked difference in the size of her breasts? Should anything be done about this to avoid embarrassment later on?

The breasts of young girls at puberty start to get larger about a year before they begin to menstruate. It is not uncommon for one breast to develop more rapidly than another and eventually both attain the same size.

Sometimes a slight difference does remain. This does not reflect any disease, nor is there need for concern. Your physician may want the opinon of an endocrinologist, or hormone specialist. He may suggest, in rare instances, the use of a hormone to help the development of the smaller breast.

We have noticed a distinctly unpleasant body odor in our fifteen-year-old daughter. She uses underarm creams and sprays but these do not seem to be effective. Can a physical condition cause this?

There truly are very few physical disorders responsible for unpleasant body odors. A general physical examination will rule out such a possibility. Cleanliness and rigid hygiene are far more important in the control of bad body odor than underarm medications alone.

A group of apocrine glands are responsible for normal, healthy perspiration. Some bacteria seem to flourish on the secretion of these glands and produce bad body odor. There is some advantage in controlling this by shaving underarm hair. On rare occasions some drugs and foods may be responsible for an odor, but this is usually distinctive from the characteristic body odor.

The most commonly overlooked reason for sustained body odor, even if cleanliness is observed, is the fact that clothes may be saturated with the odor. These should be thoroughly cleaned or even discarded.

I am eighteen and get nervous when I have to talk to anyone. My words come out so soft that people say, "What?"—which intimidates me more. I get the shakes and perspire profusely when I have to recite in school. My parents say that I will get over this. Is there anything that can be done about this medically? I have no medical doctor.

Your letter expresses what thousands of other young people feel but are too shy to articulate. In the first place, you are being deprived because you have no medical doctor to whom you can speak openly about this problem. In your city there are psychotherapists and psychologists, any one of whom could be a great help to you. The second phase of your problem revolves around your parents' belief that "you will get over this." Hope springs eternal in the human breast, but that hope and their good wishes merely delay your finding the help you need. Parents often wear parental blinders that keep them from acknowledging any possible deficiency in their children. Occasionally, parents take it as a personal insult if the suggestion is made that their child needs psychotherapy. This attitude should not exist in a world that now knows that a psychological problem is no different from a physical one. Both must, without shame or stigma, be handled early.

Discuss your problem again with your parents and I am sure that they, with greater understanding, will help you find both the doctor and the psychotherapist who will give you the emotional support you need.

My daughter is almost fourteen years old and has not yet begun

to menstruate. **Most of the girls in her class have already started and she is embarrassed because she feels she is immature and does not "belong."**

It seems incomprehensible to adults that the onset of menstruation should be so important to a fourteen-year-old girl. But it is. Most girls begin to show sexual development from the age of ten and reach maturity at fourteen. I am sure your daughter will soon begin her normal cycle. During this transitional period, it is wise that a physician thoroughly examine her for the possibility of some glandular or endocrine imbalance. There are a number of tests by which the activity of the ovaries and the other hormonal glands can be studied. Occasionally, endocrine or hormone deficiencies are evident and can be quickly rectified with proper administration of hormones. When there is no evidence of hormone deficiency and time alone seems to be the factor, then emotional support by the parents, a doctor, and a psychologist will help carry her through the difficult time she is in. And it is a difficult one for an adolescent. Patient understanding will bridge this gap for your daughter.

I have been told by the school nurse that I might have the kissing disease. Is it a venereal disease and can a test be made to prove it? I am ashamed to tell my parents about it.

Forgive me for reversing your order in answering your questions. Kissing is nothing to be ashamed of and in fact can be a pleasant part of sensible growing up. Parents were kissers, too, and yours will understand that infectious mononucleosis is not a veneral disease. A simple heterophile test is all that is needed. Parents make good friends if you let them be friends.

My granddaughter, fifteen years old, has been told by a dental specialist that she has an "overbite." He said that unless the condition is treated it might affect her ears and the permanence of her teeth. Is this possible? Will time correct it without braces?

Your orthodontist, or specialist in the straightening of teeth and the correction of the bite, is obviously well-informed. It is established that a bad "bite" can affect the entire dental structure of the teeth and the jaw joint. Bony changes within the jaw joint affect the opening and the closing of the mouth and can cause a tremendous amount of pain that can be referred to the ears.

In many instances, patients are suspected of having ear disease when in reality the jaw joint is the seat of the trouble. If you were to put your small finger inside your ear and open and close your mouth, you would feel the motion of the jaw joint. This will give you a better understanding how closely the outer ear is related to the joint and how it can be affected by it.

The correction of the malfunctioning bite will be a significant contribution to your granddaughter's dental health during this period and in her adult life. Time will make the condition worse rather than correct it.

I am a freshman at college. Many of my friends who seem to be in perfect health have colonic irrigations to clean out their "poisons." How do you feel about this?

This bit of nonsense has only recently come to my attention. Even great-grandmothers have given up this foolish pastime. A doctor may occasionally recommend a colonic irrigation, but he will critically evaluate a sick person's needs before doing so. This new college craze is fraught with danger and must be avoided by anyone with any sense of responsibility. A colonic irrigation can be far more dangerous than swallowing goldfish, overfilling phone booths or going on panty raids. Stay away from it.

Many of the girls in my daughter's high school class had their ears pierced without permission by a man who sells them earrings. Isn't this a dangerous thing to do? Shouldn't parents' permission be required by law?

It is amazing how skillful many of these jewelers are in piercing ears. Their simple methods of sterilization are effective, and infection somehow rarely occurs. However, I do believe that piercing ears must be considered a minor surgical procedure. Therefore, permission from the parents should be required by law. No operation, no matter how simple, should be performed on a minor without written parental consent, whether it be in a doctor's office or a hospital. The fact this procedure can be done in some states without that consent often tempts young girls to have it done, and then present it as a "fait accompli" to parents who might not have wanted it done. I have seen, in my own practice, a number of cases of persistent, unpleasant and protracted infections of the ear lobe following piercing of the ears.

Are there any drugs or hormones that can be safely used by a girl of sixteen who has an embarrassing amount of hair on her face?

Excess hair, or hirsutism, now responds in many instances to hormone treatment. Concentrated study of the blood and urine must, of course, be made to determine the particular hormone to be used if a deficiency exists. At the same time that these studies are in progress, epilation by the routine methods of electrolysis, waxing or bleaching continues to be helpful.

I have a terrible problem. I am now twelve years old. When I was two years old, I had an accident that left me with a dark brown scar on my face. Where can I go to find out if I'm old enough for plastic surgery?

Very close to the city in which you live there are a number of excellent hospitals with large plastic surgery departments. First, discuss your problem with your parents. They will understand why you are anxious to have this scar removed. Then they will talk to your family doctor, who will be helpful in finding a plastic surgeon who will give you an expert opinion.

My fourteen-year-old son has had a poor year as a student. The school psychologist felt that he was emotionally insecure and needed psychological help. Can a physical condition ever be responsible for failure to study and to concentrate?

There are many physical and emotional reasons for a poor study record. The period of puberty in boys and girls is always turbulent one. They are no longer children in size and they are not yet emotionally mature enough to compete in an adult world. In addition to the normal

161

problems of puberty and early adolescence there may be physical reasons for their lack of intellectual coordination. It has long been recognized that hypothyroidism, or low thyroid activity, can be responsible for sluggishness and poor intellectual attainment.

Present day psychological tests can be made to pinpoint the nature of a child's emotional problems. However, before these psychological tests are begun, a complete medical examination is imperative to rule out all the physical possibilities for his poor scholastic performance.

Fever blisters come out on my lips everytime I have a cold. This becomes embarrassing to a fourten-year-old girl because I am teased about it. Is there any way to prevent them?

Cold sores, or fever blisters, are called herpes simplex and are known to be caused by a virus infection. Small blisters appear on the skin or the mucous membrane of the lips and mouth.

It is interesting that cold sores are rarely passed from one person to another by direct contact. More often an upper respiratory infection, injury, overexposure to sunlight and emotional distress may start off an attack of them. Sometimes they come on without any reasonable cause. If cold sores are moistened or kept wet with the tongue, healing seems to be delayed. Doctors sometimes prescribe drying lotions or creams and, when necessary, use antibiotic ointments if there is a complicating infection.

I know of no way to prevent them except perhaps to keep up your body resistance, especially during the early stages of a cold. Plenty of sleep and normal diet are essential.

Can a basketball injury cause pain in the chest? It hurts when I breathe deeply.

The ribs and the muscles in between them can be injured and cause the symptoms you describe. X-rays will rule out the possibility of a rib injury or fracture. In the rest of your letter you state that you did not tell this to your coach, afraid you would be benched. This is bad judgment. All injuries must be reported.

Some of our high schools have trampolines. Can they cause in-

juries to the back? What has been your experience with this kind of exercise for elementary students?

Trampolines can be an excellent and exhilarating form of exercise. There are no more dangers inherent in the use of trampolines than there are with sports that are as apparently safe as tennis or ice skating. The rare accidents with trampolines should not keep anyone from enjoying this sport.

Safety in all sports depends on good conditioning and the understanding of one's own physical limits and abilities. If one progresses slowly and does not compete with others until in condition, this can be a delightful form of exercise.

The use of trampolines in the elementary schools should not be a great hazard. In fact, the refelxes of children are so good that the earlier they start a sport, the more proficient they become in a shorter time. Limits of safety can only be imposed on them by those who teach them this specialized form of exercise.

Is scuba diving a dangerous sport for a sixteen-year-old girl? She is an excellent swimmer, but we are afraid it is too hazardous for her.

Scuba diving, a wholesome sport and an excellent form of exercise, has attained great popularity. People of all ages are enjoying this form of relaxation. However, there are some do's and don'ts that should be considered by everyone who falls in love with this sport.

I believe that a complete physical examination with concentration on the condition of the ears, the nose, the sinuses and the heart and lungs should be done before beginning to study diving. The word "scuba" derives its name from the initial letters of the words "self-contained underwater breathing apparatus." Because it is a strenuous sport, only those in excellent physical condition should undertake it. It is especially important that only first-grade equipment be used. Less expensive equipment invites trouble. If your daughter adheres to regulations, uses excellent equipment, and is trained in the skill of skin diving, she will enjoy the sport. To deprive her of this exercise and fun will do her an injustice.

Our fourteen-year-old boy is just mad about sports, and is good

at them. My wife is afraid that he might eventually develop an athlete's heart. I don't think this makes sense. Do you?

Your wife's concern about "athlete's heart" has no medical or scientific validity. However, she needs reassurance if she, too, is to enjoy your son's accomplishments.

All muscles of the body grow larger and are benefited by exercise. The heart, a most important muscle, grows larger and stronger with sensible and controlled exercise. Professional athletes who have competed all their lives do not develop heart trouble that is attributed to their youthful activities.

It would give your wife a sense of comfort if your own doctor ruled out the possibility she fears by a complete examination. Without that, you and she may be in conflict about your boy's athletic prowess, imposing upon him an unnecessary psychological burden.

Can conjunctivitis be permanently harmful? My son is on the high school swimming team and develops this often.

Conjunctivitis is an inflammation of the conjuctiva, the delicate mucous membrane lining of the eyeball. Many people who spend much time in swimming pools, especially in chlorinated water, come out with bloodshot eyes and complain of burning sensations. Swimmers, after long exposure to chlorinated water, will be temporarily distressed. Some people are particularly sensitive to chlorine and cannot engage in any pool activity that demands underwater swimming. No permanent damage occurs to swimmers as a result of highly chlorinated water.

A number of swimming coaches have been using drops of methylcellulose to prevent such eye irritation. Of course, no drops should be used without the specific suggestion of the doctor.

Can a cauliflower ear that happened while wrestling be fixed?

I know from the rest of your letter that you are in high school and on the wrestling team. A cauliflower ear is the result of a severe injury to the outer ear which is followed by a hemorrhage into the tissue beneath the skin. The blood accumulates under a thin but tough covering of the cartilage of the ear. Unless this is emptied quickly, the ear can become severely distorted and cause permanent disfiguration. When once chronic changes take place, it is difficult to repair the ear so that it returns completely to its normal state.

It is for this reason that wrestlers and all athletes playing in contact sports must provide their ears and head with safe and adequate protection.

In a fit of anger, I slapped my teenage daughter. Soon after, her ear began to bleed. My greatest worry is that I might have injured her eardrum permanently.

Many times a slap over the ear will cause a "blast" effect to the eardrum and injure it. The first evidence of it is some blood in the ear canal. Hearing is immediately impaired. Almost always, the injury to the eardrum is temporary. Within a few weeks the ear usually returns to normal.

I assume that your daughter has been examined by a doctor or an ear specialist. This is imperative. Often people are ashamed to admit how such an injury occurred and will avoid getting the opinion and treatment by a doctor. Physicians do not stand in moral judgment in such situations and certainly would not reveal to anyone how such an injury occurred.

The chances are very great that the only residue will be your daughter's hurt feelings and your own personal guilt. Both of these can be remedied by a respectful talk about the differences that precipitated the unpleasant situation.

My son plays in a rock group. Whenever he comes home from one of their jam sessions, he can hardly speak. His hoarseness lasts for about four days. Can this be permanently harmful to his ears and voice?

There is a definite relationship between loud music and hearing. The delicate ear mechanism has some protective devices against the bombardment of sound. Despite the wonders of the ear, however, harmful changes can occur if one is exposed to the constant avalanche of high-decibel sounds in music.

The larynx, or voice-box, houses the vocal cords. When singing or screaming above the high concentration of sound, damage to the vocal cords can occur. Since it is necessary to sing above the loud sounds of the instruments in such jam sessions, injury can easily result.

Such vocal abuse can cause small hemorrhages in the vocal cords, accompanied by swelling and hoarseness. Unless there is some respect for the larynx, polyps and vocal nodules are inevitable.

I am fifteen and my best friend is sixteen. We both have terrible acne. Will it ever go away? What really causes it?

Acne continues to plague and embarrass adolescents like yourselves. At puberty more than seventy-five percent of all young people are bothered by this disorder, which needs understanding by them and by their parents for its control.

Acne occurs on skin areas where oily or sebaceous glands are most prevalent. The skin of the face, back and chest are most frequently involved. The appearance of acne suggests that it is a temporary imbalance of the hormones that causes an overstimulation of the wax- and oil-producing glands of the skin. It is this that is responsible for the acne. Infection does occur and complicates the problem.

There may be some additional factors that play a role in this annoying condition. Fatigue, vitamin deficiency, allergy, excess sweets, a poorly balanced diet and reactions to drugs may be the culprits. Emotional stress is involved in acne, possibly as a cause, but more frequently as a result.

It takes a great deal of patience to cope with acne. The fact that we all know that acne almost always disappears does not give the one who has it much encouragement. He fares better with a concrete program set down by a doctor. The physician's decision as to the use of hormones, cortisone and antibiotics depends on the individual case. His directions for diligent cleanliness and the use of non-irritating soaps may limit the extent fo the acne.

You have written about the possibility that Vitamin A may soon be used for acne. I am sixteen years old and plagued with acne. I would gladly be a subject for experiment.

I know how impatient you are about your acne—all youngsters are. We hope that soon this unpleasant condition may be prevented or cured.

A very specialized type of Vitamin A acid is being used. This is not to be confused with Vitamin A which is taken by mouth. Vitamin A acid solution is applied directly to the skin and has been most beneficial when used over a long period of time. The solution should be used only under the direction of a doctor.

It is not a cure for acne but rather a beneficial treatment. The acne tends to come back when treatments stop.

How can scarring of the face be prevented in teenagers who have acne?

Most cases of adolescent acne disappear and leave few, if any, scars, pits and depressions if the skin of the face is not roughly handled. It is when the pustules on the face are squeezed that infections may spread and leave disfigurement of the skin. The simple rules of cleanliness, using mild soaps and plenty of hot water applications, are far more beneficial than all of the expensive "magical" lotions that are sold to the desperate teenager.

A teenager deserves the opinion of a skin specialist before she embarks on treatment with over-the-counter antibiotics and cortisone creams which may be dangerous. The dermatologist can, in addition to giving psychological support, teach the young person how to avoid clogging the pores, thus complicating simple acne.

Chapter VII

Questions From The Senior Group

The process of aging is not a simple one. There are many physical, environmental, social, economic, geographic, hereditary and emotional reasons for premature aging and for delayed aging as well. The hereditary tendency toward longevity is undeniable, although not all members of a family may inherit it.

The search for youth takes many people into dangerous areas, all seeking the physical aspects of youth without ever learning that young spirits can keep time in check. Chronic diseases, excessive alcohol intake, overuse of drugs, tobacco and disrespect for body fatigue may make middle age grow sharply into old age. And hormone creams, expensive vitamin supplements and oils extracted from bats' tails do not interrupt the aging process. Instead these expensive traps cheat the buyer of his time and money and distress him without halting his advancing age.

There is an art to growing old gracefully and that art should be learned by youth in preparation for growing older. Aging becomes more apparent when one continues to live in competition with the memory of oneself, without learning the gentle joys of any age group.

One of my favorite responses about aging came from a frail but intellectually alert woman just starting her second century. She said that at no time in her life was she ever free of some problem or the need for an important decision. Facing up to them kept her young. Not for her the unrealistic attitude that peace of mind, security and health come by avoiding problems.

My mail from senior citizens is sharply divided into two distinct groups. One group, from the elderly themselves, dwells on the particular health problems that so often go with the aging process—arthritis, rheumatism, cataracts, dizzy spells, loss of hearing—along with their fears of not being able to maintain their independence or of being shunted aside by their families. The other half comes from the sons and daughters who are concerned for their parents' well-being. I don't think

I am being unfair when I say that often there is a hint of impatience, even resentment, in their letters. They can't understand why the robust parent they once knew now cannot remember what happened yesterday, why he dribbles when he eats, why she suddenly has become so mulish. They raise the question of senility, waving the word as if it were a flag of dishonor.

The fact is that only a tiny percentage of the elderly have the marked mental changes that would class them as senile. The solution lies in our developing sympathetic understanding for the elderly. None of the changes my correspondents mention are sufficient to isolate the elderly or discard them or disregard their capacity to contribute to the family society. Yes, sympathetic understanding, a respect for their present state and their past accomplishments can help the elderly live indefinitely as useful, loved and wanted citizens. Understanding their needs in particular activates them, rejuvenates them and opens their world to an all-important touch of happiness.

Is it true that elderly people become shorter in size? Do their bones actually change?

A condition known as osteoporosis is definitely linked with the process of growing older. The condition is seen rather frequently in people past the ages of seventy or eighty. As the name suggests, there is a greater porosity of the bones with a tendency for them to lose their normal calcium deposit.

This weakening of the bone structure has been identified with the menopause or "change of life" that sets in, usually, past the age of forty-five. Changes in the weight-bearing bones of the legs may result in a moderate amount of bowing which had previously not been present. Similar changes may occur in the spine and cause mild curvatures which futher emphasize the "shortening of the body in the elderly."

An interesting observation has recently called forth a great deal of enthusiasm in an effort to avoid osteoporosis or the decalicification of bones in women. It was found that women in the menopausal period could reduce the progress of this condition if they are given sustained doses of hormones like premarin.

At first this was viewed with a moderate amount of suspicion, but now the attitude is that the general aging process can be delayed if the endocrine levels are maintained both in men and women. Your doctor is always the best judge as to who is a candidate for hormone supplements.

170

Is loss of memory characteristic of old people? My mother and father are both seventy-eight. My father's memory is spectacular. My mother cannot remember anything from one moment to the next.

The blood vessels to the brain almost always become narrowed with old age. In some, the narrowing is more marked than in others. With narrowing, the amount of blood and oxygen that is brought to the brain is diminished, and the "memory center" in the brain ceases to function as it once did.

It is not unusual for elderly people whose memory is affected to remember with pinpoint detail events that happened many years ago, even during their childhood. These same people, however, may not be able to remember an incident of the night before, or even one that occurred five minutes before.

This is a difficult problem for the family to live with, and one that requires the greatest patience and understanding. It is encouraging to know that new drugs now being studied seem to hold great promise for revitalizing the "memory center" in the brain.

Should everyone as they grow older take larger and larger amounts of vitamins?

Supplementary vitamins are a good idea for those in the older age brackets.

A rather interesting report was recently released by the Gerontology Research Center of the National Institutes of Health. The preliminary study showed that one-fifth of the elderly people under investigation had abnormally low levels of Vitamin B and other essential nutritional vitamins. This was particularly surprising because most of the people under observation had been eating obviously adequate diets.

This interesting study will be expanded to learn if arteriosclerosis, high blood pressure, and other diseases may occur more frequently in the elderly because of nutritional deficiencies. Sensible vitamin additives are indeed valuable for the elderly.

When should a person who is partially hard of hearing wear a hearing aid?

171

The key word in this question is "partially." As an ear, nose and throat specialist, I am constantly made aware of the terms that people can create in order to avoid flatly saying, "I do not hear well at all times." Whether one says partially hard of hearing, partly deaf or slightly impaired hearing is not really important as a description of the severity of deafness.

There is only one real, mature, adult way to recognize deafness. When an individual has difficulty hearing sounds, full words, hearing on the telephone, the television and radio and does not have "happy hearing" at dinner parties or in the theater, they need some additional amplification of sound.

The old cliche, "It's not that I don't hear, but rather everybody whispers," is an easy way to avoid coming face-to-face with the problem.

The ideal way to handle a problem of deafness is first to be seen by an otologist, a specialist in the problems of the ear and hearing. A complete examination of the condition of the ears includes testing of the hearing with tuning forks and a pure tone audiometer. X-rays of the mastoids are sometimes helpful if chronic infection of the ears is present. When necessary the otologist may refer the patient to a nearby hearing and speech center for even more highly technical studies to determine the exact nature of the deafness.

There are now many remarkable operations which can be performed safely for the return of hearing. A specific condition called otosclerosis is a type of deafness which occurs in families and responds remarkably to an operation called stapes surgery. Other operations for the repair of perforated ear drums can now return hearing to many people who have had chronic infection.

Sometime ago you wrote that there is no hearing aid that is effective for nerve deafness. I recently bought an advertised hearing aid to cure nerve deafness and wasted a great deal of money that I can barely afford.

I have seen variations of the advertisement you sent to me. I have always resented the potential exploitation of the deaf by the sly insinuations that a specific instrument is "now" available for nerve deafness.

Almost always associated with this comes the next "tempting phrase" that their new instrument is a "scientific breakthrough that will revolutionize modern hearing aids."

"Caveat emptor!" (or "Buyer, beware!") is my warning to those who can so easily be trapped into buying expensive instruments that turn out to be worthless for people with nerve deafness.

Reliable hearing aid manufacturers and distributors usually monitor these false-claim advertisers. Better Business Bureaus try very hard to restrain overenthusiastic claims.

The best protection for a person with any kind of deafness is to follow the specific advice of an ear specialist. If there were such a thing as a "new revolutionary hearing aid," you can be sure he would be the first to know it.

The American Hearing Society has branch offices all over the United States. Its advice about hearing aids is excellent. In many instances, a deaf person himself can actually test out the efficacy of one instrument as against another. And many hospitals, colleges and universities have hearing centers where the deaf can be tested and where hearing aids can be worn on a trial basis.

Each year my husband and I go to a spa in Germany, where we drink the mineral water, get massages and mud packs, and feel extremely well for a long time after we return to the United States. Our doctor believes these trips are worthless. How do you feel about it?

I am constantly being asked about the advantages of treatment at far-off spas. In an effort to learn something more about them, I visited one in Italy where I tried the mineral water, sulphur baths and massages. After seven increasingly vigorous treatments, I found it necessary to wear a neck-collar for nine months. You can understand, therefore, that my enthusiasm for spas is at a minimal level.

The dogmatic believers in spas will be annoyed by your doctor's opinion, one that I share, that there is no great scientific substantiation of the "miracle cures" that are reported. Why, then, do I not condemn them? The reason is simple. A change of climate, rest, spa inactivity, dietary regimes and programs for rehabilitation have beneficial effects even in the absence of the "miraculous minerals contained in the waters pumped from the good earth."

There is one—and only one—way to judge the advantages of spa therapy. If you feel as well as you do after a visit there, it should be continued. For those who cannot afford such an expensive sojourn, rest, sunshine, good diet and freedom from emotional tensions can accomplish similar results much closer to home.

I've heard that people who live in warm climates live longer. Is this true?

I don't recall seeing any statistics that would substantiate this idea. I would at best be speculating if I were to suggest my own opinion. In general, I think it can be assumed that extremes of temperature whether the exceedingly hot to the exceedingly cold would be least beneficial to the greatest number of people.

After years of medical practice, I am convinced that respiratory infections and their complications occur less frequently, are less severe and are of shorter duration during the late Spring, Summer and Fall. It is well-known that there are geographical areas around the world where diseases like high blood pressure, heat disease, and even cancer are less frequent.

As you can see by my handwriting my pen shakes and gets worse as I finish the letter. I am sixty-eight. What causes this?

There are many causes of tremors such as you describe. Rather than guess the nature of it, I suggest a complete neurological examination. Many new drugs are available to control tremors.

I have a marked weakness of my bladder, and often actually lose my water during a sneezing or coughing spell. Can anything be done about this embarrassing and unpleasant condition?

Yes, there are things that can be done to help you after the exact cause has been established by examination. This condition frequently occurs in women who have had a number of children and have stretched the muscles and ligaments that support the uterus and the bladder.

A fallen womb is called a "prolapse." When the urinary bladder bulges into the vagina, it is known as a "cystocele." A "rectocele" is a bulging of the rectum into the weakened vaginal wall. These conditions can occur singly or together, and produce the symptoms you describe.

A vaginal plastic operation is often recommended by gynecologists. The results are gratifying, and the discomfort is quickly relieved. Occasionally a pessary device is used for temporary relief.

Does mental deterioration occur with Parkinson's disease?

No, there is no relationship between this illness and intellectual capacity. There is a fixed facial expression which is associated with this disorder. This masked appearance, and tremor of the hand, may give the impression of impaired mental capacity. But that is totally false.

My husband and I are both more than seventy-five years old, and we wonder if we should get early injections in the fall against the flu.

I think it's wise that you should take advantage of every precaution to maintain good health. The U.S. Public Health Service, and the local Boards of Health issue regular bulletins annually to physicians about the possibility of an influenza epidemic. I do believe that there are advantages in vaccination against influenza for certain groups of people. Certainly people in your age group, and those who have a history of chronic ailments, should be given the added protection that influenza vaccine affords.

Follow the suggestion of your own doctor about the injections. He knows best.

Is it ever possible for the intestine to become twisted and necessitate surgery?

This unusual condition is called volvulus and is seen occasionally in the end of the large intestine, or sigmoid colon. For some strange, anatomical reason there is a twisting or a torsion of this portion of the large bowel, which immediately causes swelling and interference with the blood supply and is responsible for the obstruction of the intestine.

This condition rarely occurs in young people, more often in the elderly. When the diagnosis is made, almost invariably there is an urgent need for surgery to untwist the bowel, or to remove that segment which is in trouble.

Are there different forms of colitis? Which is the most serious kind and how is it treated?

175

Colitis means an inflammation, infection, or other disorder in the large intestine, the colon. There are many types of acute, short lasting colitis and also many forms of long-standing chronic colitis.

One of the most common types is ulcerative colitis, which varies in severity from mild to moderate and to very severe. The single most common, distressing and devitalizing symptom is chronic diarrhea. This may sometimes be associated with colicky pain in the abdomen, fever, loss of weight and weakness.

The seriousness of all forms of colitis depends mostly on the degree of neglect and length of time before a patient consults a doctor.

The diagnosis can readily be made by microscopic study of the contents of the bowel and by a painless but uncomfortable examination called proctoscopy.

Chronic ulcerative colitis is a condition whose real cause is unknown. It is suspected that a virus or bacteria may be involved either as a cause or as an invader, once the condition sets in. That which is considered of major importance in this type of colitis is psychological tension and emotional upheaval, which may be responsible for the spasms of the intestine. The possibility of marked sensitivity or allergy to some foods, especially milk and milk products, is considered in most cases.

One of the characteristics of ulcerative colitis is that it may be cured only to flare up again without any known reason years later.

The treatment is usually bed rest, especially if blood is being lost through the intestinal tract. Physicians devote themselves to maintaining good nutrition and keeping the hemoglobin of the blood at a normal and constant level. Overexertion is avoided, especially when the first symptoms begin. And diarrhea is one of the earliest symptoms.

Psychological support and guidance play a most important role in the control of a single episode and in the prevention of future ones. Antibiotics and cortisone preparations are of extreme value and, when used early and vigorously, can almost always prevent the complications caused by neglect.

Antibiotics and cortisone are most effective, but the help of a psychoanalyst or psychologist must go hand in hand if these patients are to be returned to health.

———————

I am afflicted with hardening of the arteries and have a tingling sensation in my feet. I am seventy-two years old and am otherwise in perfect health. Is there any way to open the arteries?

Narrowing of the blood vessels because of arteriosclerosis occurs very often in your age group. The symptoms you describe are caused by an inadequate amount of blood flowing to the legs and feet because of the obstruction in narrowed vessels.

There was nothing in your letter about tobacco. If you do smoke, I would like to emphasize that this adds spasm to the already narrowed arteries and further reduces the blood supply to the extremities. All tobacco should be discontinued by anyone who has impaired circulation.

The prevention or retardation of arteiosclerosis starts early in life. A diet free from animal fats and high cholesterol, a well-regulated exercise program and abstinence from tobacco during adolescence and early adulthood probably can reduce the possibility of severe arteriosclerosis in the adult. When once these changes and deposits of calcium on the inner linings of the arteries occur, there is little chance of reversing the condition. A number of drugs known as vasodilators are said to widen the arteries to help increase the flow. Ask your own physician if he thinks they should be tried in your case.

Six months ago my husband had a sympathectomy operation for bad circulation, but the pain continues. He is fifty-nine years old and keeps smoking cigarettes. Can you give us any hope that his leg will get better?

Your husband is a lucky man, but a foolish one. For him to continue smoking cigarettes in the light of his poor circulation, is downright ridiculous.

Having undergone the difficult neurosurgical operation of sympathectomy, he now risks losing all the benefits of that surgery by continuing to smoke.

Sympathectomy is an operation that cuts the tiny nerve fibers that go from the spine to various blood vessels. This allows the blood vessels to dilate and carry more blood.

Cigarette smoking is known to constrict, or narrow, these blood vessels.

The only hope that can be offered your husband lies in his sensibly following his doctor's orders. And I'm certain his doctor has told him to discontinue all smoking.

177

Each morning when I awake I have a numb sensation in the fingers of my right hand. Sometimes the pain is so excruciating that I can't even pick up a cigarette. After about fifteen minutes the heavy feeling in my fingers begins to disappear and does not return for the rest of the day. What causes this?

A sensation of numbness, whether it is temporary or long lasting, is almost always due to some interference with the blood circulation. In your case, the fact that it lasts for such a short while indicates that there is little likelihood of other reasons like a pinched nerve in the armpit or at the elbow.

Sitting in an unusual position, with the arm over the back of the chair, easily explains this. Lying in bed does not usually interfere with normal circulation or cause pressure on a nerve.

Without meaning to, you tell me that you are a smoker. Tobacco, especially cigarettes, is one of the most common causes for interference with healthy blood circulation. Tingling of the hands and feet, coldness, numbness and cramps are frequently the result of spasm of the blood vessels due to tobacco.

There are, of course, other reasons. Women during the early period of change of life frequently complain of temporary periods of numbness. Early arthritis, with changes in the joints, can cause the same symptoms. The exact cause for your particular type of poor circulation should be studied so that the symptoms can be arrested.

Are there any special exercises to increase the circulation of blood to the feet?

A special series of exercises called Buerger's Exercises are done about three times a day for people with an inadequate blood supply to the feet.

First, the person lying flat on his back elevates his legs for about thirty seconds until the toes seem to become pale and blanched. Then he sits with the legs dangling over the side of the bed, moving his legs backward and forward for about two minutes until a reddish color occurs. Finally, he lies completely flat for about five minutes. This cycle is repeated again within a few minutes.

These exercises were devised by the doctor who described the vascular condition which bears his name, Buerger's disease. Before embarking on such a program of exercise it is, of course, advisable to consult with your own physician.

Why are people in the older age groups warned about hurting or cutting their feet?

As one grows older, the blood circulation to the feet becomes diminished. The blood vessels may develop small patches of arteriosclerosis and causes narrowing sufficient to impair the free flow of blood and oxygen to the tissues of the legs and feet.

If a chronic kidney condition or diabetes is present the vascular passageway is further closed. Smoking cigarettes adds to the narrowing of the blood vessels with the result that the tissues of the feet are deprived of vital blood.

Any injury with a blunt instrument, with tight shoes, or with a nail cutter can cause infection which, when untreated, may result in the death of the muscles of the toes. This is gangrene.

The basis for safety is that the feet should be cleansed and dried to prevent friction or blistering. Mild lubricants can keep the skin soft.

Nails should never be trimmed except by another person. The nails should be cut straight across. Callouses, corns and ingrown toenails can only be safely treated by chiropodists or podiatrists trained in safe techniques. The care of the feet is most important to the safety and health of the elderly.

My bedridden mother uses a hot water bottle for relief of pain in the legs. Can this be harmful?

There is less chance of your mother getting burnt if you persuade her to switch to an electric heating pad where the temperature can be constantly controlled.

What is chronic phlebitis and what causes it?

Phlebitis is an inflammation or an infection of the inner lining of the veins. This can occur anywhere in the body, but most frequently happens in the veins of the legs and the arms. Injury is one of the most common causes of phlebitis. Many of us can recall how an infection at the tip of the finger or the toe is followed by red streaks up the arm or the leg. This is due to inflammation of the veins.

Tobacco is a very common cause of phelbitis, especially in those who are highly sensitive to it.

Phlebitis deserves immediate attention. If the blood vessels are not treated with rest and antibiotics, clots can form within them and interfere with the blood circulation.

I have a momentary feeling of dizziness if I make a sudden change of position or if I get up too quickly in the morning. I am sixty-eight years old and am otherwise in good health. Can this mean that I am leading to a stroke or to a brain tumor?

In most instances, occasional attacks of lightheadedness occur at your age because the blood supply cannot quickly adjust to a change of position.

A common error is to believe that these sensations which are not really dizziness, are due to disease of the inner ear. Let me explain that the center for balance lies in the semicircular canals deep in the inner ear. These three canals can be disturbed by sudden changes of position, by drugs, and by allergies, without actual disease in the inner ear.

Your fear of a stroke or a tumor has kept you from doing the sensible thing—a visit to your doctor who could have immediately relieved you of your anxiety and made some important suggestions. By avoiding rapid positional changes, you probably will be more comfortable but this should not keep you from your real need—a complete and regular examination.

For the past two years I have had attacks of dizziness which make me reel like a drunkard although I do not drink alcohol. The condition has been diagnosed as ménière's disease by one doctor and another doctor believes it is due to poor circulation to the brain because of my age, which is seventy-six.

I don't quite know why the name ménière's disease frightens so many people, but it does. Unfortunately, some people use the term ménière's disease as a synonym for dizziness when it is not.

Ménière's disease is a very specific condition associated with sudden episodes of intense dizziness, progressive hearing impairment and noise in the head. Even naming these symptoms will, I am afraid, make some readers believe, "That's just what I have," even though it is not true.

There are dozens of causes of dizziness which have wrongly been labeled ménière's disease. Low blood pressure, high blood pressure, arteriosclerosis of the blood vessels in the elderly, drugs, low blood sugar and infections of the ear can all cause some form of dizziness. Patients themselves confuse headaches, faintness and light headedness with dizziness when they describe their sensations to a doctor. Whether you have ménière's or not, and the likelihood is that you do not, your condition can be controlled by diligently following the doctor's instructions.

How dangerous is an operation in a woman past the age of seventy?

I could not possibly deny that major surgery in the elderly does have a greater risk than in people who are younger. Yet modern day anesthesias and highly trained specialists in this field have markedly decreased the risks and hazards of surgery for the elderly.

Preoperative preparations with antibiotics and other drugs have prevented many distressing complications that previously occurred to high risk patients. Physicians and surgeons carefully evaluate each patient, the kind of surgery that is being contemplated, and the possible risks involved. You can be sure of a great safety factor if surgery has been recommended by your doctor.

Can a person over seventy safely undergo an operation for a prostate condition?

The age of a person is not the only or even the most important factor in the safety of this operation or any other surgery. It is the general condition that is important. When the heart, lungs, blood pressure and circulation are good the potential risks of surgery are reduced to a minimum. The developments in today's anesthesia are so remarkable that the elderly are operated on with almost the same degree of safety as men and women aged fifty to seventy.

Before a physician recommends surgery, all advantages are carefully balanced against any possible risk in order to insure the fastest recovery and the most successful results.

For as long as I can remember I have taken some kind of medicine for constipation. I wish you could recommend some way that I could kick the habit.

181

"Laxative hopping" is part of the great American fixation on the false mystique of "regularity."

Americans spend more than $50,000,000 a year making a ritual out of the "sluggish bowel." It seems to me that, for some diabolical reason, every TV commercial promoting the cause of regularity and explaining the mechanics of bowel movement always coincides with the dinner hour.

Constipation is a condition that can be easily controlled in most instances by proper diet and especially by a sufficient intake of water each day.

Unfortunately, there is a misconception that the whole life cycle of the individual depends on the daily bowel movement. Some people develop a tremendous sense of anxiety if their digestive system does not function on a pre-planned time schedule. Actually, a bowel movement every two or three days is normal for many people in good health.

The result is that many do exactly as you have been doing, jumping from a carthartic to a purgative, to physics, enemas, bulk-producers, and irritants, all to ensure ritualistic punctuality of elimination.

Uness your doctor definitely prescribes a laxative, try to interrupt your dependency on them. Give your body a chance to function naturally.

How dangerous are ulcers of the feet and legs?

Ulcers of the feet and legs, especially in the elderly, present a great threat unless their cause is established early. Poor circulation of the feet, because of narrowing of the arteries by arteriosclerosis, deprives the tissues and muscles of blood and the oxygen it carries. It is for this reason that people with circulatory disturbances and chronic illnesses like diabetes, must be particularly careful not to injure, bruise, or cut their feet, because healing is so much more difficult.

A technique known as arteriography now aids in better understanding blood circulation. Using this method it is possible to inject a special type of dye and follow it through the circulation of the arteries and veins in the legs and in the feet. The speed with which the dye passes through the blood stream is determined by X-rays taken at repeated intervals.

Abnormalities of blood vessels and varicose veins deep within the muscles of the leg can be readily recognized and, in many cases, repaired by surgical methods.

My feet become swollen as the day progresses. At night I can push the skin in almost half an inch. When I wake up in the morning, the swelling is gone.

Such swelling of the ankle and the feet need not be a serious condition, but certainly its cause should be found by complete physical examination.

"Pitting edema," or swelling of the legs, may be caused by simple or by complicated conditions.

Varicose veins or marked overweight, especially in people who stand on their feet all day, can cause this type of swelling.

It is also true that people who have chronic heart disease and kidney disease may have edema which is more persistent and does not vary as much during different parts of the day.

You are doing yourself a great injustice if you continue to worry about the condition without actually doing anything to pinpoint its exact cause.

My mother has just been told that she has glaucoma. The entire family has been thrown into a panic. What is glaucoma? How serious is it?

Glaucoma is an eye condition in which there is an increased pressure of fluid within the eyeball. A simple test for it can be performed quickly and painlessly with a tonometer.

Perhaps it will give you and your family a degree of comfort to know that early glaucoma, when treated intensively, can be controlled in many instances to preserve sight.

Glaucoma is not a cancer and not contagious. It has no relationship to a cataract and it does not mean that blindness is inevitable.

To understand glaucoma and to relieve unnecessary fears about it, let me describe how it is produced. In normal health the eyeball contains a specialized kind of fluid. This is constantly produced and then drained off through a delicate tube. In one type of glaucoma, the primary type, there seems to be an imbalance between the amount of fluid that is manufactured and the amount that is drained off. Fluid then accumulates in the eyeball and impairs the vision by the increased pressure. There are many different causes for the overproduction of fluid and for the poor drainage.

183

Another type of glaucoma, the secondary type, may be the result of infection, inflammation and injury to the tiny delicate structures within the eyeball. Emotional stresses and disturbances are said to play an important role in both the cause and the aftereffect of glaucoma.

The chances are good that your mother's glaucoma can be kept in control now that it is known. Special drugs and eyedrops can help relieve the pressure within the eye and can help preserve the vision. When drugs alone are not sufficient, surgery can be performed safely and with great success to insure the fact that the glaucoma will not progress.

My doctor told me a year ago that I had cataracts. It frightened me so that I never went back to him. My vision is getting worse every day. Will you please explain the operation? Will I be in the hospital long? How long will my eyes be bandaged?

It is almost painful for me to read such a letter. It is disheartening and makes me believe that doctors simply cannot overcome confusion, fear, and lack of cooperation by their patients.

You waited a year and suffered progressive loss of vision and then asked me questions which you should have asked your own doctor when he suggested surgery. Your questions are logical and understandable. Cataract surgery is painless, remarkably safe, and most successful by any of the many techniques now available.

Return to your doctor, arrange to have the cataracts removed, ask him all the questions that concern you and sensibly exercise your right to healthy vision.

Where can I get more information about donating eyes for science?

I am always touched by those who want to give sight to the sightless. Your planned gift deserves admiration.

The miraculous accomplishments of modern eye surgery have made the transplantation of corneas a reality, not fantasy. Gift corneas are indeed an unselfish humanitarian impulse and a true heritage for those who will again see.

The Manhattan Eye, Ear and Throat Hospital of New York City has been one of the driving forces in the creation and growth of the Eye

Bank for Sight Restoration, whose address is 210 East 64 Street, New York City 10021. Write to them.

After complaining for many years about weakness and nervousness, it was finally found that I had low blood sugar. Is there any special kind of diet for this condition so that I will not have the feeling that I am about to faint during the day? What causes it to begin with?

The condition you described is known medically as hypoglycemia, which means an abnormally low level of sugar in the blood. There are a number of causes of this condition which, with special testing, can be pinpointed. An overproduction of insulin from the pancreas, liver disease, hormone imbalance and infection are only a few of the major reasons for hypoglycemia. Fortunately, these serious reasons are not nearly as frequent as the others, which are more readily controlled.

If a patient goes for a long period of time without food, especially protein, he may develop a lowering of the blood sugar, followed by symptoms of rapid pulse, weakness, nervousness, headache and dizziness. These symptoms can occur with many other conditions and, therefore, should not, as I frequently warn, be used for self-diagnosis of low blood sugar.

The immediate treatment for this kind of sudden episode of weakness is to take a glass of orange juice, sugar, candy or honey. People who are supected of having hypoglycemia should not allow many hours to go by without some kind of in between meals snack.

The diet for the relief of the symptoms of low blood sugar should be high in fats, high in proteins and low in carbohydrates. Perhaps the most important aspect of the diet is that it should be distributed in at least seven or eight feedings during the twenty-four hour period. A slight snack immediately after waking and one just before going to bed should keep the blood sugar sufficeintly elevated.

What would cause a flare-up of gout after I was free of it for a year or more?

Gout is a disturbance in the manufacture of uric acid. One of the characteristics of this condition is that there can be recurrent attacks at unknown intervals.

The level of uric acid in the blood varies from day to day depending on the nature of the diet. Many patients stay in good health for months with a restricted diet and with continued use of anti-gout medicines.

Then suddenly, without any apparent reason, a painful attack of gout may strike the joints of the leg or feet. Injury, even very slight, may set an attack in motion. Overindulgence in alcohol, infection and even some drugs may induce an acute attack of gout.

Surgery performed in a person with a gout tendency may occasionally trigger a painful episode. Patients who have gout are usually instructed to take daily doses of drugs which help to prevent the accumulation of uric acid in the blood. If, despite this precaution, a sudden episode of pain and swelling of a joint occurs, the doctor should be notified immediately.

Whenever a new drug is taken and an unexpected side-effect follows it should immediately be discontinued until the condition is reported to the doctor. The early use of colchicine (taken only under doctor's orders) can very dramatically nip the attack before it sets in.

A new and remarkable drug, allopurinol, is now available to sufferers of gout. It is expected that this drug will be the greatest boon to sufferers as a preventative of acute and chronic forms of gout.

What is the cause of a persistent backache? I wake up with it every morning. It wears off in a couple of hours.

"Backache" is a very vague term used to describe every kind of pain from the neck to the base of the spine. Such pain may be caused by problems in the bones of the spine itself, or in the muscles that lie over it. The complex network of nerves that surround the back may refer pain from one place to another a distance away.

Treatment for any backache must, of course, depend upon finding the exact cause. It is unwise to speculate and lose valuable time. Too often simple backache progresses during neglect and becomes more difficult to treat and cure.

I have deliberately laid to one side the severe and often bitter acrimony that goes on between doctors and chiropractors. A great many people are fervent admirers of a chiropractor who has benefited them when all other means seemed to fail. My only plea is that people with severe backache first eliminate the possibility of important underlying cause for backache before embarking on a massage and manipulation program.

My father had a stroke and now has "aphasia." I don't understand what aphasia means. Can it be cured?

Aphasia means the inability to speak. Actually, it includes the inability to write, read, and especially, to understand.

There are many types of aphasia associated with strokes. The kind of aphasia depends on the part of the brain affected. In a right-handed person, interference with the blood supply to the left side of the brain may cause an inability to speak. The reason is that, in a right-handed person, the speech center is in the left lobe of the brain. The reverse is true in a left-handed person.

Some patients are unable to express themselves. This is called "expressive aphasia."

Others, with "receptive aphasia," have difficulty in understanding the spoken or written word.

"Total aphasia" occurs when the person can neither express himself nor understand.

It is important to realize that aphasic people are not mentally ill or retarded. There are, incidentally, many other reasons for aphasia besides a stroke. Birth defects and injuries may also cause it. How much function will return depends entirely on the severity of brain damage.

Some drugs have been effective in restoring circulation to the brain and reducing the duration of the aphasia.

All aphasia patients need a tremendous amount of sympathetic understanding and encouragement. It is enormously gratifying to help these patients learn new ways of communication. Rehabilitative programs including intensive speech therapy help make aphasic people serviceable and allow them to take their dignified place in society.

Can the use of the arm and leg return after a stroke? Is it possible to learn how to speak again?

A stroke means that the blood supply to a part of the brain has been interfered with. This may be caused by a clot, or thrombus, in a blood vessel that brings blood and oxygen to the brain. A hemorrhage of a blood vessel or a spasm of a blood vessel can do the same thing.

The extent of the paralysis of the arm or leg and the duration before recovery depends entirely on the size of the blood vessel and the particular area of the brain that has been deprived of its nourishment.

187

In a right-handed person, there is a small spot called Broca's area in the left side of the brain. The reverse occurs in the left-handed person. When the blood supply to these areas is interfered with, disorders of speech may follow. There are many types of aphasia which affect speech and the understanding of another person's words.

Recovery is a remarkable phenomenon of the body. The brain, contrary to general belief, is a very hardy organ. In fact, we who operate in the areas of the mastoid bone are often amazed at how much injury the brain can take and still survive. The recovery of speech and the use of the hand and leg depends on whether or not the blood supply can be re-established. Sometimes small blood vessels take over the job of one that was closed by the clot or by the break in its continuity. In a wonderful way the part of the brain that was deprived of its oxygen again begins to function. In fact, total recovery sometimes occurs.

Today, patients who have had a stroke, or a cerebro-vascular accident, are immediately trained to function. Specialists in rehabilitative medicine regularly encourage these patients to learn, with the help of new devices, to again take their place in society as productive people.

Is it possible for a person to have more than one stroke? What causes it in someone who was perfectly healthy up to the time it happened?

Any interference with the free flow of blood to the brain can cause a cerebro-vascular accident which is known as a stroke. There are a number of ways that the brain can be deprived of blood. A hemorrhage due to a rupture or a tear in a blood vessel is one of the major causes of stroke. Occasionally, a spasm of an artery in the brain due to tobacco or drugs can temporarily interfere with the free flow of blood. High blood pressure can be responsible for a break in a blood vessel. An aneurysm is a weakness of the wall of a blood vessel. This can resemble a bubble on the inner tube of an automobile tire. A hemorrhage results if such an aneurysm suddenly breaks.

People with arteriosclerosis have a narrowing of the blood vessels in all parts of the body. Fortunately, the process is a slow one and allows nature to build up an additional blood supply to counteract the closure of a blood vessel.

A thrombus, or clot, sometimes forms in a blood vessel that has been narrowed and shuts off the circulation to the brain. This, too, causes a stroke or apoplexy.

It is possible to have more than one stroke and recover from all of them. This is true when the underlying reason for the stroke is treated. Some patients have many "small strokes" which go unnoticed. Sometimes the symptoms are so slight that they fail to report them to their doctor. Only later, with prodding from their physicians, do they recall a vague sensation of dizziness that lasted a short while or a temporary loss of memory or even a strange behavior in an ordinary, daily experience. Physicians are on the alert to recognize "small strokes" in order to better treat a patient and prevent a serious stroke.

Your father was in apparent good health before the stroke occurred. This does not mean that the blood vessels to the brain were as "open and healthy" as they appeared.

Stroke victims need medical, nursing and custodial care in addition to psychological support. Today, the victim of a stroke is no longer kept as a chronic invalid. Physicians who specialize in rehabilitative medicine are contributing greatly to returning these patients to a happier life and helping them regain their dignity and productivity.

My fingers get stiff, especially in the morning, and I am scared that I will become disabled. Three doctors have given me different kinds of pills and still there is no change. Have you heard about a copper bracelet that prevents arthritis from becoming chronic?

You have already fallen into the trap of shopping for a quick cure for the arthritis that you may or may not have. Having seen three doctors in a short period of time you probably have not given any of them the time necessary for diagnosis and the treatment of your particular form of "arthritis." Your impatience is now leading you into areas outside the well-established practice of medicine.

So you may understand why it takes so much diligence and patience to treat arthritis and to prevent its progress, let me just name some of the different kinds of arthritis and related conditions.

Arthritis may be caused by infections, rheumatic fever, allergy, injury, gout, drugs, circulatory disease, serum sickness and even tuberculosis. It takes a great deal of effort, testing, X-rays and blood study to arrive at the exact nature of the arthritis. Not until you have continued on a diet and drug regime outlined by your doctor should you consider the treatment ineffective.

The value of copper bracelets as a defense against the onset or progress of arthritis is nil. Yet you will find some people who will "fight to the death" anyone who will dare say that copper is not the answer to forms of arthritis. If you want to wear a copper bracelet, be sure it is an attractive one so that you may have that advantage at least, even if it serves no function in the arrest of your disease. Do not waste valuable time waiting for the valueless copper to work while other more important medical treatment should be going on.

What is meant by the "gold" treatment for arthritis?

For years, many physicians have been enthusiastic about the use of gold as a form of treatment for rheumatoid arthritis. However, there are just as many doctors who lack enthusiasm for this form of treatment. Rheumatoid arthritis occurs so frequently and is often so difficult to control, that the use of gold injections has had some advantage. But not all cases of this form of arthritis should be treated in this manner, because of its side effects for certain people.

Physicians who use it keep their patients under constant observation and discontinue it if there is any suggestion of unusual toxic reation.

Gold alone is never used without all the additional forms of treatment that have some value in alleviating pain and controlling disability. Proper diet and high vitamin intake, with the use of cortisone, are used in conjunction with carefully adjusted doses of gold.

Is there any truth that some forms of arthritis can be cured by surgery?

It is most certainly true that surgery is being used in carefully selected cases of arthritis, especially those that have marked deformities of the hands. Very recently a special type of artificial joint was made out of polypropylene and inserted into deformed or partially destroyed finger joints. The results were sufficiently exciting to stimulate the interest of the doctors who heard the preliminary report. The American Rheumatism Association carefully evaluates all new procedures. It is a guiding force in the evaluation of all of the new studies of surgical correction of arthritic deformities.

Are there any new kinds of treatment for rheumatoid arthritis? I have tried almost everything, with little success.

190

The exact cause of rheumatoid arthritis, a complex disease, has never been specifically established. All avenues of scientific research try to pinpoint the cause by studying infections, hormone imbalance, allergies and metabolic disorders.

The American Arthritis Foundation and the American Rheumatism Association constantly publish reports on the progress toward prevention and control of this disorder. Only recently, a report was published about the use of an amino acid, normally found in most protein foods. This substance, L-histidine, was given by mouth to a large group of people suffering with rheumatoid arthritis. Many apparently benefited for as long as nine months. These studies are continuing, but a great deal of time will be necessary to confirm the value of this drug.

Is there a difference between rheumatism and arthritis?

Although they are technically different, these terms have been used interchangeably by the laity. The physician, however, uses it in its strict medical sense.

Rheumatism applies to acute and chronic conditions associated with stiffness and soreness of the muscles and with pains in the joints and nearby structures. Actually, this term can include forms of arthritis resulting from infection, gout or injury. There are many forms of rheumatism that so closely resemble arthritis that from the point of view of the layman the distinction is hardly necessary.

Arthritis is an actual inflammation of the joints accompanied by pain, tenderness and later changes within the joints. Arthritis, too, can be the result of infection, injury or gout.

In both conditions there are perhaps ten or fifteen subdivisions based on the suspected cause, duration, severity and the permanence of the changes within the joints.

Does bursitis occur only in the shoulder?

Many joints in the body move like well-oiled machines because of the presence of a bursa or sac. There are also bursae between muscles and joints and even between some ligaments and bone.

The purpose of these bursae is to permit free movement without pressure or friction. The bursae, soft and elastic, contain fluid to reduce the impact of bone against bone. Injury, infection, arthritis and gout may

191

cause an increase of pressure within the sac and may make movement of the shoulder, the elbow, the ankel and knee exceedingly painful.

Contrary to general laymen's knowledge the application of heat to an inflamed bursa seems to increase the pain. Icepacks applied directly to the inflamed bursa bring far more relief. Occasionally this varies and, of course the decision to use one extreme of heat or the other depends on the doctor's advice.

The swollen bursa responds best to rest. It is almost automatic for anyone suffering from this condition to keep the shoulder at complete rest by using some form of sling. Rest for other areas, too, is mandatory. Fortunately, injections of cortisone and anesthetics can bring welcome relief in a relatively short time.

Sometimes the fluid can actually be drawn out of the bursa. With it may come some calcium or uric acid crystals, because small stony deposits are frequently present as a result of chronic bursitis. X-ray therapy in some cases seems to be effective, while in others ultrasonic vibrations are used.

There are many ways of treating this distressing condition. When the acute phase has passed, it is important to find the underlying reason for the condition to avoid its repetition.

Chapter VIII

Today's Questions

Fifteen years ago, when I started to write a syndicated column on questions of health, the queries that arrived each day in the mail were as predictable as freckles on a redheaded youngster. There were the questions from women about weight problems and menstrual troubles, about varicose veins and stretch marks. Men wrote about baldness and prostate glands, hernias and hemorrhoids. Senior citizens inevitably worried about loss of memory, arthritis, insomnia and constipation. As for teenagers, the number one problem was acne.

That was fifteen years ago. Today, my mailbag has a much different look. Today's correspondents are more sophisticated; their questions far more involved and based on a broader, deeper knowledge of their bodies and of advances in the medical world. Frequently, their questions are complex. Often they echo the topics that we see day after day in newspaper headlines or hear discussed on the evening news on television. Questions about marijuana, drugs and their potential dangers, pollution, alcohol, acupuncture, euthanasia, cholesterol, nutritional deficiencies, psychological aberrations, genetic deficiencies—they're all very much on the public mind and in my readers' minds.

One reader wants to know if it is safe to take a jet plane flight if one has an ulcer; another worries about what freezing food does to its nutritive values. From a university town comes a question about tear gas and its affect on the human body; from a city reader comes a probing question on child abuse and its causes.

True, the varicose veins, the hemorrhoids, the arthritis and the insomnia questions continue to be asked, but they share the stage with questions that are typically and totally of the moment. And what's more, that handful of young people who wrote in to me fifteen years ago about their complexion difficulties have turned into hundreds of concerned young people with far different problems and questions—drugs and alcoholism prime among them.

It is good to know that, with all their modern problems, people still turn to a time-honored source for help—the medical column. I shall continue to provide them with the answers they need or at the very least try to direct them to the right sources for help.

Here are samples of the kinds of questions I find crossing my desk these days.

Recently I read something about the use of acupuncture in China for the cure of deafness. If this is true, why isn't it being used all over the world?

Acupuncture is a traditional Chinese form of treatment in which tiny gold needles are inserted under the skin. For five thousand years, Chinese acupuncture practitioners have mapped out tiny nerve areas all over the skin of the body.

Specially chosen sites for the placement of the needles have brought alleged "cures" for malaria, syphilis, blindness, cancer, tuberculosis, brain tumors, ulcers, coronary heart attacks, and even mental disturbances. And now, added to this list is deafness.

It should be noted that the reporter's enthusiasm for the story is not balanced by critical medical judgment.

It is inconceivable that scientists at major hospitals all over the world would deny the value of acupuncture for deafness if there were the slightest validity to these recent reports.

The nerve that brings sound from the ear to the brain lies deep within the mastoid bone, in an area that can be approached only with the most complex bone-penetrating instruments.

Even those without intensive knowledge of the anatomy of hearing can realize how impossible it would be to restore hearing by merely penetrating the skin over the ear with a tiny wire.

My real distress over this report is for the thousands of people with congenital or acquired deafness who might be given the false hope that they can be liberated from the desolation of silence by the magic of a gold needle.

How do doctors feel about acupuncture since it has gotten so much publicity?

In a recent column I pointed out that physicians have adopted an open mind toward acupuncture.

Even doctors who previously gave no credence to the magico-religious implications of acupuncture are waiting for more scientific evidence of its value.

At the National Institutes of Health in Bethesda, Maryland, a rather extensive program for scientific investigation of acupuncture is in progress. Its value in specific cases will be carefully studied and later presented to the world of medicine.

The newer attitudes toward acupuncture have, however, been accompanied by some dangers. This would suggest a warning against overenthusiasm at this time.

Acupuncture centers are springing up throughout the country, and are being staffed in many instances by people who are untrained in the art and science of this new and yet unproven concept of treatment.

Case reports already reveal exploitation of patients who, in desperation, are turning from orthodox medicine to the hope of acupuncture. One patient with a tumor of the spine had delayed receiving surgical treatment that might have been beneficial while undergoing an acupuncture series that lasted for four months. Grave dangers can result when a condition that might have been amenable to medical or surgical treatment is neglected. Laws are already being enacted to keep self-made specialists from exploiting the sick and the hopeful.

A large center in New York City that attracted hundreds of people who wanted to be first with a new-fangled idea was closed by health-licensing authorities when the people administering the needles were found to be medically inadequate.

Doctors and patients must wait until solid, objective studies are completed about acupuncture. Unless this is done, any potential advantages of acupuncture will fall by the wayside and become the property of charlatans and exploiters who thrive on the fears and diseases of the public. Until then, I advise my readers to proceed with caution and to continue to follow the advice of their own doctors.

Can cigarette smoking lead to disease and death?

One of the largest and probably one of the most significant studies of the effect of cigarette smoking on various causes of death has just been completed. Dr. Takeshi Hirayama, of the National Cancer Research Institute in Tokyo, released a study on more than 250,000 adults of forty years and older.

For the first time, women were studied as carefully as men in linking cigarette smoking to chronic disease and mortality. The study showed that cigarette smokers have a significantly higher mortality rate for total deaths of cancer, for arteriosclerotic heart disease, and for ulcer of the stomach.

The study is particularly important because the researchers dealt with the smoking habits of non-Caucasian people whose diets differ from those of Western people.

Female smokers were beginning to show progressively higher frequencies of cigarette-related diseases than were formerly suspected.

A very interesting outgrowth of this report is the fact that "the mortality rate for most major causes of death was higher for people who began to smoke earlier." For those who began smoking before nineteen years of age, the mortality rate from lung cancer was higher than for those who began smoking at twenty-four, and in particular was overwhelmingly higher than for those who never smoked at all.

Unless smokers read and reread these vital statistics, imprint them in their memory, and stop smoking, they cheat themselves of the true hope of modern medicine.

Can you name some of the major reasons why smoking cigarettes is harmful?

Dr. James Sterling Moran of New York City recently presented me with such a list written by the mother of a large family and the widow of three husbands all of whom smoked. She wrote this to Sir Benjamin Brodie, an English surgeon who lived in the 18th century:

1. Because it injures the curtains.

2. Because it is injurious to the furniture generally.

3. Because it is not agreeable to breakfast in the room when the gentlemen have been smoking overnight.

4. Because no man's temper is the better for it the next morning.

5. Because it keeps persons up to late hours, when every respectable person ought to be in bed.

6. Because the smell haunts a man's clothes, and his beard, and his hair, and his whiskers, and his whole body, for days afterwards—so much so that it is positively uncomfortable sometimes to go near him.

7. Because it is a selfish gratification that not only injures those who partake of it, but has the further effect of driving the ladies out of the room.

8. Because it is also an expensive habit which the ladies, not par-

ticipating in its so-called enjoyments, cannot possibly have the smallest sympathy with or appreciation for.

9. Because it has the further effect of making gentlemen drink a great deal more than they otherwise would, and so weakens their purses besides ruining their constitutions, to say nothing of the many comforts and new dresses that their dear wives and children may have been unjustly deprived of, supposing the same amount of money had only been judiciously laid out at home.

10. Because it gives extra trouble to the servants who have to clean and to ventilate the room the next morning.

11. Because how are one's daughters to get married, if the gentlemen are always locked up in a separate room paying court to their filthy pipes and cigars?

12. Because it unfits a young man, who is wedded to it, for the refining influences of female society.

13. Because it puts a stop to music, singing, flirting, and all rational enjoyments.

14. Because it is a custom originally imported from the savages.

15. Because we see the nations that smoke the most are mostly the stupidest, heaviest, laziest, dreariest, dreamiest, most senseless, and worthless beings that encumber—like so many weeds, only capable of emiting so much smoke—the face of the earth.

16. Because when a man says he is going out to smoke a cigar, there's no knowing what mischief he is bent upon, or the harm the monster may be likely to get into.

17. Because it is not allowed in the Palace, or Windsor Castle, or in any respectable establishment.

18. Because the majority of husbands only do it because they know it is offensive to their wives.

I add, 19 through 101: Because there is an undeniable relationship between smoking and cancer of the larynx, cancer of the lungs and heart, and circulatory diseases.

The original author added: "And a thousand other good reasons, if one only had the patience to enumerate them all. Pray did Adam smoke?"

How dangerous can LSD be if so many young people are taking it?

It is some years since I first wrote about the dangers of LSD, denouncing its experimental use on Harvard students. Since then hundreds of cases of severe and sometimes permanent aftereffects have been reported in young people who take "trips" in total ignorance of its hazards. In major cities, more than fifty cases a month are admitted to psychiatric wards. Many of these people may have their lives permanently threatened by the thrill of an LSD experience.

How often have we seen youngsters walking close to a third rail, tempting fate and enjoying the thrill of tottering on the brink of destruction? How often have we seen inexperienced climbers walking as close to a precipice as possible? How often have we seen swimmers hundreds of yards from shore despite the warning signals of danger? Whether or not they are motivated by the same reason as those who use LSD is not significant.

That which is important is that LSD can be a threat to the permanent health, physical and emotional, of the person tempted to use it. I have heard all the arguments of the high school students who in their ignorance "know" all the answers about the safety of pot, speed and smack. There is no more difficult problem than to combat ignorance that masquerades as truth.

LSD is available, but so are guns with which to play Russian roulette. Too often the adolescent has a simple excuse when his best friend has been killed by such nonsense. "I did not know it was loaded when we began the game" or "I'm sorry" or "We were only kidding" has never brought life back to the victim.

LSD is loaded dynamite. LSD is playing Russian roulette with all six barrels filled with lead. LSD is going over Niagara Falls in a barrel. LSD is deadly. An LSD trip is not the way for modern youth to buy itself status. Those who in their ignorance threaten each other's lives by temptations of destruction must be controlled by teaching.

And to reply to the letters that will quote the "remarkable aspects" of this drug, let me state that I know about them. LSD in the hands of highly specialized physicians and psychologists may yet open wide avenues for creativity and for the return to emotional health. These experts and only they can use this drug for specialized reasons in carefully selected cases.

"Square" parents must impress on their chrildren that the danger of LSD is as great as lighting a cigarette while filling the tank of their automobile with gasoline.

Is the mind-expanding drug STP less dangerous than LSD?

I know by your letter that you are fifteen years old and that you are in high school. I know, too, that you are not taking these drugs, but want to write an article about them. Take this line, underline it, don't forget it, and keep repeating it to your classmates: Any one of these mind-influencing drugs is dangerous, more dangerous than playing Russian roulette.

Our son, nineteen, confessed that he tried LSD four times. Since he told us that we think he has been behaving oddly and are worried that the drug may have caused permanent harm. How can we find out?

As you know, LSD stands for lysergic acid, a chemical referred to as a mind-expanding drug. Reactions to it vary to such a degree that it is impossible to say beforehand what it will do to any one person.

All sensations are said to become intensified. Colors may be more brilliant and sound may be heightened in intensity. Hallucinations and strange delusions frequently occur and may be one of the reasons why the drug intrigues those who are ignorant of its dangers.

LSD is indeed potential dynamite. Severe depression, anxiety, and uncontrolled panic may follow one or more experiences.

The chances are that your son has not been permanently affected. A doctor and a psychiatrist should thoroughly test him with the many psychological studies that are available to learn if harm was done, but more especially to learn the reasons why he took LSD to begin with.

I wonder whether you can honestly ask yourself if your son's odd behavior now is any different than it was before. The chances are great that you may have overlooked many of the symptoms of rebelliousness and not really had your hand on the true pulse of his activity. Were you in complete control of his outside activities or aware of the the character of his friends?

This seems rather harsh because you may believe that I am placing the burden of your son's irresponsibility on you. I do not mean to do this but rather direct myself to other parents in the hope that they may be spared the anguish you now are suffering. When once you find, as you probably will, that your son is not suffering from any permanent damage, you must follow the instructions of the psychiatrist and attempt to reestablish his personal values so that he will no longer be tempted to take drugs.

Why don't you try to tell people how much a drug addict needs their help when he tries to go "cold turkey" to get off the habit. I am an addict and can tell you that the fear of the ghastly pains of withdrawal symptoms makes it impossible to kick the habit.

Most readers know that "cold turkey" is a method by which the dope addict is suddenly and completely taken off heroin in an effort to break the habit and start the process of rehabilitation. This method is rarely used now because of the tortuous physical and emotional pain associated with sudden withdrawal of the drug.

"Cold turkey" is never used to break the sleeping pill or barbiturate habit. Convulsions and death are the possible results of this method and this should be known to those addicted to large quantities of these pills.

You and other addicts must be assured that the nightmare of "cold turkey" withdrawal symptoms is no longer necessary to endure. This fear must not keep the addict from seeking every possibility for the restoration of his life.

The methadone programs being used all over the country are not based on "cold turkey." This substitute drug, in combination with psychiatric help, now gives the addict his best chance to return to society.

How can one combat increasing drug use?

A new appraoch to the problem of drug addiction has been instituted at the University of California in Los Angeles by Dr. J. Thomas Ungerleider. It is known as Project DARE (Drug Abuse Research and Education).

Its prime purpose is to "Turn on to Life, Not Drugs." This vital message is being practiced and taught by a group of students who feel that they are in the best position to direct the activities of young men and women exposed to and tempted by the use of drugs.

This falls in line with an important approach to drug abuse, namely, showing young people the joys and rewards of living.

DARE members exert their greatest pressure by showing other teenagers and college students how to get "high" on life without the use of drugs.

Members spread their message through films, panel discussions, pamphlets, and in encounter groups.

In this age of social protest, rebelliousness, and drug curiosity, every conceivable effort must be made to preserve the lives of youngsters that might otherwise be ruined and devastated by drug involvement.

I was shocked to learn that some children are born heroin addicts. Does this mean that drug addiction is a hereditary condition?

Let me clarify a misconception. This is not a hereditary condition passed on through the mother's genes or the chromosomes to the child.

Women heroin addicts rarely tell their doctors about their addiction for fear of prosecution. The result is that a heroin intoxication is passed on to the unborn child through the mother's bloodstream.

It is interesting, too, that this occurs despite the fact that the mother's blood does not ever mingle directly with the blood of the unborn child's.

For years, many children were found dead in their cribs shortly after birth without any logical explanation for the calamity.

Now it is known that unexplained symptoms of the newly born child, such as poor breathing, trembling, twitching, convulsions, and rapid respirations, may be due to withdrawal symptoms of the child deprived of the heroin he was accustomed to before birth.

These children can be kept alive if the mother's heroin addiction has been uncovered before the birth of the child. Doctors are exceedingly careful in searching for evidence that the mother is taking heroin. If the mother is not an addict but the father is, the child is not born with this horrendous problem. The effect of drug abuse with amphetamines, LSD, and barbiturates is recognized as a distinct hazard to the unborn child. The danger of marijuana during pregnancy is under constant surveillance by health authorities. All drugs, addictive and nonaddictive, must be avoided as much as possible during pregnancy.

Is it possible to know, by any chemical tests, if a young adult has been taking heroin?

Addicts are overwhelmingly brilliant in the ways they devise to purchase drugs and the techniques they use to inject them so that they will not be detected. Needle marks on arms and hands are telltale evidence, but these can be avoided by other methods too disturbing to describe.

A number of tests have been devised and studied for the detection of morphine in the urine. Some of them are rapid and reliable, others take time.

An encouraging report from the Marquette School of Medicine tells of a new test of urine that quickly can detect traces of morphine and show that the person has been taking the drug.

It is hoped that along with such rapid and positive testing will come social legislation that will make urine examinations mandatory at regular intervals. Only early detection offers any hope for the control of drug addiction. And this, of course, is only second best to the need for elaborate educational programs of prevention.

My daugher was furious when she read an article you wrote called "From Marijuana to Heroin." At that time she was smoking marijuana with her friends and insisted that that was where it would stop. I am heartbroken to tell you that she is now a confirmed heroin addict. Is there no way that other children and parents can be spared this heartache?

One of the most difficult problems is to break through the barriers of ignorance about the dangers of marijuana. It is surprising how such misconceptions flourish and masquerade as truths, especially among adolescents.

Perhaps the newer knowledge of marijuana may penetrate their resistance and bring them to their senses. A university professor in California once believed that marijuana should be legalized. Now he has made a complete turnabout, based on his studies of five hundred students during the past five years.

He found that persons who used marijuana once a day for a period of six months to a year can develop chronic changes in the brain. Moreover, the impaired judgment of the marijuana smoker makes him less resistant to the blandishments of those who tempt him to go on to more potent and harmful drugs.

Parents must arm themselves with facts and must not be railroaded by the false reasoning of their children's "expertise" about marijuana. When parents suspect that their child is using drugs, they must not permit a moment to go by or leave a stone unturned to stop the addiction.

Parents too often lose the battle against their child's drug addiction by pretending to themselves that it does not exist. By bringing it out into the open, and with the help of their doctor, a psychiatrist, a religious advisor and other educators, they can stem the tide of this epidemic disease of youth.

I like your column and I really get the feeling that you understand young people like me. But I disagree with you about "grass." No one in my class at college who uses marijuana believes that you can become addicted to it. They feel as I do that it is no more dangerous than smoking cigarettes.

It is comforting to know that young readers sense the faith that I have in them. I'm impressed by their courage, their vision and their desire to contribute to a better society.

I wish I were able to convey to you that I am not on a crusade against marijuana; a crusade based on "adult morality" or greater wisdom. You must believe me when I tell you that you and your fellow students are dead wrong about the safety of this intoxicating drug.

Whether or not marijuana is addictive is a scientific problem which, before long, will be established by those who are studying its effects on laboratory animals. Until that drug's potency is definitely established, I beg you to accept the following arbitrary and dogmatic statemnt: Marijuana can cause smokers to become confused, unrealistic, and nonproductive. This has been proved repeatedly in healthy subjects tested at colleges and medical schools throughout the country.

Now, as to cigarettes—let me emphasize that they are undoubtedly responsible for some cancers of the lung, some cancers of the larynx, some cases of emphysema, and many circulatory disorders. This has been definitely and medically established. Why, therefore, do marijuana smokers offer the false and specious argument that marijuana is no more harmful than cigarettes? Both do damage to the body and mind in different ways. You cannot be allowed the false line of reasoning that the use of one justifies the use of the other. In either case, you are playing with dynamite.

I tried to sniff cocaine once. How soon can I become an addict if I do it again?

One sniff of cocaine at your age simply means you are already in trouble. You are not an addict yet but you have taken the first giant step to becoming one. Talk to your parents, your teachers or a doctor as fast as you can, so that you can be kept from falling into the trap you have already set for yourself.

Is it possible to become addicted to the codeine in the cough medicine that is sold over-the-counter without a prescription?

It most certainly is. In fact, students of the addiction problem and public health officials have sent out warnings that this occurs far more frequently than is suspected.

There are some people who become addicted to almost anything—salt, ice cream, liquor, artichokes, tobacco, and almost any substance they may eat or drink. These are addictive personalities who almost always have some deep-seated neurotic problem.

The codeine in over-the-counter cough medicines and the alcohol that they contain have turned out to be one of the easiest methods for an addict that is still within the law. Better legislation in the states that allow such sales could help prevent people from falling into the trap of addiction to cough medicine.

Parents are warned to be on the lookout for unusual behavior problems in youngsters who may be using cough medicine codeine.

How can one tell if they are having an unusual side effect from a new drug?

Many patients who give absolutely no history to their doctor of being allergic or sensitive may develop an unusual reaction to any kind of medicine that is prescribed for them. Some reactions are mild, some severe and most of them cannot be anticipated by the doctor.

Whenever a patient is given a prescription he should know what it is and for what purpose it is given. The patient should ask what response he might have to the drug and what can be considered normal. Any unusual sensation, skin rash, swelling of the lips and nausea and vomiting means that the patient is probably sensitive to the drug and that it should be discontinued until further instructions are given by the doctor.

Occasionally, there are patients who react exactly opposite to that which is normally expected from a drug. I have given patients antihistamine, or anti-allergy drugs, which normally make many people drowsy and have found some actually exhilarated by them. Drugs which are meant to be stimulating are sometimes responsible for a feeling of complete relaxation.

Knowing that any drug can cause some peculiar side effect in some people makes it important to watch for unusual reactions when any new drug is tried.

Is it safe to drink alcohol if you are taking a tranquilizing drug? Because of the pressure of his work, my husband takes a tranquilizer three times a day. At night he says he gets relaxation with a few drinks.

Generally, it is unwise to risk taking more than one drug that has a similar effect. For example, tranquilizers and barbiturates, although different, can be depressing to normal body functions when used in combination. Either of these drugs, when used with alcohol, can be reinforced and have serious consequences.

The amount of tranquilizer and the amount of alcohol your husband consumes probably are not sufficient to do him damage since he has apparently been doing this for some time. Nevertheless, the dependence on both tranquilizers and alcohol may become greater. If there is an increase in quantity of the drug and the alcohol, the combination may become hazardous.

The physician who prescribed the tranquilizer knows the dosage and is in the best position to advise you about the potential dangers.

My husband and I take two or three drinks before dinner. On Saturday night, at the club or at home, we really set no limits. We enjoy drinking and we want to know if we can coat our stomachs with something before we start our weekend.

Yes, indeed, I can make that recommendation. You can line your stomachs with milk and with soft drinks, and stay away from alcohol. I'm certain that you consider yourselves "social drinkers." Have you given any consideration to the possibility that you either are, or are on the way to becoming, alcoholics?

It is amazing how many drinkers drink themselves into oblivion. They seem to have a single purpose, and that is to saturate themselves so completely that reality will fade and they can slip into a world of fantasy.

By now you and your husband should know your own limits for alcohol intake, but you obviously choose to go beyond those limits.

"Coating" your stomach with olive oil and all the other nonsensical methods that are suggested has nothing to do with your basic problem. That is the need to find out what motivates you to drink without limits.

Have either of you considered a medical examination to find out the state of your liver? Sometimes, a serious report of chronic liver disease brings people sharply to the awareness that they are sacrificing their health and longevity to chronic alcoholism.

Now that you have brought your problem into the open by writing to me, why not continue this honesty and bring your problem to the attention of your doctor and a psychiatrist? If they agree that there is a deep-seated problem of alcoholism their recommendations can help reestablish a more sane and more mature pattern of living.

My husband and I drink a lot of alcohol but we are not alcoholics. We try to cut down but when there is any crisis in the family, we begin to drink. We have been told there is a drug that can control the urge to drink. Can you tell us about it?

Alcoholism is a disease which needs intensive treatment if it is not to undermine your life and the lives of other members of your family. If you were to trace the slow progression of the amount of alcohol you need to get through a day, you would find that you are denying to yourselves the seriousness of your alcoholic problem.

There is no drug that can control the urge to drink or reduce the amount. There is a drug, Antabuse, which is not a cure for alcoholism, but which can be used successfully in another way. It is a complex drug that affects the liver and causes chemical changes. When taking it, the slightest drop of alcohol in any form can make one violently sick. A large quantity of alcohol taken with this drug can cause serious complications and even result in death.

Consequently, when Antabuse is taken every day, alcohol must be avoided in any form. Even small amounts in cooking must be eliminated.

In order to control your problem, you must first face the truth of your situation and discuss the matter openly with your physician. There may be a need for psychological help to start you on the proper path to recovery. Personally I believe that one of the dominant forces in modern society offered to alcoholics is the program of Alcoholics Anonymous. Consult your local chapter. Later your doctor may suggest Antabuse.

Is group therapy an accepted form of psychoanalysis? What are its advantages?

All schools and methods of psychoanalysis have a single purpose and goal: to help an individual to gain a greater insight into his emotions and better adapt himself to the stresses of modern living.

Newer analytic attitudes are devoted more and more to reducing the time necessary for a patient to be relieved of his anxieties and neuroticisms.

The advantages of group therapy are many. Such sessions may even be more beneficial than individual therapy in some cases. This decision of course must depend on the judgment of the therapist and the evaluation of the patient's need.

Group therapy permits a larger number of people to be treated at the same time and thus reduces the severe and often punishing cost of modern-day psychoanalysis. The shortage of well-trained therapists in some communities may make it possible to distribute their help to many more people through group therapy.

———

Can you clarify some of the basic terms that are used to describe mental retardation?

Feeblemindedness, mental retardation, and mental deficiency generally refer to some defect in the ability of a child to understand, to learn, to progress, and to meet normal social standards of behavior.

More specifically, the term "idiocy" is considered the lowest capacity in mental progress. An I.Q., or Intelligence Quotient, below thirty, along with speech and physical coordination impairment, are included in this classification.

The term "imbecile" is applied to a higher level of mental retardation in which the I.Q. may range between thirty and sixty. Here, too, the learning capcity is very poor, but some of the lesser manual activities can be accomplished.

The word "moron" is applied to those whose I.Q. ranges from about sixty to eighty, and can be compared to the mental development of a seven-year-old child. Many of these retarded persons can function in society if too great pressure is not put upon them.

With an I.Q. of about ninety, a person can be taught to perform many tasks that will support him and allow him to live in social dignity.

The word "mongolism" had been used to describe a type of mental deficiency with a characteristic facial expression. This genetic disorder was associated with a Mongolian appearance. In essence, this is exceedingly unfair since Mongols have a high level of intelligence. Today, this condition is referred to as the Down's syndrome, a more accurate medical description.

Complex aptitude, I.Q., and psychometric tests can be performed to learn what the capacity of retarded children is. Many cases that were formerly hopeless are now frequently helped to progress beyond expectation.

Are there any dangers to watching television too much? Our teenage children spend at least three hours a day watching the tube and it is a constant source of argument.

Studies indicate that television viewing, within sensible limits, does not harm healthy eyes. In fact, the physical problems of television addiction are not nearly as great as the emotional and educational penalties.

Undoubtedly, many programs are of value when chosen with discrimination. Educational programs can contribute to the development of children, adolescents and adults.

The greatest penalty paid by your children, however, is that the time spent watching television could be used for so many other exciting and worthwhile activities. Your children will eventually appreciate the limits you establish for their development.

My son tells me that many of his friends at school buy and read pornographic books. I don't know whether my son reads them, but I do know that he is very tense when he talks about it.

Young people are in a psychological bind between sophisticated permissiveness and rigid control.

Educators, sociologists and psychologists all have their own theories about pornography and its relationship to sex urge, emotional liberation, aggression and guilt feelings. All are sure that their own concept is the total answer. I wish there was more modesty in their attitude and that they were less scientific about how parents should handle this problem.

I allow myself a personal indulgence by saying that "filthy" pictures, films and magazines are obscenities that serve no function in attaining physical, emotional and psychological maturity. Many of the experts will undoubtedly disagree. Yet as a parent and physician I deny the right of pornography to masquerade as "educational" material.

One of my neighbors mercilessly beats his children. Yet no one seems to interfere because they are afraid of his temper.

I don't know what the heartbreaking statistics of child abuse are in your city, but I am sure that they do not vary much from those in New York City. For the first six months of this year, hundreds of cases of child abuse and child neglect were reported.

Doctors familiar with this unhappy picture of the "battered child" are working hard with legislative agencies to combat the increasing evidence of violence.

All of us have the responsibility to report to local police and health agencies any maltreatment of children. Your own identity is shielded so that you do not pay a penalty for your solicitous involvement. Child abuse committees now are active in establishing laws to punish abusing parents and to remove the children from life-threatening situations.

None of us with any morality would hesitate to report a hit-and-run driver who injures or kills a child. We owe ourselves and society that same moral obligation to interfere actively in the growing epidemic of child abuse.

Whenever I take a flight of more than four or five hours my whole system goes out of kilter. Not only am I sleepy and confused, but all my body functions are in disarray. Can this be psychological?

There are indeed psychological alterations just as there are physical changes associated with the "jet lag" phenomenon. Technically this is known as "dysrhythmia." As the name implies, the timeclock mechanisms are thrown out of their normal pattern of rhythmic behavior.

One of the most remarkable functions of the organs of the body is the exactness with which our biological timeclocks work. Fluctuations of body temperature, changes in the rate of the heartbeat and urinary output are more evident when the body's timeclock goes off than are the subtle changes that occur in the liver, in the spleen, the brain, the intestinal tract, and the circulatory system.

The chemical and hormone balance, so carefully established by our bodies, and the normal flow of digestive juices are also disturbed from their familiar rhythm by the sudden change of time zone.

Many excellent surveys by the armed forces medical departments have tried to ease the disruptive effects of dysrhythmia. One of the most important contributions to those who suffer from jet lag is to try to gently ease into the new time change. On your next trip, try to let your activities conform to your time of departure rather than your time of arrival in the new place. By gradually adjusting your time clocks to the new environment you will find that your psychological and physical capacities are almost as great as they were before you set out on your dysrhythmic trip.

Is it dangerous for someone with a duodenal ulcer to travel to Europe in a jet plane?

A jet flight does not exert any special bodily stress on those people who have duodenal or stomach ulcers. Nevertheless, anyone who is in the midst of an acute attack should be wary of even this additional emotional burden. One's physician, of course, is in the best position to relieve one's anxiety in such a situation.

When I get home from work I see at least ten neighbors of all sizes and weights jogging until they're ready to fall in their tracks. Do you think that this is a good way to keep in trim?

Two axioms about exercise are undeniable: First, some form of exercise is important for everyone. And second, the nature and extent of exercise must be tailored to an individual's needs and capacity.

Jogging is an excellent form of exercise because there is no need for special equipment or special hours of the day. The stimulation of the blood circulation and the lung capacity is undeniable.

Unfortunately, many people still have not learned that even this form of exercise must be begun slowly and increased gradually, without exertion to the point of exhaustion.

This rule, of course, applies to any form of exercise. The value of exercise can be negated by punishing the body and asking it to overextend itself.

It must also be remembered that exercise alone is not a weight-reducing program. Only in conjucntion with a low calorie diet can this be accomplished.

I have heard that there are some types of eggs that are especially low in cholesterol. Is this fact or fiction?

The Department of Foods and Nutrition of the American Medical Association seems to be intrigued by this possibility.

An AMA spokesman has some interesting things to say about eggs, their color and their cholesterol content. According to him, eggs with dark shells are slightly higher in cholesterol than white shell eggs. Hens that have been fed diets containing polyunsaturated vegetable oils have produced eggs whose cholesterol and saturated fat content are almost exactly the same as average eggs.

Special claims have been made that eggs produced by the South American Aracuna chicken are particularly low in cholesterol. These claims have not been thoroughly substantiated. Until there is absolute proof, people who have a cholesterol problem should still stay away from a high egg diet.

A recent report that plastics around meat products can be dangerous is disturbing. What is the latest news on this?

Preliminary studies about the heavy plastic, polyvinyl, used to package certain foods, medicines, cooking oils and fruit juices seem to indicate that some possible danger exists in large concentrations.

It is for this reason that the Federal Drug Administration and other health-governing agencies are evaluating this and other plastics to insure complete safety to the consumer.

We seem unable to buy any food that doesn't contain an additive or preservative. I worry about this.

It is estimated there are almost three thousand different substances that are now added to food and beverages for different reasons. Many of these are used as preservatives or to enhance the flavor or to make their appearance more attractive.

The addition of preservatives is important in preventing a terrible

211

waste of food due to spoilage. It is estimated that almost a quarter of all the food in the world is lost because of short shelf life.

Ascorbic acid has been used successfully to prevent discoloration in canned vegetables and fruits. The flour and baking industries use a wide variety of bleaching agents to make their products more attractive. They also use chemicals to retain softness and to avoid too rapid spoilage. Additives are now an acceptable part of the entire food industry. As a matter of fact, the consumer benefits greatly in most instances because of the rigid control of local state and national protective agencies.

The United Nations, through the World Health Organization, keeps a constant watch on the safety of all substances added to food or drinks. Manufactureres themselves, whose destiny depends on consumer acceptance and government approval, in most instances, monitor their products for safety.

Additives are not used simply to change the character of inferior products. Such fraudulent adulteration is immediately condemned by the Pure Food and Drug Administration.

The total absence of all additives and preservatives may not necessarily give the consumer the greatest advantage. Yet it is to the credit of some manufactureres that they are able to successfully produce, market, and preserve foods that do not contain chemicals, preservatives or artificial ingredients of any kind.

We live in a university town and have had one sad experience with tear gas. Is tear gas harmful? Can it do permanent damage?

Many people, although personally uninvolved in riots, have paid a penalty by being exposed to tear gas. This irritating gas causes excessive tearing of the eyes, impairing vision temporarily. The entire lining of the lungs becomes inflamed, causing coughing and difficulty in breathing.

If exposure to tear gas occurs indoors, it may produce permanent damage to the lungs. As soon as possible after exposure, the eyes should be washed out with clear water. Rinsing the mouth will remove the chemical. For the burning or irritation of the skin, do not use any oils, creams or ointments, because these tend to seal in the irritating chemical.

Examination by a doctor, particularly an eye specialist, is important in order to make sure that there has been no injury to the delicate membrane of the eyes.

Our two teenage children are organic food enthusiasts. They want us to buy a water purifier. Is there any value to their ideas?

The growth of interest in organic foods can be traced directly to the problem of total pollution that surrounds us.

Young men and women are now reaching out for a role in preventing further desecration of the land that is their heritage. With insecticides, chemicals, smoke and refuse we have bespoiled that gift. It is understandable that organic food grown in protected soil is one of their great hopes for survival.

Water filters are devised to purify and to remove odors and bad taste from ordinary tap water. Every conceivable method that brings greater safety and protection from our indiscriminate pollution has an advantage.

With all the pollution that surrounds us is there any way to tell if a swift flowing stream is safe as drinking water? Our families are campers and we want to be sure that we are not drinking infected water.

Long before the threat of contaminated water became such an important issue, campers were constantly warned against drinking "sparkling clear mountain fresh water." There is no relationship between the appearance of such inviting water and the possibility that it might be contaminated.

Water might even taste delicious and still contain toxic chemicals that might have been poured into the stream at some distance.

In many camping sites all over the United States, the chemical contents and the bacteria count of the water are carefully studied before campers are permitted to drink it. In many instances, boiling the water is recommended as an added precaution that can prevent illness and avoid spoiling a lovely camping holiday.

Even swimming in these streams should be done only when contamination has been guarded against.

A large industrial plant continues to pour its waste products into our once beautiful river. We have begged, pleaded and threatened but get nowhere. It is a moral crime to see the inevitable destruction of our land.

213

Your expression of rightful distress adequately states the pathetic conditions that exist in communities all over America. The fact that physical beauty is being besmirched is sad enough. Now we are being threatened by health hazards, chronic disease and potential permanent damage to our genes and chromosomes.

"Wake up, world!" is only an unheard cry in the wilderness. Yet there is still hope that massive, heartless, computerized industries may be listening to the plaintive pleas of those who ask only for the right to see a cloudless sky, to breathe exhilarating pure air and swim without fear in uncontaminated waters. We have bequeathed to youth the farmlands, the forests and the waterways—let it not be said that we gave them a permanently spoiled environment. Take heed that there are thousands like yourself who want to preserve the beauty and the health that are our heritage. Our concentrated political and social effort can convert selfish pollution to environmental purity.

Chapter IX

Some Questions Of Sex

From time to time I have had occasion to see columns in magazines and in newspapers that go into great detail about sex and specific sexual relationships. Sometimes both the questions and the answers sound like the plot of a bestselling novel headed right for the movie screen.

Alas, I seem not to hear from readers with titillating sex problems. My mail seldom, if ever, reflects desperate passions. I don't know whether this could be interpreted as a comment on the way my readers regard me or as an indication of their own celibate tendencies. At any rate, I am content to continue answering a whole other area of sex-related questions, not as colorful perhaps, but just as urgent and important. Queries about syphilis and gonorrhea, about fertility and infertility, impotency, sterilization, vasectomies—these are the questions I hear over and over again.

Indeed, those who read my column regularly may wonder at the frequency with which I discuss veneral diseases. There's very good reason. The widespread occurrence of syphilis in teenagers and in young adults demands the concentrated efforts of every physician and all public agencies. Despite widespread educational campaigns, venereal disease has reached a peak even higher than before the discovery of penicillin. And it is estimated that about one in every ten girls, married and unmarried, between the ages of fifteen and twenty-five, has gonorrhea and doesn't know it. Unfortunately, the untreated case becomes complicated and may involve the fallopian tubes and the ovaries and be responsible for permanent inability to bear children. There are reliable tests which can be done within a few minutes to indicate the presence of the destructive bacteria causing syphilis and gonorrhea. It is in order to get this message across that I so often select letters about venereal disease to appear in my column.

Another question that constantly crosses my desk comes from worried parents who ask, "When should we start teaching our children about sex?" I know that I am leading with my chin when I even attempt a reply. As a physician, I learned long ago that there can be no dogmatic answer to such an important question. Some educators, parents and perhaps psychologists will, I am sure, pounce on me for my recommendation in this regard. But I firmly believe the teaching of sex should be done by qualified educators and by doctors, particularly those who specialize in adolescent medicine and who understand the sexual confusions of the young. The role of the parents is primarily to set a loving and a moral atmosphere within the home, to provide an example for their children that reinforces the image of sex as the beautiful and mutually rewarding relationship it is meant to be.

I remember that when my wife and I drove our daughter to college, my daughter asked, "Aren't you going to give me some advice about living away from home for the first time?"

I knew the kind of advice she meant and I answered, "None at all —for what can I possibly teach you about morality in 300 miles of driving that you haven't already absorbed in your seventeen years with us?"

Does every human being have both male and female sex hormones?

Both male and female hormones are present in both sexes. Estrogen is the female sex hormone. Androgen is the male sex hormone.

As the female advances into puberty and adolescence there is a slow, progressive diminution of the amount of male hormones in the blood. Similarly, there is a reduction of the female estrogen in the male as he advances into adulthood.

Hormones, both natural and synthetic, have a complexity that staggers the imagination. They play a role in every phase of health and disease. The way the body maintains the balance of hormones is intricate and mystifying.

When any hormonal imbalance is suspected, complex blood studies can now quickly reveal deficiencies and direct the path to re-establishing the hormone balance.

Many readers ask if the presence of male and female sex hormones in one person is responsible for homosexual tendencies. There may be some role that the hormones play in this alteration of male and female characteristics. But there are an infinite number of factors in the total equation of homosexuality, both physical and psychological, besides the distribution of hormones.

Can a young boy have both male and female sex hormones? Is this unusual and can it affect him in later life?

All boys and girls have within them female and male sex hormones. As the boy advances through puberty there is a decrease in the female sex hormones. Similarly, as the girl passes through puberty, there is a decrease in the male sex hormones. The correct balance between these hormones is established in adolescence. You need not have concern about this problem, but if you need added assurance, discuss it freely with your doctor.

Is there any danger in prolonged hormone therapy for men or women?

In healthy men and women the balance of hormones is maintained up until the change of life or menopause, which comes to most women about the age of forty-five. There is also a male "menopause" at about the same age when there is a diminishing of the male hormone.

In recent years there as been great enthusiasm about the idea of giving women estrogen during the beginning and end of the change of life. Its advantages have been so extolled in popular magazines that estrogen therapy is now demanded by many women.

These hormones cannot be given promiscuously to women or to men. The cases must be carefully chosen so that the over-use may not produce changes in the rest of the body that are unwanted side effects.

An enormous amount of research is being done on the relationship between male and female sex hormones and arteriosclerosis and the formation of cholesterol. It is generally accepted that the prolonged use of sex hormones should be discouraged unless the patient is under the constant guidance and study of the doctor who prescribed it.

I have been taking hormones after an operation on my ovaries. I have noticed that my voice is husky and I wonder if there can be any relationship between the two.

Cases have been reported of huskiness of the voice after taking hormones for a long period of time. This, however, is not the only cause of hoarseness. It may be a pure coincidence that the hoarseness should have occurred at the time you were taking this medication.

The larynx can be easily and quickly examined and can reveal any one of the other possible causes. A slight hemorrhage into one of the vocal cords, a polyp or a nodule may be the reason, rather than the hormone.

If the hormone is responsible, the vocal cords usually return to normal when the hormone is discontinued.

My husband and I are confused and in conflict about what to say about sex to our twins who now are twelve years old. Would it be best for all of us to have a family open forum on the subject?

I once listened to a tape recording made with the parents' permission of a family powwow on sex. It was garbled, aimless and filled with so much ignorance that I wondered if the children would ever be able to extricate themselves from the confusion that overwhelmed them.

The teaching of sex should be done by those who are specially qualified in the art and science of this most important aspect of a child's growth. I do not believe that because a patient has recovered from tuberculosis, he is equipped to teach it to medical students. Neither do I believe that because parents created their children through sex, they are the ideal educators in this matter.

I have found that most parents are exceedingly embarrassed by the so-called open discussion of sex. Many, in fact, transmit to their children their own sexual hang-ups and impose restrictions on the sensitive adolescent mind.

Educators on the other hand are able to discuss without embarrassment, with complete freedom, and with studied security, subjects that are often difficult for parents.

It has been my feeling for a long time that when children graduate from the pediatric age they should be treated by doctors who specialize in adolescent medicine. Such a person with good psychological insight can talk to his post-puberty patients and give them helpful guidance that will lead to sexual maturity. This is also a good time to teach them about promiscuity and venereal disease. I am sorry to note that the routine teaching of sex education in schools is often deficient and does not attain its real objective.

What is the span of reproduction in women?

There are cases on record of pregnancy successfully completed before the age of ten and after the age of sixty-two. These, of course, are bizarre and unusual occurrences.

The beginning of the menstrual cycle ushers in the time that the female is capable of conceiving. The cessation of the menses at the time of the menopause, or change of life, represents the end of her reproductive period.

It must be remembered that there is rarely a sudden natural change of life. Rather, more frequently there is a slow change of life, with irregularities of menstruation. During this time the possibility of pregnancy still continues.

We have been married three years and I have been unsuccessful in becoming pregnant. I have been going to a doctor who feels that he cannot go any further unless my husband cooperates and submits to tests for fertility. My husband refuses to do so because he is embarrassed. How can I persuade him?

Infertility among young couples occurs in more than ten percent of marriages. Many of these problems can be corrected. Unless there is a mature attitude on the part of both wife and husband, the possibility of success is greatly reduced.

Many good marriages are senselessly destroyed because the husband or wife accuses the other, consciously or not, of being responsible for failure to achieve pregnancy.

Frequently men behave as your husband does because, in a framework of ignorance, they confuse fertility with potency. There is no relationship between the two. An infertile male can be a perfectly normal, potent sexual partner.

Your husband can be helped to get over this embarrassment by consultation with your doctor or a psychologist.

Fertility evaluation can be done only when both husband and wife sincerely seek an answer to their problem.

My husband and I have been trying to have a baby for four years, with no success. I am perfectly willing to have any tests

done but my husband is embarrassed. Are there any out-of-state clinics where this can be done?

Although I cannot condone such a mid-Victorian attitude, I do appreciate that some people may be highly sensitive about this problem. Even if you were to have the tests done in the city where you live, it would never become public knowledge. Doctors recognize the psychological implications of temporary or permanent infertility and certainly would not want to impose a further emotional burden on either of you.

There are excellent specialists in fertility all over America who are using extensive, standardized techniques in an effort to help attain conception. Through your own physician, you can find one in your own town or outside your state who can give you the help you seek, and who will maintain the privacy that is so important to your husband.

My husband and I have finally acknowledged that we are a non-fertile couple. Artificial insemination has been suggested because I seem to be free of any problems that would prevent me from becoming pregnant. Is there any literature on this subject?

Before embarking on this project you should inquire and read about the psychological and legal implications of artificial insemination. There is a vast amount of literature in medical, psychological and legal journals that will enlighten you about this highly sensitive undertaking.

Because your husband is not fertile, it would be necessary to seek donor sperm which then would be introduced in you by your own physician. It is obvious that moral and legalistic problems may ensue. To avoid future unhappiness, the detailed discussions should take place between both of you, your doctor and even a psychiatrist. Far too many people have found that their initial enthusiasm was marred by subsequent problems that were not anticipated.

What are the most common reasons for infertility in men?

In the male, the absence of sperm, an inadequate amount of sperm, and low mobility of sperm are the major reasons for infertility.

There are some abnormalities in development that make it impossible for some men to produce sperm. Infections and inflammation of the testicles ("orchitis") may also affect male sterility.

It is interesting how much more frequently the man is responsible for infertility than is commonly supposed. It is estimated that as much as forty per cent of infertile marriages can be attributed to the husband.

In order to establish the cause of infertility, hormone studies are made, in addition to microscopic studies of the sperm. Chemical analysis and the acidity of the fluid that carries the sperm are very significant.

It takes concentrated study to find the cause and correct it, if possibilities of fertility are to be increased.

Would you tell us your reaction to reports about the hazards of vasectomy for male sterilization?

Each year since 1969, when this simple, safe operation exploded into popularity, the numbers of men choosing vasectomy as a method of contraception have been growing.

No apparent dangers were reported until recently when an incomplete report was made about the possible relationship between vasectomies and arthritis and multiple sclerosis. It was understandable that such a report would cause confusion and anxiety in those who had already had the vasectomy operation as well as in those who were contemplating it.

Two nationally important specialists in urology have stated that there was no scientific validity to reports of these harmful effects following the vasectomy. Dr. Joseph E. Davis, president of the Association for Voluntary Sterilization, and his colleagues are well aware that certain antibodies seem to increase slightly in the blood of people who have had the vasectomy operation but they believe that they are not sufficiently significant to cause concern.

Dr. Robert Rosen, of the Dover General Hospital in New Jersey, believes there is no valid reason to discontinue this operation which has been one of the greatest contributions to planned parenthood.

Both these scientists feel that until findings are definitive, this significant surgical advance should not be in any way limited. Anyone who is hesitant should, of course, follow the advice of his own physician or urologist.

I made a sad mistake when I had a vasectomy operation to avoid having more children. At the time it seemed like a good idea. But my wife died four years ago. Now my new wife would like to have a family.

My warnings about vasectomy are always directed at the possibility that a change in social circumstances may bring regrets. Also, there are reported cases of men who have suffered psychologically because of sudden loss of fertility, even though this was the object of the operation.

Surgeons are devoting themselves to finding a method by which the vas deferens, which carries the sperm, can be closed off and later reopened should the need arise. At present, the operation to reunite cut ends of the sperm-carrying tubes is not as successful as it might be. Even in cases where the tube is reunited there is some question whether the sperm is as active and capable of causing pregnancy as it was before the operation.

All surgery carries some degree of risk. Vasectomy, for those who contemplate it, must carry with it a social and psychological risk that deserves intensive consideration before surgery. Such a decision must not be an impulsive one.

I have had five children in the past seven years. My husband and I have mutually agreed that I should have a sterilization operation to prevent further pregnancies. Do you believe that there is any reason why this should not be done?

Voluntary sterilization is a complex physical, emotional, moral and ethical problem. No one set of answers can possibly be satisfactory to all people in all circumstances.

Generally, you must be warned that sterilization of the woman by tying off her tubes and sterilization of the man are not reversible. Once these operations are performed it is exceedingly rare that the tubes will once again open and function normally.

In the light of modern methods of contraception, it hardly seems sound that you and your husband should embark on the road from which there is no return.

The American College of Obstetricians and Gynecologists has recognized that there may be special reasons for sterilization of the female. If a possible pregnancy can threaten the life or the mental stability of a person, the operation should be considered.

It would be exceedingly presumptuous of me to believe that I could answer a problem of such importance to you and your husband. My only contribution can be to urge you to speak the entire matter out with your own doctor, and take a long time before undertaking an operation that is so unalterable.

I have been reading your columns consistently and have not read anything about contraceptive pills. Are they safe?

Physicians all over America are being asked many questions about the oral contraceptive hormone commonly referred to as "the pill." Physicians custom-tailor their answers to the specific needs of their individual patients.

There is no blanket statement that can answer all the physical, emotional, cultural and religious aspects associated with this form of family control. The American Medical Association has published a report on "The Control of Fertility." In it they state: "The effectiveness of the oral contraceptive is virtually one hundred percent, certainly the highest of any method."

The United States Food and Drug Administration has given its stamp of approval for safety to many different contraceptive products. They state that "there has been no evidence to support the belief that hormone contraception has an adverse effect on menopause." They do suggest that, while further studies continue, the pill should be prescribed only to patients who remain under the direction and supervision of their physicians.

A terrifying article on birth control pills appeared recently in a magazine. Are we really risking death or permanent injury by taking these pills?

Unfortunately, some eager writers, with little or no scientific knowledge, find that the greatest impact can be made by emphasizing fear rather than hope in their writing. I disagree completely with this destructive attitude.

Before contraceptive pills were distributed to the general public, untold control studies were done to be sure of their safety. This is one of the great responsibilities of governmental health agencies which constantly protect the American people from the overenthusiasm for new drugs by their manufacturers.

All drugs may have some potential danger. Even the most innocuous drugs can call forth an unusual reaction in a highly sensitive or allergic person. It is with this understanding that your doctor prescribed the birth control pills. The advantages and disadvantages are carefully

223

weighed in the choice of these pills. You can be certain that all these considerations were appreciated by him for you.

There are some risks in everything we do. We must not permit ourselves to be terrified into believing that our health and lives are in jeopardy every time we read scare statistics that have no solid basis in scientific truth.

When is the fertile period of the month? When is the least fertile period?

The fertile period is the time when ovulation takes place. This is when the ovary produces the tiny egg. In women who have a normal twenty-eight day cycle, the most fertile period occurs about twelve to sixteen days after the onset of the mestrual period. The barren period occurs about seven to nine days before the onset of the menses, continues during the menstrual period, and lasts up to five days afterwards.

Since the menstrual cycle of women varies so widely, there can, of course, be no definite schedule.

Can you list the causes of impotency that occurred to me in my late forties? Could mumps at the age of sixteen cause this?

A list of the causes would serve no function other than to have you choose one and believe it relates to your problem. Many men write to me rather than discuss this with their physician because they feel there is some shame attached to the condition. There is not.

Your doctor must first rule out the presence of a physical or organic disorder that may account for the sudden onset of impotency. It is only when this is completely ruled out that the possible psychological basis is considered. And this is most important because there is a tendency to avoid coming face to face with the reality that the emotions play a vital role in the onset of this condition. Unless this is studied in detail both by the physician and the psychologist, anxiety begins to mount and only tends to further magnify the problem. Mumps may affect fertility, but rarely is responsible for impotency.

Is homosexuality inherited?

There is no evidence that homosexuality is transmitted through the chromosomes and genes. Many complex factors are at work, in the home and in the environment, that may be responsible for homosexual patterns that may begin very early in life.

"Beyond Sexual Freedom," by Dr. Charles W. Socarides, is one book that may clarify some of the aspects of the problem for you. In your letter you intimate that such a problem exists in your home. Seek the advice of your physician and a psychiatrist or psychologist. There is a tendency to pretend that a problem does not exist and, by doing so, much valuable time is wasted if any form of treatment is needed.

My wife expects to give birth in four months. I never knew that we had so many scientists in our family. They all have definite opinions about the value of circumcision. What is yours?

You will find that much of the debate revolves around the fact that circumcision has some religious, cultural or ritualistic implication. It is true that some religious and some social groups insist on circumcision when a male child is born. But in modern society, circumcision is performed frequently without any relation to religious beliefs or customs.

Basically it is done for better hygiene. Boys who are not circumcised may develop a condition known as "phimosis." This is a tightness of the foreskin over the penis which may be painful and difficult to keep clean.

The decision should be made by you, your wife and your physician.

Is there any danger in circumcision in an adult? Why are some children circumcised at birth and others not?

Circumcision was once considered to be identified with religious sects and tribal customs. The procedure as a ritual has been traced to tribes as far back as 1000 B.C. Even in uncivilized remote areas, the procedure was practiced as a health measure at birth and at puberty.

Today circumcision is almost a routine health measure performed on most children shortly after birth. It is an accepted fact that hygiene and cleanliness are made easier in boys who are circumcised.

The operation is not a dangerous one for adults and can be performed without any unusual risk.

My husband has been having trouble with his prostate gland. He is concerned that it may have to be removed by an operation. I have been told that such surgery can make a man impotent and that he cannot fulfill his marital relations or have children. Is this true?

The prostate gland, found only in males, is about the size of a large plum, perhaps two inches wide. Its three lobes surround the urinary bladder. The important function of the prostate gland is to produce the fluid which carries the sperm cells. The gland itself does *not* produce sperm cells.

For some unknown reason this gland tends to become larger during middle age and sometimes causes frequency of urination and may obstruct the flow of urine from the bladder.

Surgery of the prostate has progressed tremendously in the past twenty-five years. An operation can now be performed painlessly without an incision through the urethra using an electrocoagulating instrument. The operation is also being done with cryosurgery, a deep freezing method which is reported to be highly successful by the surgeons using it.

Sexual activity is rarely affected by the removal of the gland alone for a simple ordinary enlargement without complications. Marital relationships, in fact, often improve after such surgery because of the better health of the man after complete recovery.

The removal of the prostate gland would not, by itself, be responsible for the inability to have children. The sterility that so often follows prostate removal is due to another reason. When the gland is removed, a small tube, the vas deferens, is often tied, thus preventing the male sperm from passing through it.

Techniques of surgery and improved methods of anesthesia have considerably reduced the risk of prostate surgery. The use of antibiotics before, during and after surgery has cut down infections to a minimum. Your husband should see his physician or a urologist for diagnosis.

Would you explain what is meant by the different stages of syphilis? Does the germ that causes this affect any particular part of the body?

Syphilis is an infectious veneral disease caused by a germ, a spirochete known as the treponema pallidum. The course of this severe and complicated disease is usually divided into three stages. The first is when a chancre or ulceration appears on the skin of the genitals or on the mucous membrane lining of the mouth, lips and genitals.

Unfortunately, many of these chancres are painless and therefore are frequently overlooked and neglected. Healing may take place in a few days without any treatment, leaving little or no scar. Yet syphilis remains.

The second stage may suddenly erupt from one to three months after the disease is contracted. Now there may be a variety of symptoms which may resemble other illnesses and may not even, at first, be considered as syphilis. Sore throats, a skin rash, low-grade fever, or aches in various parts of the body may be the apparently simple symptoms that later are found to be syphilis.

The third stage of untreated syphilis may occur virtually at any time in life and produce the most bizarre and uncharacteristic symptoms. No organ in the body is exempt from the catastrophic effects of untreated and neglected syphilis. The brain, the spinal cord, the liver, the heart, the eyes, the ears, the blood vessels, the kidneys and every large and small organ can be damaged.

Children born of syphilitic parents can carry the sad stigmata of their parents' carelessness in avoiding treatment. They may be born with a variety of congenital handicaps.

Premarital testing has largely been responsible for wiping out inherited syphilis. Routine hospital admissions insure that all adults will be tested even in the absence of any history of syphilis. But the world-wide epidemic of syphilis will increase in geometric ratio unless intensive education will lead to prevention and earliest possible treatment.

What organs of the body can be affected by syphilis?

The heart, the blood vessels, the liver, the brain, the spinal cord, the nervous system, the skin (the largest organ of the body), the glandular system, and every other organ can be affected by the third stage of syphilis.

It is for this reason that syphilis must be actively treated at the first sign of the disease. The initial "chancre," or "ulcer," of syphilis spontaneously disappears after a brief period. Careless or uninformed people may believe that the disease, too, has disappeared. Therefore, they do not seek immediate medical help. The primary infection then progresses to the secondary stage and eventually to the third, or "tertiary," stage, slowly and insidiously producing disorders that seriously affect health.

Can syphilis be transmitted through the blood from a pregnant mother to her unborn child?

It most certainly can be, and when it is, the baby is frequently born with definite evidences of it.

Syphilis, unrecognized and untreated, can impose great heartaches on parents and their children. I must again emphasize that veneral disease is now at a level of epidemic proportions in the teenager and the young adult. Unfortunately, it is in this age group that a sense of responsibility is diminished. Fear that their parents may learn of their infection keeps these youngsters from revealing it to their doctors.

Only with proper and intensive sex education can young men and women be taught the need for immediate treatment if exposure to venereal disease becomes known.

My uncle is fifty-four. He was in perfect health until recently when he was told that he has syphilis in its "chronic" stage. Is it possible for someone to go through life and have this disease crop up suddenly?

Syphilis is one of the strangest diseases that affects man. In fact, it is an axiom in medicine that if you know all about syphilis you know all about man's entire range of diseases. Syphilis can resemble and mimic almost every other known condition in the body.

One of the serious aspects of syphilis is that the initial sore of the mouth or the genital area may heal and disappear without any treatment. Consequently, a person can harbor syphilis for many years without any subsequent symptoms. It is for this reason that health officials have embarked on such an active campaign to induce exposed people to have treatment immediately.

One of the great social contributions has been the requirement that all people have a test for syphilis before marriage. This is a compulsory way to detect the disease and thus prevent the havoc and catastrophe of neglect. Your uncle could have been harboring this condition for many years. With active antisyphilitic treatment, he may yet return to good health.

Is it possible for syphilis to show up suddenly in the spinal cord in someone who has never had any symptoms of it? A friend of mine who is forty-seven years old was just told that he has this disease.

The key word in your question is "suddenly." I doubt that your friend's condition, which is known as tabes dorsalis, developed that quickly. More realistically it can be assumed that he had syphilis at some time in his youth and it was not adequately treated then. It may take many years before syphilis affects the brain or the spinal cord after having been dormant.

One sad aspect of syphilis is that the sore on the mouth or in the genital area may disappear of its own accord after a few weeks. Disregard of this sore can mean that syphilis is overlooked and not treated in its early stages. Many years later the calamity of advanced syphilis may occur with total loss of the memory of an previous exposure to the disease.

Can an infection with syphilis during my youth show up in later years? I now am married and have two children and even though my blood checks out normally each year, I continue to worry.

Since you are married and have normal, healthy children, there is hardly any chance that your original infection may show signs now or as you get older. I assume that at the time you were infected, you were actively treated to be sure that the disease was completely controlled.

Your concern may be coupled with guilt that you might have transmitted syphilis to your children. This, too, is a negligible possibility. Yet for their sake and the rest of your family, blood studies will put your mind at rest. These tests can be done on them discreetly in cooperation with your doctor who, too, wants to spare the family emotional stress.

You are one of the fortunate ones who sought treatment for your past disease and obviously have been completely cured. It is pathetic that so many thousands of young people develop venereal disease and fail to seek treatment. These are the ones who pay a penalty in later life, when syphilis crops up in some unexpected way.

Is gonorrhea classed as a venereal disease? Can it be responsible for sterility in later life?

Gonorrhea is most certainly a venereal disease. The nonsense passed around in sheer ignorance by many adolescents that gonorrhea is a "cold" of the genital region that can be easily cured must be strongly discounted by parents and educators.

Gonorrhea, a highly contagious disease, occurs in both sexes and is caused by the gonococcus germ. Promiscuity is the basis for the transmission of gonorrhea, which most certainly can later produce sterility in both the male and the female.

A mistaken notion exists that this highly active venereal disease cannot affect other parts of the body when it remains untreated. In the male, chronic infection of the prostate, special types of arthritis and even inflammation of the lining of the heart or endocarditis may complicate this condition.

In the female the germ may cause severe disease anywhere along the urinary, vaginal and uterine tracts. Many cases of sterility have been traced to an infection that may have been untreated and even casually neglected.

I thought gonorrhea was a temporary illness that caused no complications. I now know better—it has left both of my knees crippled for life.

I'm sorry that you had to learn this the hard way. Despite exhaustive public health campaigns for young people, many still believe that gonorrhea is a simple "youthful experience" of no importance.

With active treatment immediately after exposure, the gonococcus germ can most often be kept under control. When neglected, this germ can invade the joints of the knee, the wrist, and the ankle, and can cause a permanent "frozen" immovable type of arthritis in both men and women.

Young girls often have extension of the gonorrheal infection to their tubes and ovaries, and thus may give up the possibility of bearing children later in life.

When I was eighteen I was infected with gonorrhea. I was treated and told that I was cured. Now, at twenty-eight, I'm seriously thinking about marriage. Can I still transmit this disease to my future wife?

Your sense of responsibility is admirable. Unfortunately, there are far too many young people who, having acquired a venereal disease, do not seek treatment. Consequently, they spread their disease to others.

Since you were effectively treated for your gonorrheal infection, there is little reason to suspect that any remnants of it remain. Nevertheless, an examination with smears and cultures should be done to give you the added assurance you seek.

A premarital blood test for syphilis does not indicate the absence or presence of gonorrhea. It is for this reason that a complete physical examination by the physician is one of the great gifts that a young couple can give to each other before marriage.

Does a discharge from the vagina in a healthy married woman mean that there may be a venereal disease? What is the cause of it and can it be cured?

The most frequent cause of a vaginal discharge, or leucorrhea, is a protozoa, a small cell which resembles a fungus. The condition it produces is called trichomonas vaginalis. This condition is a common one and is a nuisance rather than real trouble.

The exact diagnosis is made very easily by microscopic examination of the discharge. Treatment today is effective with a variety of new drugs. The condition clears up spectacularly after a short while with the concentrated use of drugs and with rigid personal hygiene.

In order to be certain that the condition will not recur, the husband, too, must be considered as a possible cause for reinfecting the wife with the protozoa. This disorder is not a venereal disease.

Can the germ that causes syphilis be responsible for other illnesses that are not venereal diseases?

A special germ is the treponema, or spirochete, a threadlike organism responsible for a wide variety of non-venereal diseases in addition to syphilis. One particular spirochete, the pallidum, is the definite cause of syphilis. Ordinary trench mouth is caused by one of the non-venereal varieties. Yaws is an infectious tropical disease caused by a related organism. Pinta, called azul or carate or spotted-sickness, is another strange variety of illness that is not venereal. Swineherds disease and relapsing fever are two other strange diseases caused by one of the many forms of spirochetes.

Names like rat-bite fever, famine fever and small garapata disease are found where hygiene is poor, water polluted and in parasitically infested underprivileged countries.

Can a venereal disease be transmitted through kissing? My daughter insists that this is not so.

Syphilis is a disease caused by a germ. This germ can be transmitted from one person to another during intimate contact, if a person is infected with it.

Many young people have developed the sore, or chancre, on the lips by kissing a person who is in an active phase of this dread venereal disease. Your daughter and all other young adults should know that there is a tremendous new wave of venereal disease. Parents and educators must teach them that their entire lives are threatened by promiscuity.

Is there a vaccine for venereal disease?

Unfortunately, no vaccine is available for gonorrhea or syphilis. The present massive epidemic of venereal disease, especially among teenagers and young adults, has spurred scientific research to find such a vaccine.

At one time, gonorrhea was considered almost a controlled disease and no longer a public health menace. In 1957, rapid treatment centers for syphilis were being closed across the country. Antibiotics seemed to have conquered both syphilis and gonorrhea. But by 1958, the bubble of optimism burst. From then on, there has been a rapid rise in the frequency and severity of venereal disease.

There are a number of reasons for the current epidemic, among them sexual promiscuity, the contraceptive pill, a diminished fear of venereal disease and "reduced interest in the problem."

The hope for an eventual vaccine must not dissuade public health officials from educational campaigns directed at the young. Parents, in cooperation with education and health officials, can be the greatest force in solving this problem.

Chapter X

Concerned About Cancer

I am overwhelmed by the number of letters that come to me from both men and women who live in terror of developing cancer. One woman from Chicago wrote a poignant letter in which she said, "Every morning and every night of my life I examine myself, seeking a lump in my breast. It has wrought havoc in my life and yet my fear grows worse and I don't know where to turn for some sense of peace."

Like so many others, this woman is overreacting to the stories she hears day in and day out in magazines, newspapers, on television and radio about cancer. True, it is important that we know all we can about this age-old scourge, that we be kept up-to-date on the complex jigsaw of its causes, its diagnoses and treatments. The fact that thousands of research scientists around the world are constantly exploring every lead in the hope they will uncover the mystery of cancer deserves to be told and retold. And yet, the lay observer bombarded by statistics and pronouncements and predictions about cancer feels a sense of hopelessness and fear, very often translated into personal terms.

What disturbs me deeply is the fact that so many of my correspondents who are fearful of cancer are reluctant to talk to their own doctors about those fears—or that they suspect their doctors are hiding the fact of cancer from them.

The woman in Chicago may continue to feel her body for lumps for the rest of her life and never find one. Yet a small lump may be present—a cystic change in the breast that so frequently happens in adult females, especially during menstrual phases and even during the menopause. But can she convince herself that anything she feels is not a cancer? Obviously, she is in a trap from which she cannot extricate herself without the help of an understanding physician.

Certainly it is true that cancer can be a devastating disease. Yet it is also true that when cancer is recognized early and treated intensively the cures are often spectacular and long-lasting. But to impress on people the need for constant examination and observation of one's body

233

serves only to magnify their expressed and unexpressed fears. How much more encouraging it would be to induce people to have regular medical examinations of their general health rather than "cancer checks." The key to the cure for cancer and hundreds of other illnesses lies in the early recognition of diseases and the early start of treatment. To delay that early examination is to invite conversion of simple problems into complicated ones.

Incidentally, progress has been far greater in the battle against cancer than is commonly suspected. There are new methods for early recognition of tumors, cysts and other types of body thickening that can be cancerous. The concept that the body itself can build its own defense mechanism against malignant cells has been found valid in some instances. New information about female hormones is accumulating, new vaccines are being tried. There is hope on the horizon that cancer in many forms will soon be controlled. It is this hope I try to convey in my column.

My husband and I suddenly realized that all we know about cancer is that it is a fatal disease, but we have no inkling what makes it so. Before our high school children ask us about it, we would like to arm ourselves with your knowledge.

It is a delight to know that there are some parents who do not know everything about everything, and openly say so. I frequently teach my resident surgeons in ear, nose and throat disease that the essence of maturity is to be able to say, "I don't know, but I will find out."

Now let me immodestly tell you all I know about cancer. There is a tremendous amount of information that is rapidly accumulating about the cause, the early diagnosis, the treatment, the control and even the cure of many different kinds of cancer. There is probably just as much information that has yet resisted discovery.

Every organ in the body—heart, lungs, breast, skin, bones, kidneys —is composed of hundreds of millions of tiny cells. These are the architectural blocks on which the body is built.

The cells can only be seen and studied under a microscope. Their size varies but most of them are no larger than 1/5000ths of an inch. Each cell contains a fluid called protoplasm and is contained within a membrane.

The wonders of the cell are immense. The fluid contains proteins, fats, sugars, minerals and countless other substances that play a role in health and disease. In the center of the cell is a nucleus which contains the genes that determine heredity and body characteristics.

The chemical DNA also present here is highly important as a factor in cancer. Normally, all cells multiply and divide in a very exact, well-regulated way. They stay within the confines of their own territory in every organ.

A change in the regulating mechanism of each individual cell may be the beginning of a cancer. The cells begin to divide peculiarly and change the appearance of the nucleus and affect the fluid protoplasm within it. Suddenly, the pattern becomes chaos and the cells find their way into territories where they do not belong.

This abnormal growth of cells becomes a tumor. It may either be a benign or safe tumor that does little damage to its neighbor or a malignant tumor or cancer that destroys its neighbors and invades tissue.

There are hundreds of forms of benign and malignant tumors. Some can be recognized by the naked eye. All must be verified by microscope examination.

Can a person who has all the "danger signs" find out if he has cancer? For the last year, I have had all the symptoms listed by the Health Department.

You are one of many who confuse educational advice by interpreting all signs and symptoms as ones that you have. People who read their own illness into every symptom are not benefiting from the educational material they read. Not only are you worrying about symptoms that probably do not apply to you, but you have failed to take advantage of advice available to you. You have failed to see your doctor to discuss any of the real or imagined symptoms that frighten you.

"See your doctor" is the basic rule that must be followed after you detect any danger signals. A year is a long time to live with unnecessary fear.

I have been deathly afraid of cancer all my life. Our neighbor just came back from the hospital after surgery for a cancer. Can a cancer be contagious?

Cancers are not contagious. They cannot be passed from one person to another even in close contact. However, the fear of cancer is definitely

235

contagious and can be passed on from person to person and to immeasurable harm to the emotional stability of those who "catch" this fear.

You obviously are one of the many people who live in terror of acquiring a disease that may never afflict you. It is a shame that so many people go through life missing many of its joys because of uncontrolled anxiety about this disease. When you live in such a state of constant fear, it is inevitable for you to contagiously spread your fears to those who surround you. Before long, the rest of your family will become "infected" by anxiety and then spend their lives perpetuating the same unfounded fears.

I have just returned from the doctor's office and absolutely forgot his explanation and the instructions he gave. I don't know what to tell my husband and I'm too embarrassed to call my doctor and have him repeat what he told me. I have a cyst of the ovary and want to know if this is or can become cancerous.

Let me assure you that a cyst of the ovary is not malignant. Changes do occur in size and character and it is for this reason that doctors suggest repeated and regular examinations in order to follow the condition. Your concern that it might be a cancer undoubtedly had been increasing for weeks before you consulted your doctor.

When you finally presented yourself at his office, you were probably breathless, teary and perspired freely. This the typical picture of anxiety.

I once made the observation that new patients usually sat at the edge of their chair when first they consulted me. It was only later when their fears were assuaged that they actually took a deep breath, leaned back in the chair and listened to my instructions.

As a mature adult you can call your doctor, who will understand that your original anxiety about your condition confused your listening ability. Ask your questions and write down the answers so that you can repeat them to your husband. Many patients wisely write out their complaints and questions. If they are not all answered by the doctor, they then can be asked of him.

For the past three years I have coughed up a small amount of

blood every morning. My wife wants me to have a test for cancer or tuberculosis even though I am in excellent health.

Even small amounts of blood coughed up every day for three years certainly must be considered abnormal. Hemoptysis, or coughing blood, does not always mean tuberculosis or cancer, but its origin must be found.

In most instances the cause of the bleeding is unimportant. It may come from the teeth, the gums or a break in the tiny blood vessels in the back of the nose or throat. The blood vessel may be broken by active hawking or violent blowing of the nose. Both are common to many people during the early morning clearing-up process. Allergies, chronic bronchitis and tobacco irritation may be responsible for slight bleeding.

Your wife is justified in prodding you into a physical examination. The cancer or tuberculosis test needn't be any more elaborate than the routine X-ray of the lungs. Examination of the throat may show the exact bleeding point and relieve your family's anxieties about this condition.

Is a cyst of the lung the same as a cancer of the lung?

No, a cyst of the lung is not a malignant cancer. Usually, these cysts are considered birth abnormalities. They rarely cause any symptoms unless they become enlarged and put pressure on the surrounding organs. When they do, the surgical removal of them is safe and successful.

Is it possible to tell if a small growth in the breast is cancerous without removing it?

A tumor, or growth, in the breast has certain characteristics which indicate to the doctor the possibility that it might be either benign or malignant (cancerous). When there is the slightest suspicion that a growth may be troublesome a number of examinations can be performed to determine its exact nature. One technique which is becoming more and more valuable is the sensitive study of the temperature of the skin surface. By this method the possible presence of malignant tissue under the skin can be revealed.

The one positive way to know the exact nature of a growth is to remove a part of it and send it to a laboratory where the exact nature of the cells can be seen and studied under a microscope. This biopsy method also determines the need for more extensive surgery.

When are X-ray treatments used in a patient who has had a breast removed for cancer?

X-ray radiation and cobalt radiation are frequently used as an added precaution when a breast has been removed for cancer. The safety of the skilled use of cobalt is great and gives added assurance that cancer cells that may have escaped even the most careful inspection by the surgeon are destroyed.

X-ray treatments have added immeasurably to the permanent cure of patients, especially in those whose condition was discovered early. Unfortunately some women delay their visit to the doctor for fear of "what he will say." The fear is understandable but realistic and mature judgment dictates an early examination by the doctor. Only in this way can the spectacular successes that surgery and X-ray therapy have brought about be continued.

Can a man develop a breast tumor? A small lump appeared in my breast and then disappeared without any treatment. Does the fact that it disappeared mean that it is of no importance?

Tumors of the breast, cancerous and non-cancerous, can and do occur occasionally in men. They are comparatively rare as compared with the frequency with which they occur in women. The fact that it disappeared in your case suggests, of course, that you may have been mistaken and that it has no meaning. Nevertheless, an examination by your doctor can give you greater peace of mind.

Young people occasionally develop a swelling of the breast which lasts a short while and then disappears without any treatment. Occasionally, a young boy may have an enlarged breast which may cause him marked embarrassment. This is known as gynecomastia, and may or may not be associated with glandular or hormone imbalance. It is most important that this enlargement be treated and even surgically removed to spare the boy the psychological handicap that may accompany it.

If your lump reappears, by all means have it looked at immediately by your doctor.

Recently I developed a tenderness around the nipple of my left breast. As far as I can see, there don't seem to be any lumps in the breast. I would like your opinion, however, before I go to the doctor.

The chances are great that you do not have cancer. Yet you do yourself and your family a disservice by delaying an immediate examination by your own physician. I understand why you want my opinion: You hope to be relieved of the anxiety that oppresses you. Now that you have it, be sure that you see your physician immediately.

There are many excellent tests that can quickly establish a diagnosis to determine the exact form of treatment. Let me stress that no newspaper or magazine article can substitute for the knowledge of your own physician.

I have been told that I have chronic cystic mastitis of both breasts. I am frightened that this might be cancerous. Is surgery performed for this condition?

Chronic cystic changes in the breast are not, in themselves, malignant. This does not mean that the condition should be disregarded.

Cystic disease of the breast is considered to be the result of some imbalance of the female hormone estrogen. The breasts undergo some slight changes each month, before, during, or after the menstrual cycle. The cystic condition is also observed during menopause.

Had your physician suspected the possibility of an underlying, more serious condition he would have used any one of a number of new techniques for furthering the diagnoses. Cysts can be painlessly emptied under local anesthesia. The soft breast tissue can be X-rayed by a technique known as mammography. This new method is truly a remarkable advance for distinguishing cystic disease from other growths. Sometimes a small piece of tissue is removed and examined under the microscope. The biopsy method of examination is definitive and indicates the nature of the medical treatment or the need for surgery.

Often hormone therapy is sufficient to relieve some cases of cystic mastitis. Support of the breasts before the menses relieves the tenderness and soreness. Surgery is performed only if there is a large cyst or if the physician suspects the possibility of a more serious condition.

239

What determines a doctor's decision as to whether to treat a cancer of the breast by surgery or by X-ray?

The size of the growth, the location, its duration, the appearance and the relationship to the underlying structure of the breast is of extreme importance in the clinical diagnosis. Special X-rays of the breast known as mammagrams are very significant.

Tumors are frequently removed, even when the doctor suspects that they are not cancerous, for the purpose of detailed study under a microscope. This biopsy study is one of the most important factors in the decision about the course of treatment.

There are many grades of severity of cancers. Some of them seem to be localized while others may invade adjacent tissues. These are important considerations in the doctor's decision.

There is no medical dispute between surgery and X-ray or radiotherapy. Each individual case determines its own treatment. No two are alike. Unfortunately the patient does not have any choice in this decision. It is purely a medical one.

The extent of the surgery can only be decided at the time of operation and depends entirely on the findings and surgeon's judgment. Sometimes even after extensive surgery, X-ray treatment is used to further insure total and complete recovery. In some instances X-ray treatment is used before the operation. With so many combinations of approach to the cure of breast cancer, there cannot be a single answer for all cases. The combined judgment of the surgeon and the physician can be depended on for the ideal choice.

Can a cancer of the breast be caused by an injury?

I doubt that injury is commonly accepted as the cause of breast cancer. Sometimes injury may cause the rupture of a blood vessel, and a collection of blood (hematoma) may give the appearance of a tumor.

One of the reasons why some women attribute a breast cancer to an injury is that it was the injury that made them inspect their breast more frequently. An undiscovered lump is thus brought to light.

Can polyps of the intestine become cancerous? What causes them?

A polyp is a tumor that results from chronic infection or inflammation. It can occur in the intestines as well as in the nose, the ear, the rectum, the womb and the stomach. A polyp is a benign, non-cancerous tumor which may bleed easily and over a long period of time may become large in size.

Despite the fact that a polyp is a non-cancerous condition it is watched very carefully for changes that may occur in the cells. It is for this reason that physicians carefully observe the growth of polyps and when there is the slightest suspicion that there may be malignant or cancerous degeneration, removal is suggested. There is no need for living with the threat that this will occur. A large percentage of polyps never change their character and stay perfectly benign.

Can a tumor of the intestines ever be non-cancerous? I had one removed and was told this, but I don't believe I am being told the truth because a small part of the intestine was removed with it.

Non-cancerous, or benign, tumors of the intestinal tract most certainly do occur, and when removed there is a complete cure. There are many benign types of polyps and myomas, or muscle tumors, that fall into this classification.

The fact that a small part of your intestine was removed should not induce the fear that you are being lied to. Very often, the surgeon decides to perform this type of operation rather than try to remove the tumor alone.

You do yourself a great injustice by disbelieving your physician, and by living in a state of anxiety because of it. Discuss this freely with your doctor. Perhaps he has not been aware of your fear and has not gone into sufficient detail.

I have a strange cyst of the ovary known as a luteum cyst. Can it lead to cancer?

Let me immediately assure you that the universal fear of cancer should not enter into every medical problem that arises. Cancer is not the inevitable aftermath of every disease of the body. The fear of cancer seems to dominate the lives of many people and can, if unchecked, be more destructive than the disease they may have.

When a woman produces an egg in the ovary, a small sac or follicle is present. This sac disappears in most instances. Occasionally it becomes enlarged and forms a corpus luteum cyst of varying size. Only when the cyst becomes markedly enlarged or becomes complicated is surgery necessary. The chance that a cyst will become malignant is highly improbable. These cysts, when followed regularly by the doctor for any changes in size, are usually safely controlled.

Are there different kinds of fibroid tumors of the womb? Is one more dangerous than the other? How long can I wait before surgery is necessary?

A fibroid tumor of the womb or uterus is a benign or non-cancerous growth. There are no different kinds of fibroid tumors, but their locations can be different.

Some of these are attached to the outer covering of the uterus, while others grow on the inside of the womb. The largest number grow deep within the powerful muscle of the womb.

A benign, non-cancerous tumor is not dangerous. When they grow to unusually large size, these tumors may cause pressure on the bladder or on the large bowel. Many instances of infertility are attributed to fibroid tumors. It is astonishing how large these can grow before being troublesome.

When once a fibroid tumor is found, the doctor keeps the patient under observation and watches for signs of rapid growth or for pressure symptoms. The exact time of surgery depends on the doctor's judgment and evaluation of the symptoms. The kind of operation depends on his findings when once he sees the uterus. Sometimes a fibroid tumor can be shelled out without removing the womb. When once the decision for surgery is made, delay can only lead to complicating a safe operation.

I follow my doctor's advice and have a Pap test done every year. I have been very curious about what the word "Pap" means and why the test is done so frequently.

"Pap" is short for the name of Dr. George Papanicolaou, the scientist who discovered the test that has saved the lives of thousands of women. How is it done and why? A cotton swab gently scrapes cells from the vaginal wall or from the cervix of the uterus. The cells are smeared on a glass slide, stained with a special dye, and then examined under a microscope.

242

Cancer cells are readily distinguished from normal cells by pathologists who specialize in the study of tissue and cells and can determine the degree of severity of cancer, if it is present.

The Pap test is a painless one and, in fact, can be done by the woman herself. At the Johns Hopkins Hospital, a special kit was devised and distributed to women in outlying rural areas. These women, who cannot easily get to a doctor, were able to take the specimen according to directions and mail it back to the hospital for examination. If performed at regular yearly intervals, the Pap test can detect early cancer and can be responsible for a tremendous increase in the number of permanent cures.

I have been told to watch a white patch in the inside of my mouth. Even if I do watch it, how will I know if it ever becomes cancerous?

You have just hit on one of my favorite targets. I, too, do not understand what is meant by "watching a white patch." These are called "leukoplakia" and have been given the frightening term of "precancerous."

I have known patients who were so terrified by the notion of precancerous white patches that they have laid out their entire lives around the inevitability that they will die of this disease. The term "pre-cancerous" serves no function. It only frightens and terrifies people who would fare much better with an attitude of reassurance.

You are quite right. How would you know if the white patch ever did become malignant?

It is for this very reason that I believe that all observation should be done by the doctor or the dentist at regular intervals. Why burden the patient with a suspicion? If and when any procedure has to be done, that is the time for the patient to play an active role in the problem.

However, if a white patch is due to excessive tobacco, pipe smoking or a jagged edge of a tooth, the patient should do his part to avoid further irritation.

Is chilosis a dangerous condition of the mouth? Can it be cancerous if neglected?

I assume you refer to a medical condition known as cheilosis. Cheilosis is a disorder of the lips and the angles of the mouth associated

243

with small cracks and scaling. Sometimes it is due to a Vitamin B deficiency. It is frequently seen in children who lick their lips a great deal and in those who have a tendency to drool saliva. Adults who wear badly fitting dentures may be burdened by this unpleasant, but usually not serious condition. Sometimes a fungus infection may be responsible. Rarely, if ever, is there a possibility that this condition will become cancerous, especially in the young. Yet a rule of medical safety suggests that treatment of a condition, rather than neglect, is wise.

I have a hard lump in the middle of my palate. It doesn't hurt but worries me even though I have had it for a long time. I am sure I have a cancer.

And like so many people you are doing nothing about finding out if your suspicions are right or wrong. Living with your fears means living with an emotional burden that you don't deserve.

The bony "lump" you describe is probably a condition known as torus palatinus, which is due to improper development before birth. Rarely do these grow large enough to interfere with swallowing and almost never do they affect health. Only in rare instances is surgery necessary.

These bony tumors sometimes interfere with the use of dental plates and therefore surgery may be suggested. Those of us who see this condition rather frequently always advise people not to drink fluids that are too hot because this area of the palate is less sensitive and the delicate covering can be easily burned.

I assume that you have a torus and certainly it is not cancerous. To be absolutely sure that another condition does not exist, by all means do the sensible thing and have it examined by your doctor.

How do people learn to speak when their voice box has been removed by surgery?

The vocal cords are two strands of muscle that come together when we speak and separate when we breathe. They are about an inch long and lie in the larynx or voice box. The Adam's apple that one feels in the midline of the neck is part of the larynx that houses the vocal cords.

A cancer of the larynx that involves only one vocal cord can be removed without taking out the entire larynx. When a cancer is more extensive and involves both vocal cords or the surrounding tissue, it may become necessary to remove the entire larynx to save the life of the patient.

When this operation is complete the patient breathes through a small hole in the neck through which the air passes directly into the lungs. This is known as a tracheostomy or tracheotomy, both meaning an opening into the trachea or the tube just below where the voice box originally was.

The operation is an extensive one but has been remarkably successful in saving many victims who might never have survived without it.

Speech therapists are now able to teach many of these patients to swallow the air and actually learn to speak in an easily recognizable way by "burping" the air through the esophagus. The sound is usually a flat, monotonous one, but this is hardly important to these patients who luxuriate in the fact that they have been given this second chance of living.

By what method can a skin cancer of the cheek be removed so that the disfigurement is not bad?

Skin cancers of the face are cured in a high number of cases and when found early, the results are astonishing. The choice of the method of removal, of course, takes into consideration the best cosmetic result. However, the prime purpose of any procedure for cancer is to cure it permanently. Therefore, the ideal method of treatment is one that cures.

There is danger in choosing a method based only on appearance. Surgery, chemical and electrical cauterization and surgery by freezing are only a few of the available techniques. The decision must be left to the judgment of your doctor, who will not sacrifice safety for appearance. A scar is a small price to pay for saving your life.

Can too much sun cause skin cancer or early wrinkling of the skin?

Concern about two such widely different problems cannot be bunched together. In one instance, the serious danger to health involved in cancer of the skin must be considered. The other, wrinkling of the skin, is of course, a matter of vanity.

More and more specialists are suggesting the possibility that intense over-exposure to the ultraviolet rays of the sun can produce severe burns and may be responsible for cancer of the skin.

Concern and fear have deprived many people of the pleasure of sunbathing because of these imposed "statistics." Some people with dark-pigmented skin can tolerate long exposure to the sun without danger;

others with pale, translucent skin are overexposed by even a few minutes of the sun's rays.

Unless there is advice against it by the doctor, sunbathing in moderation gives many people a glow of good health.

The problem of wrinkling has been studied for years, and the general feeling is that overexposure to sunlight dries the skin and causes other changes that hasten the aging process. In addition, the brown liver spots that come out during middle age are attributed to the sun. These are known as lentigines.

There you have the calculated risk of exposure to the sun. I believe that fear should not deter sunbathing. Only if your doctor specifically suggests that there is an extra hazard should it be avoided. As for wrinkles, you must balance advantages against disadvantages and come to a conclusion free of anxiety.

A safety factor can be added by using some of the better creams and lotions that act as protective filters against sunburn without interfering with tanning. Starting exposure for a few minutes and increasing it at regular intervals can prevent painful burns.

Are all forms of leukemia fatal? Can it be considered as a cancer and what new treatments are hopeful?

Leukemia has been called a cancer of the blood, mostly because certain cells run wild and invade normal body tissue. Actually there is a technical distinction but both are malignant and dangerous diseases.

There are many different kinds of leukemia, two of which are the most important forms. There is a myeloid and a lymphatic type. The signs and symptoms are somewhat different but the distinction is made by the complex microscopic examination of the blood. Some cases of leukemia have been kept in an arrested state for many, many years. They pass through a time of marked activity and then into a period of remission. There is no universal law about the behavior of this serious disorder of the blood cells.

Viruses have been incriminated as the cause in some cases. But this, too, does not apply to all forms. Leukemia, undoubtedly, is a highly dangerous condition but hope must not be abandoned.

Scientific studies are progressing toward a better knowledge of its cause and its eventual control.

Are skin cancers as dangerous as other cancers?

The rate of cure of skin cancer is especially high, especially when it is recognized and treated early.

Any open sore on the skin surface, even if it is only the size of a pea, should be carefully examined if it fails to heal within a reasonable length of time.

Is it possible to survive a brain tumor operation with no after-effects?

Yes, it is possible. Some non-cancerous tumors may arise in a part of the brain that is referred to as "silent areas."

When there is no pressure on the areas of the brain responsible for memory, speech, sight, hearing or other vital functions, recovery can be complete and permanent.

Every time I have a general examination, my doctor always does a rectal examination. Could he be looking for or suspecting a growth?

No general examination is ever complete unless a rectal examination is included. This especially holds for adults. Your doctor shows great wisdom, because the early detection of a growth means the greater possibility of recovery. He is not looking for a growth, but if it is there, he wants to know about it.

Is sarcoma a form of cancer or is this a word that our doctor used because he did not want to tell us the truth about someone he is treating in the family?

A sarcoma is one of a group of malignant, or cancerous tumors. They can occur in the bone and in the cartilage. Another type of tumor of this nature is the lymphosarcoma. This, with Hodgkin's disease, is classed as a lymphoma.

Rapid strides are being made in the treatment of these conditions

247

with complex chemicals and X-ray radiation. More and more of these highly malignant tumors, when discovered early, can be treated in this way.

When physicians are confronted with such serious problems they have no choice but to tell some member of the family the severity of the condition. This term is never used to bypass the truth.

A swelling on my wrist has been growing larger and I am beginning to get that uncomfortable feeling that this may be cancerous.

The best way to rid yourself of such a fear is to come face to face with the reality that your wrist should be seen by a doctor.

I do not mean to be presumptuous when, without examination, I suggest that you probably have a cyst or a ganglion that so commonly occurs on the wrist.

These are benign, non-cancerous conditions which usually cause no interference with the function of the wrist. Rather they are a nuisance, and cosmetically disturbing.

Are there doctors who specialize in the treatment of cancers?

It is a general misconception to believe that doctors specialize in the medical or surgical treatment of cancers.

Cancer surgery is performed by surgeons in all specialties. For example, the general surgeon may treat a cancer of the larynx. There are some hospitals that devote themselves to the medical and surgical treatment of cancers and have special equipment and nursing facilities available for that purpose.

A few weeks ago I noticed a small lump on the back of my daughter's neck and took her to the doctor for an examination. When he left the room, I read a note he had written on the chart. It said, "Mass on back Lipoxia." I can't tell him I read it. Can this be cancerous?

Concern, rather than curiosity, frequently motivates people to peek at doctors' charts. Then they are usually more confused and anxious than ever because of their inability to understand or interpret technical terms.

The handwriting of most doctors being what it is, it is reasonable to assume that what your doctor wrote was not lipoxia, but "lipoma" which is a benign fatty tumor. It is not cancerous.

The assurance your doctor gave you should have relieved your anxiety. You will probably feel better if you tell him that you read the chart so that he can clarify his findings for you.

Our four-year-old son seems to be inclined to growths. He was born with one on his lip. Now he has one on the back of his neck. We are terrified that this is cancerous.

There really is no "inclination" to growths that could explain the two that have occured in your son. Undoubtedly, the double presence is mere coincidence. "Watching" any growth can become a full-time occupation and devastate the emotions of a family.

How much wiser it would be to have this growth removed, and thus free all of you from the unnecessary anxiety expressed in your letter.

You can be certain that if there were the slightest suspicion of cancer your doctor would not allow the growth to remain. This is an important obligation that a doctor has to a patient and to himself.

There is a sad aftermath to this kind of concern. Almost invariably, the child senses the anxiety of the parents and reflects it in later life. This is far too great a penalty for what seems to be a relatively insignificant problem.

I have heard that saccharin can give you cancer of the bladder. I worry because I diet with foods and drinks that contain it.

I, too, saw a premature report on the possible relationship between saccharin and cancer of the bladder in experimental animals. Nevertheless, I feel that your concern at this time is unnecessary. If, however, you persist in worrying a great deal about this, why not simply stop? There are many other ways to diet without the burden of your fears.

The Pure Food and Drug Administration is the alert guardian of our health. When there is the slightest suspicion that any such substance can be harmful, intensive studies are made and revealed to manufacturers and to the general public.

249

My mother and two sisters all had enlargements of the neck and needed surgery for a goiter. It has now been suggested that mine be removed. I fear it may be cancerous.

A goiter is an enlargement of the thyroid gland. Almost always it is benign (non-cancerous). These enlargements are not hereditary.

It is assumed that your family members live in the same area and that they drink the area water. This is the key for the formation of goiters. They are most frequently due to a lack of iodine in the water. A deficiency of this chemical does occur in inland areas.

When this was recognized, iodized salt was increased in the diet and iodine added to some reservoirs. The result has been a marked reduction in a number of cases of goiter.

Sometimes goiters interfere with the proper activity of the thyroid gland and must be removed. In most instances the reason for surgery is a cosmetic one. Only rarely does a goiter become cancerous.

Chapter XI

The Disease Has A
Strange Name

According to our patients, we doctors speak a strange language. Oddly enough, although they don't always understand what we tell them, they wait until they get home, then decide for themselves exactly what it was we said to them—a kind of belated self-translation which is not exactly the ideal way to understand an illness.

Take the patient who has been told he has blepharitis, for example. In the consultation room, he accepts the term calmly, non-commitedly. Once home, he begins thinking about making a will and the high cost of funerals. Blepharitis has such a dire sound to him that he may be convinced he has a very short time to live. If only he had expressed his puzzlement to the doctor, he would have discovered that what he really has is an unimportant, treatable condition that produces sticky or dry granules on the eyelids.

I once taped conversations with fifty random patients, all adults, during which I carefully explained my medical findings, my diagnosis, my reasons for medical or surgical treatment and the prognosis. I deliberately reiterated all this and encouraged questions about any detail that might be unclear or confusing. One-half hour later, my nurse-technician taped another conversation in which each patient recapitulated my message to their spouses. And, after another half hour, I taped a third series of sessions during which the spouse relayed to me as many details as he or she could recall without being prompted or directed by me in any way.

The messages that were finally relayed back to me were, in many instances, almost unrecognizable. They were misquoted, garbled, exaggerated and misconstrued.

It was clear to me that anxiety, despite my efforts to eliminate it, was the dominant element that interfered with complete understanding between me and my patients. (I cannot say the same for the spouse-to-spouse communication—there the diagnosed illness was often elaborated and magnified for some special interpersonal reasons.)

But the lesson is clear. Communication between doctors and patients must be kept totally free of vagaries. Every word must be spelled out —literally. If the disease has a strange name—at least one that sounds peculiar to the patient—it should be identified in layman's language. Pharmacological terms and Latin labels mean little to a man or woman who is worried about his or her health and how it will affect working capacities. When the lines of communication are wide open, when there are no more unfamiliar terms to make a patient's heart skip a beat, a milestone will be reached. And when that comes to pass, my mailbag may be free at last of letters that ask: "Is psoriasis always fatal?" or "I have ridiculitis and it isn't funny at all."

For years I have been complaining of pain in the neck always worse in the morning. Recently, I have been told that I have ridiculitis and that I must learn to live with it. I really don't mean to be funny when I say this, but I haven't been able to tell my husband the name of my condition because I know he won't believe it.

The condition you have is radiculitis and, for the record, there isn't anything funny or ridiculous about having it. Anyone who has ever suffered from this painful affliction will testify to that.

Radiculitis is an inflammation of the nerves that come from the spinal cord in the area of the neck. There are many reasons for it. Arthritis of the spine and a dislocated disc may cause pain in the neck which may radiate down the shoulder, back and the arm. Sleep and rest are interfered with and the slightest movement of the neck is distressing.

X-rays of the cervical or neck portion of the spine and a neurological examination may show the exact cause. With drugs, collars and stretching of the neck relief can be obtained and the condition frequently arrested.

I know that a sarcoma is a dangerous form of cancer. Recently, a member of my family was told that he has sarcoidosis and I wonder if this is just a word that the doctor uses to avoid telling him the real trouble.

The words seem sufficiently close in sound and spelling so that your confusion is understandable. They are not the same. Sarcoidosis is a chronic disease first described by a Scandinavian doctor. The condition bears his name, Boeck's sarcoid.

At one time, this condition was thought to be related to tuberculosis because so many of the symptoms resembled it. The disease is still rather a mystery, even though its seriousness is relatively minor and recovery frequently occurs even when untreated. A strange relationship has been suggested between sarcoidosis and the pollens of pine trees because it occurs more frequently in those people who chew the resin of pine trees in some parts of the world.

Can poor posture during childhood cause a condition which has been diagnosed as "scoliosis?"

Scoliosis simply means a curvature of the spinal column. Poor posture is not responsible for scoliosis. More likely the cause was a birth defect that later produced poor posture. "Lordosis," or sway-back, is another anatomical variation from the normally straight spinal column.

All these conditions vary in degree and severity. They call for extensive X-ray and clinical examination by an orthopedist, or bone specialist, to reach a decision about proper treatment. Corrective exercises, casts, and surgery as well as the ideal time for any of these treatments depend, of course, on the exact diagnosis and the judgment of the surgeon.

Have you ever heard the term "Commando Operation?" What does it mean?

I don't know how the term came to be applied to surgery but such an operation does exist. In essence it refers to a very radical and courageous operation for the removal of an extensive cancer of the neck. This daring surgical technique is responsible for saving many lives that might otherwise have been lost. Such surgical procedures on the neck are now performed with transplants of tissue to make speech and swallowing again possible.

Have you ever heard of St. Gervasius' disease?

About fifty diseases have been identified with religious figures. Many

253

of these have interesting historical backgrounds and have been identified with saints. St. Gervasius' disease is the name applied centuries ago to the disease now known as rheumatism.

I have recently been discharged from the hospital after septicemia. Now I worry if it could happen again.

Septicemia is the technical term for blood poisoning. When bacteria or their poisonous products enter into the bloodstream they multiply and circulate throughout the body. High fever and chills are the predominant signs.

Since the discovery of antibiotics, the extreme danger associated with septicemia has been diminished.

The exact bacteria responsible for blood poisoning are discovered by cultures from the bloodstream, and then are bombarded by massive doses of a specific antibiotic known to be destructive to them.

The fact that you once have had septicemia does not mean that you have an unusual susceptibility to it.

Have you ever heard the expression "a mask of pregnancy?" My daughter, pregnant with her second child, was told that she has it and that it will never go away.

A brownish discoloration occasionally occurs on the cheeks of women during pregnancy. The medical term for this is "chloasma." It is thought to be caused by some temporary hormone imbalance. Almost always the discoloration disappears as soon as the child is born. So rarely does it persist that your daughter and you should not be distressed during this happy period of her life.

I recall when I was a child that my father and mother always referred to any stomach aches as "dyspepsia." My wife insists there is no such condition, that "dyspepsia" is my family's fantasy.

Dyspepsia simply means poor digestion. The word originates from the Greek, *dys* meaning bad and *peptin* meaning digestion. Dyspepsia is not a disease, but rather a descriptive symptom of a variety of illnesses or disorders. People have used the word to describe any stomach upset associated with nausea, vomiting, stomach cramps, or a sense of fullness.

The term is often used as a substitute for acute indigestion, upset stomach, and acidy stomach. "Biliousness" is another loose term that some apply to these symptoms. Both of these terms are occasionally used to lightly dismiss symptoms that deserve more recognition and investigation.

Diseases of the gall bladder, the pancreas, the liver, the stomach, and the intestines may present early signs of "biliousness' and "dyspepsia." Self diagnosis can lead to neglect. Only the discriminating judgment of a physician can distinguish, by the history of dyspepsia, its true importance.

What does a doctor learn by the examination of the spinal fluid? Is it a painful operation?

A spinal tap to remove fluid for examination is not a painful procedure. It is not an operation and is done in a very few minutes. The fluid is examined for bacteria, abnormal amounts of sugar and protein, and for its cellular composition. The pressure in the spinal column and these other findings are most important in many neurological problems.

Does the condition St. Vitus' Dance still exist? I remember it a great deal as a child.

St. Vitus' Dance is a nervous affliction which is associated with aimless and purposeless movements of groups of muscles that control the arms, hands, legs and head. It is technically known as chorea and is related in some ways to rheumatic fever.

It must by emphasized that simple nervous tics must not be confused with St. Vitus' Dance unless the diagnosis is definitely made by a physician. The condition still occurs but far less frequently because of better preventive medicine and the use of antibiotics, which today diminish the frequency of rheumatic fever and its complications.

A fellow teacher in my school was on sick leave because of an "echo virus." I am intrigued with the name. Would you explain it?

The letters E.C.H.O. stand for Enteric Cytopathogenic Human Orphan viruses. This special brand of virus occurs in epidemic form and can cause infections of the lungs, the intestines, or the nervous systems. These seem to affect children more than adults and cause many symptoms that resemble other viral or bacterial infections. It takes a great deal of detailed scientific study to really come to the conclusion that someone has an E.C.H.O. infection. Recovery is rapid with simple treatment.

Is narcolepsy similar to epilepsy?

There is no relationship between these two. Narcolepsy is a condition whose origin is still unknown. The major signs of this rare illness are attacks of sleep and sudden loss of muscular tone. Sleep may come on at unexpected intervals and may last for a few minutes to many hours. There is almost no control over the desire to sleep. The person wakes completely refreshed but may fall asleep again in a very few minutes. Although the condition responds moderately to modern medicines, this strange illness may persist throughout the individual's life span.

My daughter has been told that she has endometriosis. She is sure she has cancer. Can you tell us something about this condition and how we can help her?

Endometriosis is a condition whose cause is yet unknown even though many theories exist. The lining of the uterus is called the endometrium. Occasionally the cells in this lining are implanted in other areas that surround the female organs. They may be found on the outer surface of the womb, on the ovaries, the fallopian tubes, and even around the lower intestines. These are not malignant cells. They do not cause cancer.

Your daughter must be reassured about the non-malignant character of this disease. It may take a concerted effort of her doctor, her gynecologist, even a psychiatrist to replace her fear with a feeling of encouragement and hope.

What is salpingitis? What causes it, and can it leave any permanent damage?

Salpingitis is an infection of the fallopian tubes. These tiny tubes are the ones through which the female egg passes from the ovary on its way down to the uterus, or womb. It is caused by some form of bacteria. The gonococcus germ that causes gonorrhea is a great offender, especially in those with promiscuous sexual tendencies. The streptococcus and the staphylococcus, and even the germ of tuberculosis, can also cause salpingitis.

The seriousness depends, of course, upon the severity of the infection and the degree to which treatment has been neglected. For this very reason educational campaigns plead for early consultation with the doctor at any symptoms that might suggest venereal or non-venereal infection. The most serious result of neglected salpingitis is the sterility, or the inability to have children, that can accompany this condition. Sometimes surgery is necessary to remove the infected tubes and the tissue that surrounds them.

Have you ever heard of a medical condition known as "devil's pinches?"

"Devil's pinches" is a charming name for the tendency that some people have to bruise easily. In such people the slightest unusual pressure or injury to the skin seems to break a superficial blood vessel and black and blue marks appear.

Fair-skinned people with translucent skin seem to have this harmless disorder. It is said to occur in members of the same family and therefore has some hereditary factor. Blood studies rarely show any abnormality in clotting capacity or make-up of the blood or blood cells.

The name "devil's pinches" originated because the injury that caused the black and blue mark was usually insignificant and not remembered. The devil was therefore considered to be the culprit.

My husband was told he has "the Eisenhower disease of the intestines." We thought you might be able to clarify what the doctor meant.

Undoubtedly, your doctor told your husband that President Eisenhower had a similar intestinal condition to his. The medical term for this condition is "ileitis," an inflammation of the ileum or the end of the small intestine where it joins the large intestine. It is also known as

257

"regional enteritis" or "Crohn's disease" (Dr. Burhill Crohn is one of the pioneers in the study of the nature and control of this intestinal disease).

The diagnosis of this illness is confirmed by X-ray studies. Early and intensive treatment can usually keep it under control. Surgery is performed only if simple conservative measures are unsuccessful.

I am worried that I am suffering from Paget's disease. How can I know if I have it?

I am curious to know why you chose this particular disease to worry about. Paget's disease is a comparativley rare condition associated with a thickening of the bones of the skull. For many years, I have stressed that the descriptions of symptoms too often instill unnecessary fear in readers. As you have done, many people are quick to think, "That's exactly what I have." Usually they are completely wrong. In such instances, fears can mount and cause emotional stress. In your case, all you have to do is see your physician. He will X-ray your skull and, undoubtedly, relieve your anxiety about a condition that most likely does not exist.

What is a glucose tolerance test?

This is an important diagnostic test for many medical conditions. After a period of fasting, the patient is given a small amount of sugar by mouth. Blood samples are then taken at fixed intervals to measure changes in the quantity of sugar in the blood.

What is a chalazion? Can it be prevented? One was removed from my eye and left it blackened.

A chalazion is a type of cyst of the eyelid. Sometimes it is referred to as a benign tumor, which sounds more formidable than it really is. Beneath the skin in the area of the eyelid are many tiny glands that secrete a lubricating fluid. When the opening to these glands is closed, the material dams back and a chalazion results.

Perhaps poor hygiene around the eyes or overuse of cosmetics may be the cause. If this is corrected, there may be less chance of a recurrence.

The seepage of blood near the eye after removal of a chalazion is a common occurrence.

Our small child had a serious operation for a condition called "intussusception." Is there a chance that this might occur again when he gets older?

Intussusception is an unusual condition best described by the visual picture of one portion of the intestine telescoping itself into an adjacent part. Usually, this occurs at the site where the small intestine joins the large bowel. As with your child, surgery is necessary to relieve this intestinal obstruction. Once the condition has been satisfactorily repaired by surgery, there is no reason to expect that it might occur again.

I am interested in the term "collar button abscess." Is this a real medical condition? What is its origin?

It is an interesting descriptive term. One's first reaction is that it is an abscess in the center of the neck caused by pressure of a collar button. This is not the case. A collar button, if you recall, has one large flat surface connected to a small area by a thin rod. A "collar button abscess" is one that has two compartments under the skin, a large one and a smaller one, connected by a tunnel. It can occur anywhere in the body but is most frequently seen in the webs between fingers. Unless both pockets are cleaned out, the infection persists.

What are the Heberden's nodes of arthritis?

These nodes are hard, firm enlargements of the fingers, seen in advanced cases of osteoarthritis. They tend to occur more frequently in women and the disorder seems to run in families. Injury to the fingers can also produce these nodes. This doesn't mean that progressive crippling from arthritis will follow. The use of cortisone has been beneficial, especially during the early stages of the node formation.

Is arteriosclerosis the same as atherosclerosis?

Atherosclerosis is actually a subdivision of arteriosclerosis. Arteriosclerosis is the term applied to many changes that affect the inner lining, the muscle wall or the outside of the arteries. Atherosclerosis specifically refers to the thickening of the inner layer of the blood vessel with the formation of plaques that interfere with the blood supply to all organs.

What is Dupuytren's contracture?

A strange contraction of the hands which causes the fingers to be drawn into the palm is known as Dupuytren's contracture. It is named after the French surgeon who described the condition more than one hundred years ago. Following injury or infection, and frequently without any reason, changes occur around the tendons and muscles of the fingers and, unless checked, can result in severe incapacitation. Dupuytren's contracture responds remarkably well to modern surgery especially if the condition is recognized early.

What is "bronze diabetes?"

Bronze diabetes, or hemochromatosis, is a rare disease. It must not be confused with the oridnary diabetes melitus. This unusual disorder is one in which iron-containing pigments are deposited in the liver and the pancreas and cause a peculiar bronze color of the skin. Its cause is unknown.

My mother-in-law has been told that she has Hashimoto's disease. I noticed, when filling out her Medicare form, her doctor checked "No" in answer to the question, "Is the patient cured?" We are concerned.

Hashimoto's disease, named after the man who described it, is a very special type of disorder of the thyroid gland.
Goiter, an enlargement of the thyroid, or hypothyroidism, are associated with this condition.
There are a number of excellent ways of treating it with dessicated thyroid and other drugs.
The reason that your mother-in-law's doctor said "no" in answer to

the printed question is because lifelong treatment is necessary to control this disorder.

My uncle has been told that he has polycythemia. Can you explain this condition?

Polycythemia is a disorder in which there is a marked increase of red blood cells that circulate in the blood. Its exact cause is unknown; it seems to affect males more than females.

Various treatments, including radioactive phosphorous, are used. In addition, blood is removed at regular intervals to relieve the excess. This is a treatment known as phlebotomy. People with this condition can be sustained in good health when they are under constant supervision.

Can you explain what purpura is?

Purpura is the general name of a condition in which the platelets, an important constituent in the blood, are markedly reduced. There are various types of purpura, some associated with acute infection, others due to toxic drugs. Because the platelets are important in the coagulation of blood, sometimes small black and blue marks of hemorrhages occur under the skin after slight injury. While treatment for this platelet deficiency is carried on with drugs, and in severe cases, with transfusions, the basic, underlying cause must be established to attain complete and successful control of this disorder.

Where can I obtain more information about Tourette's disease? My eight-year-old boy always seemed overactive and jumpy. We just assumed that he would grow out of it. Now we have been told that he has this condition.

The Gillis de la Tourette syndrome is named for the man who first described it in 1885. It is now being given greater recognition in an effort to pinpoint the reasons for the eye twitching, the jerking of the head and shoulder, and the facial grimaces that are occasionally seen in children. These signs and symptoms closely resemble many other neurological and emotional disorders. Tourette's disease must be differentiated from others if the child is to have successful treatment. The Gillis de la Tourette Association can be reached at Box 3519, Grand Central Station, New York City. Educational material is available to give you greater insight into the problem and to guide you in helping your son.

I had an infection on my skin which the doctor called "Air Sipolis." Can you explain this to me?

I am intrigued by your spelling of erysipelas, which is an acute swelling and inflammation of the skin caused by a streptococcus germ. Most often it occurs on any part of the skin surface that has been broken and invaded by this particular bacteria. Prior to the antibiotics, this was a very severe condition. Today, it is controlled miraculously by penicillin and the mycin antibiotics.

What is Kwok's disease?

It has been found by sad experience that peculiar symptoms of all kinds appeared within a half hour after eating in Chinese restaurants. Those of us who love Chinese food must respect this discovery. Some people found that they developed a peculiar sensation of numbness in the back of the head and shoulders that extended down the arms and caused a feeling of tremendous weakness.

When this condition was traced to an overuse of monosodium glutamate (MSG), a common additive in Chinese food, the world of the Chinese gourmet seemed ready to collapse.

These findings were substantiated in all parts of the world by people who use this taste intensifier in cooking. It now seems that the Sunday night disease may be an all-week disease when MSG is used in large quantities. It is surprising how many people, despite this new bit of information, are willing to accept these strange sensations for the sheer joy of bird's nest or won ton soup.

Is a "cluster headache" one that affects different parts of the head at the same time?

No. A cluster headache is a type of migraine headache. It refers to the frequency of attacks rather than to the location in the head.

Is sprue caused by a vitamin deficiency?

Sprue is a strange chronic disease usually associated with an inability to properly absorb nutrients from the intestinal tract. There are a number of related disorders like celiac disease which are characterized by weight loss, weakness and an inability to absorb vitamins.

There are two common forms of sprue, the tropical and the nontropical. Both have some form of anemia because vitamin B-12 is poorly absorbed. Almost always there is a deficency in animal foods and folic acids.

Few diseases have as many diffuse and unrelated symptoms. It is therefore a mistake for anyone to speculate as to whether or not they have it.

Active treatment with folic acid and Vitamin B-12 is now supplemented with the use of cortisone with remarkable success when the condition is recognized early. In areas of the world where health, hygiene, and good nutrition is available, sprue is rarely encountered.

Would you please write about a condition in the mouth called "leukoplakia?"

Leukoplakia are painless white patches that frequently appear on the tongue or the inner lining of the cheeks. The name simply means "white patch." It is usually caused by badly fitted dentures, sharp-edged teeth and, occasionally, by poor hygiene of the mouth and teeth. Chronic irritation by hot smoke, especially from pipes and cigarettes, may also be a cause.

Unquestionably, all the obvious causes of leukoplakia should be removed if found. Like all changes from the normal in any part of the body, leukoplakia should be checked at regular intervals by a physician.

Could you explain what myofibrositis is?

Myofibrositis, or its reverse fibromyositis, is a group of illnesses which are associated with stiffness in the muscles and the joints. Pain and tenderness are characteristic of the condition. Infection, strain, exposure to cold and dampness may produce changes in the muscles of the back and neck, the shoulders and thighs. Occasionally, tiny nodules that trigger the pain are present over the muscles.

The condition must be differentiated from many other disorders with

263

similar symptoms. Treatment of myofibrositis consists of heat, rest, massage and drugs such as procaine and cortisone. Treatment is started only after the exact diagnosis is confirmed.

What is meant by a Morton's toe? I have been told I have it and find it exceedingly painful to walk.

Morton's toe, named after the man who first described it is a painful condition that affects the space between the third and fourth toes. It may be due to a fallen arch and a neuralgia in that area, or to a small tumor of a nerve. X-ray may point to the exact cause and may show the need for special types of treatment which now include cortisone. When the pain is very severe and incapacitating, surgery may be necessary.

Chapter XII

Doctor, About My Heart . . .

For years I have been intrigued by an expression that is consistently used by people who have recovered from a heart attack. Almost invariably the person refers to the time that he "had his coronary." Most people have very definite landmarks in their lives that identify happy and unusual experiences. Not so the individual who has recovered from a coronary.

"I gave up smoking when I had my coronary." "I began to cut down on my office activities when I had my coronary." "I eat very little since I had my coronary." These are typical expressions which indicate a time of rebirth because they have survived the impact of a heart attack—and rightfully so. "My coronary" should be a significant milestone because in many instances it brings a new lease on life for those who were desperately ill.

Preventive medicine aims at avoiding a coronary heart attack but physicians everywhere know how difficult it is to put sanity and moderation into the lives of men and women "who have no time for such nonsense." Thousands of lives might be spared if these same individuals could readjust their lives and change that much-used expression to "I'm planning to avoid a coronary."

Actually, the prevention of heart attacks should start virtually in infancy. The overfed plump child almost always becomes the fat adolescent and the overweight adult who for years has been planning his heart attack. He has laid down the blueprint for it and followed the patterns that lead right to it with overindulgence in fatty high-cholesterol foods, cigarette smoking, little or no exercise, physical and emotional fatigue, and the total neglect of body complaints.

A complete physical examination may give some warning of an impending heart attack. It is not commonly known that many people suffer a slight barely recognizable heart attack that passes unnoticed until an electrocardiogram may reveal it. When chest pain and bouts of unexplained indigestion occur repeatedly in an overweight, hard-driving smoker with high blood pressure, further neglect of such warnings is unwise. If the warnings are heeded, many deaths would be prevented.

Incidentally, a lazy heart in a lazy body adds its contribution to heart attacks. Exercise is considered so important that even those who have recovered from attacks are encouraged to follow a carefully established program of active and passive exercise.

Your heart is your faithful servant through life. Sometimes its wonders are taken for granted because of the punishment it can take from an overweight body, lack of exercise, excess fatigue, alcoholism, tobacco, overindulgence in high-cholesterol foods and emotional tension and stress.

But there is a limit to the reserve of the heart to handle these abuses. Ask yourself if you abuse your heart in one or more of these ways. And do schedule the complete physical examination that you have been postponing for so long. Only then can your physician outline a program for total health that may help to prevent a heart attack. Sparing the heart need not be a full-time preoccupation. All that is necessary is your sensible awareness of the gift of good health.

My newborn baby was born with a heart murmur and we are terribly upset because there was nothing unusual about this, my third pregnancy. We have been told that this is a functional, rather than organic, murmur. Nevertheless, we wonder whether it will affect our boy's life as he grows older and possibly make him an invalid.

Let me immediately put to rest any feeling of guilt you may have about anything you did or did not do during pregnancy. These functional murmurs frequently occur without any abnormality in the heart muscles or in the valves that separate the four chambers of the heart. This is the distinction between a functional and an organic murmur which is based on some structural abnormality. Modern surgery can now correct most of the simple and many of the very complex heart abnormalities that are organic.

I am quite certain that your anxiety prevented you from really hearing the assurance your own doctor undoubtedly gave to you. The result is that you are magnifying the importance of this murmur and unless your fear is checked, you will reflect this anxiety on your boy as he gets older. This must be avoided. Children with functional murmurs are not handicapped in any way and can take part in the most active sports without any limitation. Unless you completely understand this, you will find yourself imposing limits on him and converting a perfectly normal, healthy child into a potential physical and emotional invalid. Many children born with a murmur of this kind lose it after a few years and grow into adulthood with the normal expected longevity.

When I first get out of bed in the morning I have a sudden feeling of dizziness which lasts about a minute. Sometimes I feel it when I lie down. My blood pressure is low. Could this be the cause?

The complaint of short-lasting dizziness may very well fit in with the story of low blood pressure. Frequently a sudden change of position from lying to sitting to the reverse may produce a variety of symptoms before the circulation of the blood finds its true level.

There are, of course, many reasons for low blood pressure, many of which can be corrected when the exact cause is found. In uncomplicated cases of hypotension, or low blood pressure, a few suggestions may help. Try not to make sudden, rapid changes in position. Elastic stockings and a moderately tight abdominal corset may be an advantage. Avoid long periods between meals. In some instances drugs are used to stimulate circulation and temporarily elevate the blood pressure.

What causes a large artery to "blow out" suddenly?

The condition described as a "blow out" of a large artery is known as an aneurysm. The best description is that it is much like a large bubble on the inner tube of a tire. The cause is almost always a weakness of the muscular wall of the blood vessel. This weakness may be the result of some congenital or birth deformity or can result from one of many illnesses.

The wide variety of aneurysms and their relationship to injury, infection, and hereditary weaknesses are very often recognized by some of the symptoms they present. An aneurysm of the aorta, the largest blood vessel in the body, which leads directly from the heart, may cause pressure pains, chronic cough, and difficulty in breathing and swallowing. It must be emphasized that one or all of these symptoms may be caused by dozens of different medical conditions and therefore should not be interpreted by readers as being "exactly what I have."

X-ray studies and angiograms, highly technical methods of studying blood vessels, can now show the size of the aneurysm and its exact location. Recent advances in heart and vascular surgery make it possible to cut out the weakened part of the blood vessel and replace it with grafts of preserved or banked vessels. Dacron sleeves are successfully used to replace the bubble, both to relieve symptoms and to prevent the possibility of rupture with serious consequences. These operations are now being performed almost routinely with great success.

My new business will take me to a high dry climate. Is this safe for someone who had a mild heart attack ten years ago at the age of forty-five?

Most people adjust very quickly to changes in altitude when they move to new climates. When one has been completely free of symptoms for such a long time as you have it can be safely assumed that your heart is virtually normal. Indulging as you do in all activities, at work and at play, substantiates this. Nevertheless, I would suggest a complete reevaluation of your general health before you move to the higher altitude. Frequently doctors suggest that people try a new altitude for a while before making a final decision to live there. By doing so, you can learn more about the climate and how well you can adjust to it.

I live in a high-altitude area. Since my blood pressure is higher than normal, would I benefit by moving closer to sea level?

Many years ago, a study seemed to indicate that the blood pressure in adults was lower in tropical and sea-level areas. I don't think this has great validity, since high blood pressure does occur in these areas, too.

My suggestion is that you continue active treatment with your own physician. A trial period in a sea-level area, under a doctor's supervision, might be beneficial. But a definite move to a distant climate may be disappointing and only serve to further increase stress and tension.

How much blood is necessary to sustain life in a healthy person? What are some of the less important contents of the blood?

It is estimated that an adult has about one quart of blood for every thirty pounds of body weight. A normal healthy man weighing one hundred and fifty pounds would have about five quarts of blood. A quart is 1,000 cc. A good illustration of body needs for replenishing blood is the fact that a transfusion of 500/cc. or a pint of blood is the usual amount given.

The composition of blood represents a complex organization. Physicians who have a daily need to study blood contents never take for granted the delicacy of the balances of all the elements in the blood. There is no one single element that is more important than the other. Each serves its own purpose. The red blood cells contain hemoglobin that transports oxygen and carbon dioxide from one part of the body to the other. The white blood cells act as the first line of defense against invading bacteria.

There are dozens of protective antibodies and hormones which control the function of many of the organs of the body. The blood contains protein, phosphorus, iron, calcium, sodium, and other minerals.

There is perhaps no more delicate system than that which is responsible for the clotting of blood when it comes in contact with the air. Just as remarkable is the subtlety of the mechanism that keeps blood circulating as a fluid in the body. The blood and its contents truly are beyond belief.

Would you explain the term "blood pressure." I hear it used often but do not understand it.

Blood pressure, normal, high, and low, is of great interest to readers as evidenced by my mail. Many want to know what the numbers represent. Others are interested in the different types of high blood pressure, their causes and treatment.

Blood pressure readings are always referred to as one number over another. The upper number is the systolic blood pressure; the lower is the diastolic.

Systolic indicates the blood pressure in the arteries at the instant your heart beats and pumps blood into them. Diastolic is that pressure in the arteries between beats of your heart. The relationship between the two blood pressure readings is actually more important than the numbers themselves.

For this reason, patients themselves cannot evaluate their condition by the reading of numbers alone. Numbers can be frightening if their real importance is not understood. If you were to trade numbers with

269

your neighbors or friends, 160 over 80 would have no meaning by itself. The numbers are important only in relation to your age, body build, weight, and depend on the condition of your heart, lungs and kidney.

Now, about the types of high blood pressure. One form called "organic" can be caused by endocrine gland imbalance, by heart disease, by chronic kidney disease, and by arteriosclerosis of the blood vessels. This type of high blood pressure, or hypertension, tends to progress unless it is actively treated and the underlying cause is controlled.

The second type is called "essential" (or "primary"); this is still obscure. But more and more evidence suggests that heredity plays a part.

It must be understood that high blood pressure is really a symptom rather than a disease itself. Therefore, intensive studies must be made to find the cause, treating it actively in an effort to eliminate it, and using some of the remarkable drugs now available.

Alcohol and tobacco are usually eliminated from the treatment regime. Alcohol stimulates your heart and tends to pour more blood into the arteries. Tobacco narrows your blood vessels and interferes with the free flow of blood through the arteries. This further increases blood pressure. Excess weight adds a burden to your heart and circulatory system. Emotional tensions play an important role in the general picture of high blood pressure.

All treatment includes proper retraining of the personality to lessen those tensions and stresses. The key to successful treatment lies in continued observance by your doctor.

Whenever I ask my doctor what my blood pressure reading is he just says, "It's good," without telling me the numbers. Why is this kept as a secret?

I've said before that a doctor can't always win in his relationship with his patients. In some instances he is wrong when he is right and in others he is right when he is wrong.

When the doctor tells the patients the "numbers" they often complain that they were unnecessarily terrified. When he does not tell them the numbers then they are "scared to death" because they believe they are so sick that the doctor does not want them to know about it. I wonder what patients would do if they had to make the decision to tell or not to tell.

The fact that your blood pressure is good should in itself be a sufficient source of comfort to you. You can be sure that if high blood pressure were not responding to medication your doctor would be the first to tell you that something more drastic should be done.

Many people are confused by blood pressure readings. There is nothing mysterious about it. Blood that is circulating through the arteries of the body is being pushed with each pump of the heart. After each beat the heart then relaxes for a moment before it again begins to pump the blood through the arteries. Under normal circumstances arteries are very elastic and expand with each beat of the heart. The blood pressure reading at the time that the heart beats, or pumps is known as the systolic blood pressure. The blood pressure reading at the moment that the heart relaxes is known as the diastolic pressure. It is for this reason that blood pressure readings are described as one number over another. A high top, or systolic number, does not necessarily mean trouble. In fact, in many cases the lower, or diastolic number, is even more important as a guide for the doctor in the control of certain kinds of high blood pressure.

It is apparent, therefore, that the discussion between you and your physician should center about the cause of and what is being done to control the high blood pressure, rather than around numbers that really have no basic importance to you.

What is the normal pulse rate for an adult?

The pulse rate, which is identical with the regular heart beat, varies between sixty-five and seventy-five beats per minute in a normal healthy man. The pulse rate in a healthy woman is higher. Under emotional stress, and after exercise, the pulse rate increases rapidly, then slowly returns to normal. There are great variations in the pulse rate of people with every conceivable kind of illness, and even in normal health.

Taking one's own pulse can be confusing. In fact, it is known that when people take their own pulse and try to count it, anxiety develops and the pulse rate goes up. Tobacco, coffee, alcohol, and drugs all can cause variations of the pulse rate.

Is there any type of heart surgery that can increase the circulation to the heart muscle itself? You once mentioned that the blood supply to the heart was not as perfect as in other organisms of the body.

271

Although the wonders and the wisdom of the body are great, the two main arteries that bring oxygen and blood to the heart muscle really are not adequate when the arteries are blocked by disease. These coronary arteries are the life line to the healthy activity of the heart.

A number of remarkable operations are now being performed to bring additional blood to the heart when it needs it. So enthusiastic are we now about the safety of many of these operations that it is hoped they will be life-saving in early cases of severe coronary artery disease.

What is the normal blood pressure, systolic and diastolic for young, middle-aged and older adults? Does it vary with age?

Blood pressure readings are calculated in millimeters of mercury. The average systolic blood pressure in healthy young adults is about 120. The average diastolic pressure is about 80. These numbers are usually referred to as 120 over 80.

Variations do occur with aging. The pressure at age sixty may normally rise to 150 over 88.

The numbers themselves are not the only important representation of health or disease. If there is any personal anxiety about blood pressure, it is wise to have a checkup, followed by a frank discussion with your doctor of any emotional concern about the meaning of the blood pressure reading.

How often should the blood pressure be taken?

Unless there is unusually high blood pressure, which needs constant supervision, it is sufficient for the blood pressure to be taken only at the time of the yearly general examination.

My husband has had one slight heart attack from which he has completely recovered. Occasionally he develops pain in his chest, especially after a heavy meal. How can we be sure that his symptoms do not mean another heart attack?

It takes a great deal of medical acuity to be able to tell the difference between the symptoms of overeating and those related to the chest pain of a heart disorder.

After dietary indiscretion and emotional distress many people complain of chest pain even though their hearts are normal. Specialists in heart disorders refer to these chest pains as neurocirculatory asthenia only after they have completely studied the heart to be sure they are not overlooking a real heart condition. Neither you nor your husband can come to any conclusion about the reality or the fantasy of disease. Your doctor is the only one who can be depended on to make such a decision. It may need many visits for your husband to be convinced that he is not living on a keg of dynamite that will explode into a full-blown heart attack. Psychological guidance and tranquilizers used under the direction of the doctor may reduce these frightening episodes. Heavy meals before sleep most certainly place an additional burden on the heart and other organs, even in those people who have never had a heart attack.

Do heart attacks occur more frequently in active business executives?

Stress and emotional upsets are not the only factors that cause big business moguls to have heart attacks. Diet, heredity, cholesterol in the blood, high blood pressure and overweight are some of the other reasons. Narrowing of the arteries by tobacco is a most important factor.

A very interesting study was performed on monks, considered to lead a most placid tranquil existence. They seem to be free from the problems of everyday living and tensions. Surprisingly, this is not so.

Both in the Benedictine and Trappist orders which were studied, an interesting conclusion was arrived at. Those monks who were in the most responsible positions were found to have almost three times as many heart attacks as were those who had little or no additional responsibilities.

Diet seemed to play a most important role in this study. The Benedictines eat food high in fats and their diets are almost the same as those outside of the monastery. The Trappists are vegetarians and, therefore, had far lower cholesterol in their blood. The Trappists had a lower rate of heart disease than did the Benedictine monks.

It is obvious that there are many physical aspects to heart disease besides the serenity of an occupation.

Does a chronic cigarette cough add any special strain on the heart?

Cigarette smoke acts as an irritant. The lungs explosively try to get rid of the irritation. This constant hacking most certainly can put extra pressure on the heart.

How can I avoid a heart attack?

The American Heart Association stresses the following rules to reduce the danger of a heart attack:
1. Maintain a normal body weight.
2. Eat foods low in animal fats and cholesterol.
3. Stop smoking cigarettes.
4. If you have high blood pressure, you should be under the constant supervision of your doctor.
5. Some form of exercise in moderation is extremely beneficial.

Is it possible to have a heart attack without knowing it? A recent electrocardiogram showed some scar tissue in my heart, although I had no memory of any symptoms of a heart attack.

We have all had the experience of being awakened in the middle of the night with strange unexplained distress in our chest or upper abdomen. In most instances, it is truly the indigestion we assume it is. Sometimes, however, these little attacks may actually be very mild heart attacks. As a result, small areas of scar tissue may form in the heart, to be picked up later by a routine electrocardiogram.

Now, what should this teach all of us? To panic with every attack of indigestion? Decidedly, no. For the chances are small indeed that a bout of indigestion is a heart attack.

A very severe episode of so-called indigestion, however, especially in a cigarette smoker who is overweight and past the age of forty, should be brought immediately to the attention of a doctor.

One of the great advantages of early examination is the possibility of avoiding a severe coronary attack. If indeed the "small' heart attacks were recognized early, far more severe coronary heart attacks might be prevented.

As a wife of a middle-aged man I would like to play a part in keeping him healthy. How can I help prevent his having a heart attack?

The best candidate for a heart attack can be described as a "sedentary, flabby, middle-aged male given to excessive cigarette smoking and to meals high in animal fats, sugar and cholesterol." All of these factors can be reduced or diminished with discipline. Added to this heart attack profile is a family tendency towards diabetes and gout. A good look in the mirror can tell your husband if he fits into the distinct picture of the candidate for coronary heart disease. If it looks familiar to him, he can immediately begin to cut down on his diet, free himself of cholesterol foods and begin a planned program of exercise.

You know the dangers of smoking tobacco as well as he does. Cutting down on his weight and the elimination of tobacco is most significant. The fact is, persons who resemble the composite coronary candidate have a thirty times higher chance of suffering a heart attack than adults who do not resemble this picture.

With a history of heart attacks in my family how can I, at the age of thirty-eight, plan my life to avoid a heart attack? I feel that this is a responsibility I owe to my wife and children.

You are wise to plan now. Additional years of life may be your dividend for such careful planning.

Heart attacks can, in a measure, be predicted. In fact, there are now many computerized studies that give the major causes of heart attacks, and show how they can be prevented.

There is little that you can do about your genetic background and your family tendency towards heart attacks. Perhaps, before long, the genes and chromosomes will be manipulated so that this factor, too, may be controlled.

Till then, however, let us examine some of the main factors that contribute to heart attacks:

1. It is generally accepted that smoking cigarettes plays an important role in narrowing the blood vessels that supply the heart muscle with blood and oxygen.

2. Uncontrolled and untreated high blood pressure increases the risk of heart attacks.

3. Fatty foods high in cholesterol and other liquids, or fats, are distinct forces in the development of arteriosclerosis and narrowing of the blood vessels.

4. Extra weight certainly adds an unnecessary burden on the heart, and adds a further risk of heart disease.

Now, what do all these factors have in common? All of them can be eliminated, avoided or controlled. Herein lies the sad story behind many heart attacks. Emotional pressures in the home and in business can also be factors in potential heart attacks.

I am a tense person, and every once in a while, I get a fluttering sensation in my heart. Does this mean that at the age of forty-four I am heading towards a heart attack?

The heart has a wonderful, delicate mechanism that acts like an electrical switch to keep the heart rate regular and normal. When special demands are made on the heart to beat faster during physical activity or times of emotional distress, the heart beat suddenly increases. This mechanism can be compared to the electric valve in the fuel system of the home that keeps the heat at a constant level.

Every once in a while the heart pacemaker becomes disturbed by alcohol, caffeine, drugs and emotional tension, and an extra beat disturbs the regular rate. Many people describe this by saying, "My heart jumped into my mouth," or, as you do, as a fluttering sensation.

Almost always there is no important reason for this. It does not mean that you are heading for a heart attack. It does mean, however, that you should have a complete general examination, including an electrocardiogram, to assure yourself that there is nothing radically wrong with you.

I have recently recovered from a heart attack and am now able to spend half a day at work without becoming overtired. I am irritated because my doctor believes that driving my automobile to work in downtown traffic can be harmful. Do you agree?

If ever there was a loaded question, yours is. You are seeking an opinion, hoping to find one that will satisfy your desire and need to drive your automobile. Certainly, you are not seeking an opinion that will substantiate your own doctor's judgment.

The fact that you have successfully recovered from a heart attack is an excellent indication that you are on your way to complete good health. The fact that you are still limited to one-half a day of work means that you are not yet ready to take on the stresses and strains of full occupation. Your doctor's advice, up to now, has been valid. Why should you now undermine your relationship and possibly threaten your health by not continuing to take his advice?

***

My husband has recovered from a heart attack. Yet he has seemed to lose all interest in living even though the doctors have assured him that he can return to full activity.

Many patients remain emotional invalids for months or even years after complete recovery from an illness.

It is not unusual for a man who has recovered from a heart attack to live in the shadow of fear that another attack may occur. "Coronary anxiety" needs the greatest sympathetic assurance by you and your physician. Prodding or shaming him into activity before he is psychologically ready may prolong his emotional convalescence. You may need the help of a psychiatrist to get him to return to his full dignity as a human being.

***

Is angina pectoris a dangerous disease? My husband has just been told that he has it and refuses to believe he should limit his activities.

Angina pectoris is not a disease in itself. Rather it is an uncomfortable, painful sensation in the chest, and an important warning that there may be narrowing of the blood vessels that bring blood and oxygen to the heart muscle.

Anginal pain means that the heart may need more rest, or drugs to increase the circulation. This symptom is the body's cry and when neglected, can lead to troublesome heart problems.

It is most unwise for your husband to stubbornly refuse to recognize the importance of his doctor's warning. Often with proper rest, avoidance of emotional tensions, reduction of weight and the removal of all tobacco, this early warning symptom may be reduced in severity. The heart deserves more consideration rather than such obvious neglect.

***

What is responsible for a sudden fluttering sensation in the heart?

The rate of the heartbeat is controlled and governed by a delicate mechanism. Occasionally it is disturbed by drugs, caffeine, tobacco, infections, injuries and periods of stress.

The fluttering feeling can be terrifying when it first occurs. When one or more of the causative factors are removed, the sudden changes in the heart rate almost always disappear.

A condition known as tachycardia is a sudden increased rate of the heartbeat which presents symptoms not unlike the fluttering feeling. The causes of this condition are usually unimportant. However, if a rapid rate persists, clinical examination and study with the electrocardiogram pinpoints the cause and outlines the treatment.

Occasionally, the steady uninterrupted regularity of the heartbeat is broken by an "extra" beat or extra systole. This means that the heart has taken one or more extra beats in between its regular normal pattern.

With rest, a sudden spell of rapid heartbeat can usually be made to subside. There are many drugs, including quinine, that can break the disturbed pattern of heartbeat and help return it to normal. The fluttering beat can often be stopped by gentle pressure on the side of the neck or mild pressure over the eyeballs. Frequently the rapid rate stops just as suddenly as it occurred, even without treatment.

After a heart attack, I was told to stop smoking. Although I have never been a drinker, I have taken to having one drink before lunch and one before dinner. Is this harmful?

The wisest thing you have done, of course, is to have given up smoking absolutely and completely. There is no doubt, scientifically, about the extra hazards of tobacco in people who have had a coronary heart attack.

About alcohol: There was a time when small quantities were actually thought to be beneficial. In fact, many physicians for many years have recommended small amounts of alcohol with the idea that the blood vessels to the heart and the rest of the body would be dilated by the alcohol.

This universally accepted idea has been denied by several leading specialists who believe that even small doses of alcohol can be harmful to cardiac patients. Because this idea is such a radical departure from that which was formerly believed, I suggest you discontinue alcohol until you discuss this thoroughly with your own physician.

278

Two years ago, I recovered from a severe heart attack. I am still taking blood-thinning medicine, and wonder if I will have to continue taking it for the rest of my life.

If, after two years, your mind is still filled with anxiety about another attack then you really cannot say that you have completely "recovered."

Recovery from any illness, especially a heart attack, is complete only when a person ceases to concentrate on his former illness and enjoys the blessing of renewed health.

The fact that you have been taking a blood-thinning drug for two years does not necessarily mean that you will have to take it forever. Your doctor, by tests of your blood, will decide when this and other medication should be stopped. You must adjust yourself to the fact that you have completely recovered. If you stay within the limits established by your doctor, you will flourish in health, without psychological anxiety.

While I was attending a prize fight, my heart began to pump violently. Could nervous excitement do this?

The excitement associated with some sports most certainly can produce the kind of palpitation you describe. In most instances this is not serious, yet its cause certainly should be tracked down. A drink or two before the match, increased consumption of cigarettes during the match, and emotional tension, could well be responsible for the palpitation. Even high-spirited card games can cause this "pumping" action of the heart. A heart and electrocardiogram examination would give you reassurance.

What does a pacemaker do when it is placed under the skin of a person with heart trouble? I have been advised to have one but I don't believe in it.

A pacemaker is a lifesaving electronic device implanted under the skin of the chest wall to maintain a regular heartbeat. Normal, healthy hearts have their own remarkable mechanism for keeping the heartbeat steady. When, because of some heart condition this mechanism is thrown out of order, a pacemaker is used to electrically stimulate the heart muscle. Working as it does on a battery, the instrument may have to be replaced to keep up its lifesaving properties.

When you question its value because you "don't believe in it," you are inviting trouble. A pacemaker is not a religion or philosophy to be believed in. You have no choice if you want to take advantage of one of this era's greatest scientific advances. Just believe in this concept. You will be benefited, and you will bless the day you followed your doctor's advice.

My husband at forty-six plays handball for two hours a day and is sometimes so utterly exhausted that he cannot have his dinner. Is there any way that I can convince him that this is dangerous to his heart?

The benefits of exercise are admitted, but overdoing it, as your husband apparently does, is folly. The advantage of a sport is the enjoyment of it without the exhaustion your husband feels.

Your desire to convince him must be based on reason. Do not suggest a hazard to his heart. Your own doctor can, after careful examination, present a realistic picture to him so that he will continue his exercise in moderation and without the fatigue you describe.

You must remember that if you pressure him, he may be rebellious because his masculinity is being questioned. Allow him the right to come to his own conclusion without nagging or shaming him into conforming with your wishes, sensible as they are.

Can the heart itself become infected?

Infection, degeneration and tumors can occur in the heart as in any other organ. The heart muscle, or myocardium, can develop an infection after a severe bout of rheumatic fever, diphtheria and other infectious diseases. Sometimes an infection of the kidneys may be responsible for an inflammation of the heart muscle.

The outer lining of the heart or percardium may be infected in people with severe tuberculosis or uremia and following injury.

A fine delicate membrane called the endocardium lines the inner surface of the heart. An infection of this membrane is called endocarditis.

Years ago when the diagnosis was made of endocarditis because of bacteria in the bloodstream the chances of survival were poor. With the advent of penicillin and other antibiotics coupled with blood-thinning drugs like heparin, many patients now survive these infections. Infections of the heart muscle, the outer covering and the inner lining are now treated effectively, returning health to many who might otherwise have perished.

Recently a doctor told me that I have cardiospasm but after all kinds of tests and X-rays, I was assured I had nothing wrong with my heart. Someone is not telling the truth. Doesn't cardio mean heart?

You are confused and frightened by a term that would have been explained to you if you had asked your physician. Cardio does refer to the region of the heart. Cardiogram is a test of the heart.

There is, however, another meaning for cardio. This is the area of the esophagus which leads into the stomach. This is called the cardiac opening. Here, therefore, is the reason for the misunderstanding of your condition.

That which you have is a spasm of the muscle which leads from the esophagus to the stomach. The result is that the esophagus fails to open and, therefore, there is a retention of large quantities of food in the esophagus.

The cause of this is generally unknown. The symptoms of spasm may be belching, nausea and vomiting along with a feeling of fullness in the lower chest. These symptoms may be similar to a condition which is called hiatus hernia which occurs in the same area.

You would have spared yourself a great deal of concern if you had only asked your doctor about the exact meaning of cardiospasm.

How high should the cholesterol be in the blood before it is considered dangerous?

Numbers themselves can only be confusing and may induce fear where it should not exist. A great many other factors besides the amount of cholesterol in the bloodstream determine health and disease. Some people with a very great amount may be in better general health than those with a small quantity, depending on the condition of the other organs of the body.

The normal amount of cholesterol ranges between 150 and 250 milligrams in 100 cc. of blood. Since normal variations of this amount do occur, patients must not base their health on the number alone. It is for this reason that physicians so thoroughly discuss the meaning of cholesterol, blood pressure and sugar "numbers" in relationship to general health.

There are definite diets that seem to reduce the amount of cholesterol in the blood. This is now considered most important in the prevention of narrowing of the arteries to the heart, the lungs and the brain.

Are there some personalities more prone to having strokes than others? Two members of my family suffered strokes and of course it is a source of concern to me.

The fact you cite does not necessarily mean that all other members of your family are candidates for the same thing. There are a great many factors involved in causing strokes and heredity is probably the least important.

The American Heart Association has pointed out some "risk factors" that make a person more prone to strokes. High blood pressure, unrecognized and untreated, is probably the most important. Some heart conditions, marked hardening of the arteries, excessive smoking of cigarettes, obesity and a high cholesterol level in the blood stream are also identified with greater frequency of strokes.

It is interesting to note that many of these are preventable and correctable. For this reason regular health check-ups are valuable in early diagnosis of these high risk factors.

Is it possible to recover completely from a stroke?

Recovery depends entirely on the severity of the condition and the part of the brain involved.

In general the term "stroke" refers to some interference with the blood supply to the brain. Medically, the stroke is referred to as a cerebro-vascular accident. The all-inclusive term of "stroke" is used to describe a broken blood vessel in the brain (hemorrhage); a clot (thrombus) which clogs a blood vessel; or a spasm of the artery that brings blood to the brain.

The brain itself is divided into many tiny segments. One area is responsible for hearing, another for sight, others for balance, speech, and movement of the hands and feet.

The symptoms of stroke vary, depending on which particular blood vessel is involved and where it normally brings blood to the brain. It is interesting that in a right-handed person the speech area is situated in the left side of the brain. In a left-handed person, the speech area is located in the right side of the brain. This becomes an important guide to the doctor in deciding what part of the brain is affected by a stroke.

Today, immediate and intensive care greatly enhances the chances of recovery. The victim is no longer allowed to vegetate. Besides receiving medical attention, the patient is encouraged to embark on a program of reeducation of his muscles and speech while nature itself is working its own wonders. The new blood vessels seem to spring up in the area of the artery that had the vascular accident. Through these small blood vessels, blood is brought to the part of the brain that is deficient to help in a more rapid and complete recovery.

Chapter XIII

Under D For Diet

I have discovered something about dieters. They love to talk about their diets and, when they cannot find a listening audience, they write letters—very often to me. My correspondence on the subject of fad diets, water pills, vitamins, calories, massage and vibrating machines runs very high indeed.

Alas, there are no short cuts or fancy fads or special fat burners that take the place of calorie counting. Diet pills are only a temporary method to start weight reduction. They do not compensate for will power and an earnest desire to acquire and maintain a weight loss.

We've got to be truthful with ourselves when we do count calories. Somehow the massive number of peanuts with that daily cocktail gets lost in the tabulation. A few hundred calories here and another few hundred there can add up at the end of a day to a sizable amount —sometimes the very amount sufficient for the total daily intake of all foods. We need to master the art of "banking" calories. When we eat too much one day, we should limit ourselves the next.

A whole new approach to the problems of obesity, weight loss and the maintenance of weight loss is now being evaluated by a group of behavioral psychologists. Their methods are based on the fact that individual and family eating habits reflect in great measure one's past experiences and total environment.

New eating habits must be encouraged to replace the old ones. For example, many overweight people tend to eat by the clock. Their hunger needs must be satisfied by time pressures rather than an inner need for food. Other fat people live for sweets and rich desserts which they consume at an alarming rate. The fat child becomes the fat adolescent and the fat adult. Eating habits stay.

Would-be weight losers in all new programs restructure their total environment. First, their eating patterns are reviewed, starting with the buying, storage, preparation, serving and eating of foods and even the cleaning-up afterwards. Professional interpretation helps them discover exactly what unfavorable factors are influencing their eating habits. The system has had good results. Clearly, this kind of self-study rather than temporary adherence to a gimmicky diet, may be the real answer to permanent weight control.

Would you explain just what a calorie is and why the calorie count is so important in diet?

Every machine depends on some kind of fuel to keep it functioning. Gasoline and oil provide energy for technical machinery. The body, too, is a machine and depends on food for its fuel to maintain its vital functions, growth, repair and energy reserve.

The unit of heat that is created by the burning of this fuel or food is the calorie. Some foods produce more calories than others. A pound of fat, for example, produces about 4,000 calories. A pound of sugar produces about 2,000 calories.

The "fuel" needs, or caloric needs, of an individual vary with his size, weight, occupation, state of health and even climate.

A lumberjack expands a vast amount of energy; therefore he requires a high caloric intake to supply sufficient food to his body machine. An office worker, using mental rather than physical energy, needs fewer calories to sustain him.

The body has an intricate banking system that balances the calorie intake against the caloric need. If you consume more calories than your body requires for fuel, you will gain weight. If you consume fewer calories than your body requires for fuel, you will lose weight.

What are the basic contents of a balanced diet?

There are four basic groups of which, when included in the diet, can be considered nourishing for the normally healthy person:
1. Milk, butter and cheese
2. Meats and eggs
3. Fruits and vegetables
4. Breads and cereals

Such foods will usually contain all the daily minimal vitamin requirements for the adolescent and the adult. The growing child will (especially during the winter months) need the advantage of additional supplementary vitamins. The elderly and the infirm will also benefit from additional vitamins and minerals.

When these basic foods are used the need for expensive supplementary powders, tonics, elixirs and "magic" blood builders are unnecessary.

If there is a known deficiency your own physician will be the first to recommend additional food substances.

When I finally was able to give up smoking, I gained twenty-two pounds in six weeks. I suppose it is due to the nibbling I do in between meals as a substitute for smoking. Isn't excess weight as dangerous to a person's health as tobacco?

It is not unusual for people who stop smoking to gain weight. There are some doctors who feel that tobacco may depress the appetite. There are others who suggest that there may be some metabolic change that temporarily occurs when one stops smoking.

All agree, however, that the most important reason for the gain of weight is the uncontrolled intake of additional calories. There is a set standard rule for gaining weight in otherwise normal healthy people. When the number of calories that are consumed are more than the calories that are used up there will be a gain of weight.

Excess weight or obesity does place an added burden on the heart, lungs, and circulatory system. The disadvantages of obesity are probably less than the disadvantages of tobacco, but they cannot be compared and measured exactly.

With a sensible regime the weight you have gained will be lost and you will have the double advantage of being free from both of these unnecessary hazards to your health.

Do you have any thoughts about the need to increase roughage in the diet as a method of preventing disease of the intestines?

There has been a revival of interest in the relationship between high roughage or high fiber diets and chronic diseases, even cancer, of the lower intestinal tract.

A group of British and American physicians is concentrating on this problem. They suggest that many conditions of the large bowel would be eliminated if more fiber were included in the daily diet. "We could put the laxative industry out of business by restoring the roughage to our food," says one physician exploring this theory. "Whole meal bread is very coarse and very dense. Eating whole meal bread might do as much for health as giving up smoking."

Most physicians believe that there is great validity to this approach to eating. Yet, it must be emphasized that people with chronic intestinal problems should not, without the specific advice of their doctors, undertake a high roughage dietary regime.

Why do intelligent people simply refuse to admit that sixty-five extra pounds is a dangerous burden to their hearts? My husband is one of those who can't be convinced.

A psychiatrist may use the complex theory of the death wish to explain such problems. Perhaps it does exist, yet I am more convinced that there are intelligent people who refuse to recognize the extra load those sixty-five pounds are putting on their hearts.

It takes no particular brilliance to appreciate the fact that pounds of fat around the heart, blood vessels, liver and lungs do an injustice to the wonderful functioning of these organs. Doctors are amazed that patients who cannot give up tobacco, excess alcohol and who cannot learn to modify emotional stress find they can do so after they have had their first heart attack.

Hard-driving unreasonable people seem to be miraculously converted into angels once they have been stricken by coronary heart disease. They quickly learn that they are expendable in their businesses and that tobacco, alcohol and dietary excesses can be controlled.

It falls within the province of the physician to bring a greater awareness to people like your husband of the need for reevaluation of his total health picture.

Is there any value to massage as a way of losing weight?

It is a misconception to believe that excess poundage can be "rubbed off." Pockets of fat may be redistributed, but cannot be lost with active or passive massage.

There are, however, other advantages to good, sensible massage. It tones the muscles, and gives one a sense of well-being and invigoration.

One must not delude one's self into believing that massage is a way of avoiding calorie counting. The single accepted law of weight reduction is based on reducing the calorie intake. When the calories we eat are greater than the calories we require for our daily activities it is inevitable that a weight gain will follow.

Are vibrating machines good for reducing? I want to buy one, but my husband says they can't help.

Vibrating machines give good tone to the muscles and firm the body, but they are no substitute for a rigid diet. Unfortunately, there is no easy way out. But keep in mind diets and machines of any kind should be used only when recommended or approved by a physician.

My husband has been placed on a low protein diet. Can you suggest where I might find such a diet and one that will be tasty for him?

Low protein diets are available but are usually given to patients by the doctors who suggest them. There are many medical reasons for which protein free and protein low diets are suggested, usually involving diseases too important to be casually treated by haphazard diets. In general, these diets are aimed at reducing the formation of urea, potassium and other chemicals. Diet suggestions taken from anyone other than your physician would be a mistake. He knows the problem, the special needs of the patient and how long the diet should be maintained.

How can a soft diet be made nourishing?

Soft diets are usually recommended to patients with stomach and intestinal disturbances or those with general weakness. Sometimes people who have no teeth and cannot chew normal food are given these easily digested, low residue but highly nourishing diets.

There is fine nourishment in cooked fruit, potatoes, rice, bananas, milk, cheese, puddings, custards and eggs. Well-ground beef, fowl and fish contain all the important ingredients for a nutritious diet. A good vitamin supplement can add sufficient minerals and vitamins and furnish all the needed calories until more food is included in the diet as the patient progresses.

Why must one drink a great deal of water with a high protein reducing diet?

The high protein or "ketosis" diet is said to cause the accumulation of substances which must be flushed out in the urine. It is for this reason that large quantities of water are suggested.

There really is nothing new about this diet which has been known to doctors for many years. Its greatest popularity lies in the fact that weight reduction occurs rapidly and encourages the dieter to continue his efforts.

I believe this particular diet should never be started without your own doctor's sanction. Many problems can arise if it is undertaken by people with an imbalance of minerals or electrolytes in their body.

Why are minerals so important in the diet? Are there diseases which are caused by a deficiency of them?

One of the most remarkable mechanisms in the entire body is known as the electrolyte balance. This is a sensitive relationship between the fluid and the mineral content in the body.

Under normal circumstances there is a vast network of communication from one organ to the other to keep this balance intact. Under special circumstances this balance is disturbed and may in itself be responsible for disorders in various organs of the body.

Electrolyte balance is carefully watched following operations and in those whose illnesses affect the retention or excretion of fluids. Long periods of vomiting in children can cause acidosis. This is a temporary imbalance in the relationship between fluids and minerals. The same can result in adults from long bouts of diarrhea which leave them depleted of fluids and minerals.

When electrolyte metabolism is disturbed after severe burns or following chronic kidney disease, the physician depends on detailed study of the chemistry of the blood to reestablish a normal, healthy balance. Fluids in special concentrations, depending on the specific needs, are given into the vein to replace sodium, calcium, phosphorous, magnesium and other minerals and to establish an exact relationship between all of them.

What foods are high in Vitamin B?

Vitamin B is a very complex one, with twelve or more subdivisions. The foods high in most of these are milk, meats, liver, nuts, soybeans, green vegetables, and whole grain cereals.

Thiamin, one of the factors in Vitamin B, is found in the above foods and in fruits, egg yolks, and brewer's yeast.

Riboflavin, another important subdivision, and nicotinic acid are found in pork, fish, poultry.

Folic acid, another of the Vitamin B factors, is found in leafy vegetables, organ meats, lean meats, veal, and wheat cereals.

It should be noted that excessively high heating of foods for two to four hours, and the addition of soda in cooking may destroy some of the subdivisions of Vitamin B.

Should vitamins be taken all year round?

There is a need for vitamin supplements in the elderly and in the chronically sick, throughout the entire year. Young infants and growing children should be kept on small amounts of vitamins in addition to their nourishing diets.

Adequate, well-balanced, nourishing diets rarely need any supplementary vitamins unless there is a known deficiency of a particular one. The need for vitamins diminishes towards the end of springtime when the sun's rays begin to be concentrated. This lasts until fall sets in. With a nutritive diet and the help of the sun's rays, the body manufactures its own Vitamin D. If fruit juices are part of a well-balanced diet there rarely is need in the adult for any of the expensive food supplements and vitamin additives.

What is your feeling about health foods and natural vitamins?

I know that some of my readers will resent my personal feelings about the health food "industry." My experience in the practice of medicine has been that these highly overpriced foods are bought mostly by people who are least financially able to buy them.

I once entered into a discussion with two proprietors of health stores and came to the conclusion that they both had an encyclopedic ignorance of foods, their function and value and of nutrition. I found, too, that the cost of their products was double the ordinary price of perfectly good vitamin-laden and mineral-adequate foods.

There is nothing mysterious about good nutrition. There are some who manufacture their own "personal scientific discoveries" in order to increase the sale of an ordinary product. I have seen rice that's un-

291

polished, polished, scrubbed, lacquered and coated with "ingredient X" sold at prices that are unconscionable.

Now you know how I feel about "natural" vitamins and health store supplements. My advice is that a perfectly normal diet which includes fruit juice, sugar, proteins, fat, steak, poultry, fish, potatoes, green vegetables and milk distributed over an entire day can make your own kitchen your personal health store. If you must, you can add special wheat germs, but I suggest that you save your money and put it in simple foods.

My whole family is diet conscious. Everything that we eat or drink has a sugar substitute. Can this be dangerous to our health?

It is not unusual for a complete family to be overweight. Eating is a pleasurable experience and when the food is good, as it must be in your house, overindulgence results. Children follow the eating patterns of their parents and, before long, everyone is entrenched in the trap of obesity.

Sugar is an excellent food with relatively few calories. If a sensible diet is eaten by all of you, these few calories put on no additional weight. Sugar may even give a little extra energy to help burn off some of your calorie intake.

The Pure Food and Drug Administration has established that some sugar substitutes are potentially dangerous. Its advice should be respected.

I've noticed that every time my husband has had a heavy snack before going to bed, he is sleepless and restless. I can't convince him that this is bad for him.

Most intelligent adults recognize that there are certain foods that are harder to digest and therefore should be avoided before going to bed. A sensible, light snack in moderate quantity is usually conducive to good sleep for many people.

I recall a study done on a group of volunteers who ate a 300 calorie snack before going to sleep. For one week their sleep was studied. The next week the snack was eliminated. The researchers concluded that there was no difference in the character or the depth of sleep, whether they ate or did not eat at bedtime.

In your husband's case, he has a simple choice; a restless night after a heavy snack, or a restful sleep after a light one. Each individual is his own vigilante.

We read and hear about enzymes in our foods, in our detergents, and in our toothpastes. Yet, somehow, we never hear exactly what enzymes are. Are they good? Are they bad? Or are they just a sales promotion idea?

Enzymes are complex chemicals that play an important part in the functioning of many cells, tissues and organs in your body. An enzyme is involved in all body processes, but in itself remains unchanged. Each group of enzymes has its own function. The entire digestive process that brings nourishment to your body depends on one of the many enzymes that exist in the body.

They are important in evaluating heart attacks, liver disease, disorders of the pancreas, and certain types of cancer. It is now even possible to measure their quantity and add to them when they are deficient.

However, the proteolytic enzymes used in detergents are another matter. Such enzymes may represent a threat to health. Until this is disproved, their use should be discouraged. Also keep in mind that your dentist should be consulted about the use of any toothpaste that contains enzymes or any other unusual ingredient.

Do the emotions play an important part in the process of digestion? I made this point to a group of friends and was astonished to find that they disagreed with me.

There probably is no physical functioning of the body that is not intimately related to the emotions. If I had to choose one particular phase of body activity that is affected most by the stresses and strains of modern living, it would probably be digestion.

It has always been surprising to me that someone can gobble his food rapidly under stress and expect to thoroughly digest it without any physical distress. For this reason, I recommend learning the art of leisurely eating, even if it's only a sandwich for lunch.

Mealtime, unfortunately, has become the period when children are chastised for their behavior and when tense emotional problems are discussed. This invariably upsets the digestive tract and interferes with the true solution of family problems.

Moreover, heartburn, excess gas, belching and general discomfort can frequently be attributed to the emotions. Before this diagnosis is considered, however, a general physical examination must be made to rule out the possibility of an underlying disorder.

Why do doctors recommend black coffee with every diet they put you on?

The emphasis on black coffee is to eliminate the extra calories from sugar and cream. I doubt that black coffee is much of an appetite depressant. Certainly it plays no role in helping you to lose weight.

I have enrolled in a weight-reducing program and I have been successful in losing fifteen pounds. My health is good, but I am concerned that the diet I am on may eventually be harmful.

The fact that you have been successful in losing weight on the dietary regime that has been advised for you is an excellent testimonial to you and the organization you have been working with. My own experience has been that the nutritive elements, minerals and vitamins sufficient for normal daily requirements are contained in these diets.

The great single advantage of all supervised weight-reduction programs is the added motivation given by physicians or by weight-control organizations.

There is no need to fear the threat of malnutrition during any short period of weight reduction. If any fear is to be associated with obesity, it is that markedly obese people are more prone to physical disorders than those whose weight is normal.

I am more than a hundred pounds overweight. I have read about the famous rice diet used at Duke University. Can you give me some idea of the method they use, how long it takes, and how successful it is?

Recently, one of my patients decided to visit the Duke University Medical Center in Durham, North Carolina, to take the "rice cure." This rice diet has aroused international interest as a treatment for high blood pressure and for the massive reduction of weight.

I was fascinated by the detailed account of my friend's experience at Duke University and I think you may find his story helpful. He lost eighty pounds.

Patients must be prepared to devote three or four months to this carefully controlled regime. For the first four days my friend underwent a thorough medical examination, including tests which provided the doctors with a complete profile of his physical and psychological make-up. Then the objectives of the program, underscoring the hazards of obesity, were explained.

The program begins with a two-mile walk. Breakfast consists of one-half a grapefruit, a bowl of salt-free rice and tea. The menu is the same for lunch and dinner, with two ounces of fruit added. Later, depending on the progress of the patient, two ounces of chicken, veal or fish are added with small amounts of squash, asparagus, onions or green pepper. On this minimal caloric intake, weight reduction and control of high blood pressure begin almost immediately.

Obviously, there are other ways of losing weight and controlling blood pressure. None, however, can be successful if you are not properly motivated. It must be emphasized that such a rigid diet must never be attempted without the constant supervision of a physician.

Two of my friends have tried crash diets and were successful. Their weight loss lasted only three weeks after they stopped dieting. What interests me most is that one of them who is a placid person became extremely irritable. Could this be related to the diet?

The value of any diet is two fold. The first is the loss of weight. The second is how long the extra poundage can be kept off.

The typical crash diet aims at the speed of reduction. Many of these diets are unsound nutritionally and may be as dangerous as the overweight that one is burdened with. One cannot count calories for three weeks and then rest on one's laurels and expect the temporary weight loss to be maintained. Consistent, sensible dieting over a long period of time is the only way to maintain a permanent weight loss.

Some crash diets that depend on high protein intake may be responsible for the accumulation of toxic products in the blood. Unless these are washed out with enormous quantities of water, distinct personality changes can occur. Marked irritability, fatigue and underachievement at work are common.

There are no short cuts to sensible dieting. Consistent, medically sound, well-planned diets are not as dramatic, but are far safer and more effective in the long run.

Two of my children are hamburger and hot dog eaters. I worry particularly about the frankfurters and how nutritious they are. Is there any information about this available?

A recent report issued by a consumer group showed that today's frankfurters contain about twenty-eight percent fat, and less than twelve percent protein. This is not a good record for a meat dish. Over the last twenty years, there has been a marked increase of fat, and a lowering of the value of the protein content in frankfurters.

You may not be able to take away the frankfurter from your children's meals, but you will be able to supplement other protein foods in their diet, such as meat, fish, milk, eggs and cheese.

I have asked my doctor to give me water pills to lose weight. He refuses. Many of my friends take them and lose as much as four pounds a day. I am jealous.

Ask those same friends if they don't regain the weight within 48 hours after they lose it.

Then you will understand why your doctor refuses to fall into the trap of the nonsensical use of water pills, or diuretics, for the permanent loss of weight.

Diuretics are very valuable tools in modern medicine. They are carefully chosen for very specific conditions. They are not used by doctors for patients who simply refuse to accept the fact that they are taking in more calories by eating than their bodies need for fuel.

Is there any new and effective way to reduce weight without taking pills?

It must be completely apparent by now that weight watchers and weight gainers have no choice but to count calories. There are no short-cuts, with or without pills.

There is a simple law that is unalterable and that is if you consume more calories than you spend in daily activities a weight gain must follow.

One other factor in the control of weight is important and that is the possibility of some underlying general medical condition. Low thyroid activity can produce overweight. Fluid can be retained in the body tissues under some circumstances. All such possibilities must be checked out before any diet regime can be established.

The notion that some people come from a "fat" family is false. There are no direct hereditary tendencies to overweight. People living in the same family acquire the same poor eating habits and gain their weight by the uncontrolled intake of calories.

The psychological causes for overeating are well known to physicians. Patients must become psychologically ready to lose weight and to keep it off. New fads, special pills and complex machines only help to avoid coming face-to-face with the truth that most of us "just plain eat too much."

I can always tell when my wife is taking diet pills. The slightest infraction of the family rules by one of our children causes a flare-up of anger. She insists the pills have nothing to do with it. How do you feel about taking pills for long periods of time?

Most diet pills, in addition to curbing the appetite, are stimulating, often to the point of causing irritability. The feeling of well-being that accompanies the "pep"pills is often missed even after the regime of dieting has long been forgotten.

Apparently, this is what happened to your wife. She has grown to like that strange false sense of exhilaration and probably persists in taking the pills—which are now no longer diet pills, but rather "pep" pills.

Unfortunately, people can become addicted to their use. If one really wants to quibble about the word "addiction," then perhaps I should say they become dependent upon them. They can and do activate a great many people and cause them to become irritated with little or even no provocation.

I have been taking a small amphetamine tablet every day to suppress my appetite. Can its use over a lengthy period of time be habit-forming?

297

Amphetamines are classed as dangerous drugs. Many people, stimulated by their effects, grow dependent on and even addicted to them. Unfortunately, addictive people usually ultimately increase the amount of amphetamine necessary for the sense of well-being. I emphasize that it is a dangerous drug and you should stop taking it unless specifically ordered by your doctor.

I have been trying desperately to gain weight. I weigh less than one hundred pounds soaking wet. I stuff myself at each meal until I am distressed, yet I cannot gain.

I know that at the age of fourteen you are impatient about your progress in body building. Stuffing yourself to the point of being uncomfortable is a foolish way of trying to gain weight.

There are high calorie diets which, along with food supplements, help people to put on extra pounds.

There are a great many reasons why some people fail to gain weight. An overactive thyroid gland may be responsible for using up many of the calories that one consumes in food. A general physical examination, therefore, is the proper way to find out why the diet you are now eating is not effective in helping you put on those extra pounds.

Is there a high calorie diet for people who are underweight?

Breakfast can consist of fruit juice, hot or cold cereal with cream and sugar. If the eyes and the stomach can take it, scrambled, fried or poached eggs with bacon are exceedingly nourishing. Hot buttered toast and coffee with cream and sugar complete the breakfast.

Lunch can consist of meat, fish, vegetables, potatoes, spaghetti, bread, butter and dessert.

Dinner can be a modification of lunch. To this can be added the midday snack of an ice cream soda, malted milk or some other nourishing dessert. If you wish, you might also have a midnight snack.

This should put on weight on any one who is undernourished. May I suggest that if you are on such a diet you do not mention it to any of your friends who have been reducing all their lives. There is no better way to convert friends into enemies.

Is red meat harmful to people who have high blood pressure? Is there a need to avoid this or any other types of food for this condition?

The myth about red meat as a cause or as a harmful factor in high blood pressure has long been discarded. Red meat, when taken in moderation, contains many valuable nutrients. But its high protein content is essentially no different from the protein in other foods.

The treatment for high blood pressure, or hypertension, found new dimensions with the discovery of valuable drugs for the reduction of pressure in certain of its types. Less and less attention, therefore, is devoted to fancies about food in relationship to the problem.

There may be other reasons why a physician may limit certain foods, because of high salt content for instance, or high caloric content, or high fat content. These suggestions, in addition to modern drugs, have been remarkably effective in the control of many types of high blood pressure.

Can vitamin pills help to increase weight in a very thin person?

Vitamins themselves do not carry sufficient calories to increase weight. A nourishing, high caloric diet will help you gain weight.

What foods should be avoided by people who have an ulcer tendency?

People who suffer from indigestion, stomach disorders, peptic ulcers and intestinal complaints usually know the foods that set off an unpleasant attack.

Most patients feel more comfortable if they avoid fried or greasy foods, concentrated coffee and tea, chocolate and soups made from meat extracts. Alcohol and beer should be reduced to a tolerable minimum. Spices, gravies, pepper and highly seasoned food must be avoided.

All the foods on the "unwanted" list are there because they all tend to produce a large amount of stomach secretions, especially hydrochloric acid.

As the lining of the esophagus, the stomach and the small intestine become healed and less inflamed the diet may become more liberal. Add-

299

ing new foods and watching for reactions is the best way to avoid recurrences of healed ulcer-wounds.

What foods should be avoided in a salt free diet?

There is a difference between a salt free diet and a low salt diet, the one most frequently recommended. It is virtually impossible to eliminate all salt from all food and therefore we must seek foods which are low in salt and do not lose their total palatability.

Salt is a chemical, sodium chloride, which is found in many preserved foods. The sodium is really the salt which is used in the cereals, breads and pretzels that are made with baking powder. This is a hidden source of sodium. Meats like bacon, sausages, brains, kidneys, and most smoked meats contain large quantities of sodium. Shellfish, canned fish and spicy sauces should be eliminated in the low salt diet. Sauerkraut, catsup, horseradish are banned too.

At first people are distressed by such a diet, but soon learn to adjust to it, especially with the new salt substitutes. When the health purpose is attained by the use of such a restricted diet, it is not too great a burden.

How low is a low salt diet? Under what circumstances is it recommended?

There are a number of specific reasons why a physician may suggest the use of a low salt diet. People with high blood pressure, some types of kidney disease, heart failure and during intensive treatment with cortisone are placed on such a diet because of the need to reduce water retention. Salt is, chemically, sodium chloride. The sodium portion of this salt is responsible for the accumulation of fluid.

The nature of the condition suggests how drastic the salt restriction should be. This depends entirely on the judgment of the physician who suggests it. Under some situations like very hot, humid weather, there may be an additional body loss of salt and a depletion may produce strange symptoms. The doctor, therefore, balances the salt intake and may use chemical studies of the blood to guide him in increasing or decreasing the salt intake.

My sister is on a kelp diet kick. This is about the tenth gimmicky diet she's tried.

Kelp is a seaweed known to be highly nutritious and very low in calories. It is often an important part of the regular diet in Far Eastern countries. Kelp has captured the attention of a great many health enthusiasts and actually has been used successfully for many people who are trying to lose weight.

However, a problem has come to light that should be brought to your sister's attention. About five percent of the American people seem to have unusual sensitivity to iodine. Since kelp contains a large amount of potassium iodide it would pose a potential health risk for these people. It is true that this percentage may seem small. Yet, for those who have this sensitivity, complex problems, centered around the thyroid gland, might result.

I therefore suggest that, before anyone plans an extensive period of kelp-supplemented diet, their thyroid function be investigated. Then, with permission of the doctor, this diet could be considered safe.

I read a great deal about iron deficiency and really don't know what it means. Are any special foods used to prevent this deficiency?

A very special type of anemia is referred to as iron deficiency anemia. The only way to determine an iron deficiency anemia is by specialized studies of the blood. The size, shape, and number of the red blood cells indicate to the physician the possibility of iron anemia.

When the condition is present, a well-balanced diet with iron supplements can usually improve the condition. Iron deficiency is commonly caused by chronic loss of blood or severe malnutrition.

There now is a tendency for manufacturers of expensive food supplements to suggest that everyone has an iron deficiency and needs their products as preventives. This promotion is aimed particularly at women, with the suggestion that menstruation is always responsible for iron deficiency anemia. It is not always true and merely induces in many women another sense of anxiety that they do not need. Your doctor is the only one who can make the diagnosis of this condition and suggest treatment for it if it exists.

I am twenty-five pounds overweight. The doctor said I couldn't diet because I am anemic. Is it possible for someone who eats as much as I do to be anemic?

Obese people can also be anemic. There need not be a relationship between overweight and the blood contents. There are dozens of different kinds of anemia which may not be in any way related to dietary intake.

Only a detailed study of the blood can indicate the exact type of anemia that one has. Treatment is then directed at the control of and cure of the condition.

Are there special foods that help children to develop high I'Q.'s? Someone in my high school class said that fish is called a "brain food."

Somehow, there is a mistaken notion that fish, sweetbreads and brain itself have a special importance in the intellectual development of man. There is no scientific truth that any one food is a stimulant to intellectual growth.

The brain is an organ that flourishes and grows on good nutrition as does every other organ of the body. A well-balanced nutritional diet that supplies carbohydrate, protein, fat, minerals and vitamins will sustain good health to all parts of the body.

Intellectual development is the result of reading, studying, and exposure to the sciences and to the humanities. Many young children and adolescents are learning that there are many joys and rewards associated with the processes of learning.

If an infant is allergic to milk and is given milk substitutes, does it interfere with its growth and normal development?

It is said that cow's milk is one of the most totally nourishing foods for the growth of children. Yet many newborn babies who have a special allergy to cow's milk thrive and develop normally and are as resistant to infections as are other infants.

There are excellent substitutes for milk and milk products which

302

supply all the energy that an infant needs. Goat's milk and synthetic "bean" milks contain sufficient nutritives for the child's growth.

It is not unusual for some cases of allergy to disappear when the child is two or three years old. Certainly, there is no reason for your concern; your child undoubtedly is under a doctor's supervision.

Is it possible to become allergic to a food you have eaten all your life?

The complexities of allergic responses are many. I have a patient who cannot tolerate milk at different times of the year. It turns out that he is sensitive to the type of grass that the cow has been feeding on. If you know you are allergic to a food, new or old, the sure cure is to avoid it.

I have had all sorts of intestinal complaints and have consulted many doctors without any real relief. My present doctor suggested that I give up milk and milk products. I can't understand how this can help since I am not allergic to anything.

Your physician wisely suspects a condition known as "lactase deficiency." More and more patients are found to have this condition which is not in any way related to allergy.

The condition is created by a peculiar intolerance to lactose, the most important sugar or carbohydrate in milk. Lactase is an enzyme that is normally found in the small intestine and is the one that digests lactose. When there is a deficiency of lactase, the sugar (lactose) passes on into the small intestine in an undigested state. This can be responsible for abdominal cramps, gas accumulation, and other intestinal symptoms.

Nutritional experts all over the world are now recognizing lactase deficiency and nutritive substances are being sought that will offer the nourishment of milk without the possibility of intestinal distress.

I have eaten eggs two or three times a day for years. Is there any reason why I should stop. My friends tell me that eggs are dangerous for middle-aged people.

I'm afraid you'll have to join the not-too-exclusive club of middle-aged people who have cut down almost completely on this pleasurable food. Your friends are right: The yolks of eggs can contribute markedly to the formation of cholesterol and its accumulation in the blood. Moreover, cholesterol may be responsible for arteriosclerosis of the blood vessels.

You are wise to listen to your friends; you will be even wiser to consult your doctor.

Are stones in the gall bladder caused by diet alone? When should they be removed by surgery?

Some people are more prone than others to form stones in the gall bladder, and in the ducts that lead to and from it. Diet undoubtedly is one of the important contributing factors but infection, too, plays a role. Women tend to develop stones about three or four times more often than men. Pregnancy, with its hormone and perhaps dietary changes, may be a partial explanation for this.

Small stones in the gall bladder may lie dormant for many years without giving any symptoms and may be found during a routine X-ray taken for a totally different reason.

Unfortunately there are no known ways to dissolve stones by drugs. Surgery therefore becomes the safest and simplest method of treatment when distressing symptoms are present. Repeated attacks of indigestion with painful spasms and distension should not be tolerated when once the diagnosis is established by the study of the gall bladder with X-rays and with dyes. Sometimes stones can be removed from the gall bladder or from the ducts without removing the gall bladder itself. Such decisions depend entirely on the judgment of the surgeon and the condition that he finds at the time of operation. Deliberate delay of sugery when it is distinctly indicated invites unnecessary trouble.

I am planning to travel to Mexico and I wonder how I can avoid the intestinal disturbances that so many of my friends have had.

Any change to a tropical or subtropical climate, with new water and new foods, may cause some intestinal or stomach disorders. Mexico cannot be singled out as the only area where salmonella and amebic dysentery are present.

A good safe rule is to use bottled water in any country whose water supply is even vaguely suspicious. In these places, vegetables should be avoided unless they are thoroughly cooked. Fruits with a heavy peel, like oranges or bananas, are safe. Other fruits should be peeled or at least thoroughly scrubbed to make sure that there is no residue of insecticide on them. Only reputable restaurants should be patronized. Standards of hygiene and cleanliness should be of utmost importance in choosing a restaurant. And, for the first few days in new lands, it is best to avoid overindulgence in unfamiliar food.

Are some people more sensitive to foods that contain garlic, onions and alcohol? Why does the odor of garlic, for example, last longer with me?

There is no hereditary or bodily structure or physiological mechanism that makes one person retain the odor of these distinctive substances for a longer period of time.

Garlic leaves its characteristic odor in the following way. After it is eaten the garlic is later absorbed from the stomach and goes into the blood stream. Here is circulates until it gets to the lungs and is exhaled. When the chronic garlic eater exhales it in the pathway of another person, he knows it.

This happens with many other substances and has been responsible for a scientific study called circulation time. In an effort to learn whether or not the blood circulation is normal, a chemical is injected into the blood stream in the vein at the elbow. With a stop watch, "circulation time" is measured from the moment of the injection until the odor of garlic is detected in the breath.

Nature has a wonderful protective device for garlic eaters. They never can get a whiff of their own breath and thus go their way oblivious of the fact that their friends and neighbors know they are garlic eaters. The nose and throat doctor has learned to duck the exhalations of these gourmets.

Chapter XIV

The Troubles With Skin

The skin is the largest single organ of the body. Unlike other organs that have always been recognized for their special importance, the skin was once thought of merely as an envelope or at best, a protective covering.

At last the skin is getting credit for its importance in many body functions. It keeps the body temperature stable; it is a shield against injury; it retains body fluids; it keeps out foreign substances; it protects against invasion by germs; it helps to regulate the flow of blood; it cools the body; it protects against the ultraviolet rays of the sun; it distinguishes individuals by texture and pigment and even distinctly identifies them by the patterns of the finger prints.

Probably the most remarkable faculty of the skin is its ability to heal its own wounds. This self-repair mechanism rivals the wonders of all the other organs of the body.

The skin consists of three layers. The outercovering is the epidermis. It's the epidermis that has the ridges and whorls that make each human being distinctive. This outer layer sheds its scaly dead skin which is then replaced by newly formed cells.

The middle layer, the dermis or true skin, and the subcataneous or deep layer harbor the real wonders of the skin. Sweat glands, sebaceous or lubricating glands, tiny muscles, arteries, veins, protective fatty tissue, hair cells and pigment are all housed in the skin structure, the wonders of which defy the imagination.

The skin is in a constant state of change, repair and regeneration. It varies in texture from infancy to maturity. It adapts itself almost miraculously to changes of humidity, temperature, exposure to cold, heat, frost and rain.

Would you believe that one square foot of skin contains almost twenty feet of blood vessels which open and close to meet the immediate demands of the body. Tiny nerve endings can, in a millionth of a second, send a message to the brain and make the hand quickly withdraw from a burn or injury. Probably the greatest wonder of the skin is its intricate mechanism for healing a burn or any type of wound.

During infancy and early childhood the skin is delicate, velvety-smooth, clear, free of hair and blemishes. During puberty and adolescence, the hair cells become larger, and the sweat and oil glands more active. The skin loses its early softness as it is more and more exposed to climate and injury.

Miraculously, the skin adapts itself to changes in size and shape throughout life. Despite exposure to frost, rain and sun, heat, humidity and dryness, the skin carries on its remarkable functions, protecting the body against external conditions, injury and invasion.

Troubles with skin? Yes, there are. Ask any teenager with a face full of pimples or the fashion-minded young woman with a bad sunburn rather than the bronzy tan she sought, or the individual with very dry skin. And again, let me remind you that the skin withstands more abuse than any other organ. As long as there is life, the skin continues its wondrous process of regeneration and remains the prime line of defense of the body.

What is acne?

Acne is a condition that affects the skin in areas where there are numerous oily, or sebaceous, glands. The skin of the face, back, and chest are the most common sites for acne.

Acne is of course, most common at puberty and is said to affect almost eighty percent of all adolescents.

Why does acne occur particularly during adolescence?

In boys and girls at puberty there is an alteration and imbalance of the sex hormones. It is believed that this temporary change in the hormone balance overstimulates the sebaceous glands and causes them to produce an excess of oily wax.

Are there different types and grades of severity of acne?

There is no definite classification, but acne is considered as being of two types, simple acne and the more complex variety where infection is predominant.

There are also vague gradations of acne. Grade 1 is the type that does not last long and does not leave any severe aftereffects. Grade 2 is slightly more severe but does not leave any noticeable scarring of the face. In Grade 3 and 4 there is severe inflammation and irritation of the skin and underlying tissue. If neglected, permanent scars and pits of the skin result.

What are some of the causes of acne?

There are many associated reasons for this condition. Fatigue, vitamin deficiency, drugs, excessive sweets, allergy, emotional stress and a poorly balanced diet can help an attack of acne to flare up.

Sometimes there is a temptation to pick and squeeze blackheads and pimples which then form small cysts and pus pockets. The staphylococcus germ that normally lives on the skin invades the tissue hurt by squeezing and only complicates acne with infection.

Can acne be prevented?

Diligent cleanliness, using non-irritating soaps, is an excellent preventative. Warm applications to small cysts, pus pockets and blackheads are soothing and far less irritating than vigorous scrubbing and squeezing.

How can acne best be treated?

Patience, perseverance and gentleness are an ideal combination. Over-the-counter or mail order "secret, special and magical formulas" are expensive and harmful because they delay seeking the advice of a physician. Hormones, cortisones and antibiotics must be chosen with special care for the needs of each individual patient.

Anti-bacterial soap can be soothing and help to destroy some of the bacteria which complicates acne. Dermatologists, specialists in skin diseases, sometimes use small doses of X-ray to reduce the activity of the oil producing glands. They are careful to use it only in cases where the need is particularly great.

Can the scars on the face caused by severe acne be removed by operation?

There is now a very successful technique for acne scarring called dermabrasion. As the name suggests, the skin is planed with a rapidly rotating brush until the surface around the "pit" is level. The skin is first anesthetized so that the procedure is really a painless one.

There are other techniques that must be avoided. A number of non-medical people have been using a dangerous "phenol" method for scars and wrinkles. Severe burns of the face have resulted from this method which has been classed by the American Medical Association under the heading of "Quackery."

Skin specialists have improved the abrasion technique as a substitute for surgery so that the results are now remarkably successful and gratifying. Scars that were unsightly are now made barely visible. In some cases, it is necessary to repeat the abrasion in order to obtain a perfect result. Doctors are exceedingly careful to choose only the cases most suitable for this method.

What is the best way to treat unsightly warts?

Unsightly is the ideal way to describe warts. It may be that a virus is responsible for this piling up of excess skin, but the exact one certainly has not been found to teach us how to prevent them.

For some strange, unaccountable reason, most warts disappear in a year or two if they are left completely alone. It is said that after three or four years almost all of them are gone.

When the warts cause pain because they are inflamed, it may be necessary to consider removing them. There are a number of techniques, including burning them with painless applications of trichloracetic acid, or freezing them with liquid nitrogen. Another method is by the use of electrocoagulation, using anesthesia that makes it painless to the child. When they are made to understand exactly what is being done, even small children become remarkably cooperative.

Can you tell me everything that is known about moles? Are they dangerous and what can be done about them? When do they become worrisome?

In essence, that which you want to know about moles is whether or not you can tell if they are dangerous by their appearance. You cannot.

A mole is a discolored spot on the skin usually elevated above the surface and almost always present at birth. The exact cause is usually unknown. Every conceivable scientific approach has somehow failed to answer all the questions about all moles.

Most of them are harmless unless they are irritated, picked on and made to grow. A mole that changes in size, shape, or one that begins to bleed, most certainly needs the attention of a specialist either in the field of plastic surgery or in skin diseases. Even highly trained specialists sometimes cannot tell whether a mole is benign or dangerous. They carefully inspect it with high powered lenses and frequently remove a portion or all of it, for special microscopic study.

The vast majority of skin moles are harmless and should not be a source of concern.

I get many small pimples at the edge of my nose. Then my nose blows up like a comic cartoon. Can diet be responsible?

I doubt diet is in any way related to pimples in the nose such as you describe.

Severe malnutrition, especially in the elderly, may weaken body resistance and make any area of the body more vulnerable to infection.

At the very tip of the nose, where the skin and nasal lining join, protective hair cells are present. Sometimes, too vigorous wiping of the nose may tear out the hairs and open avenues for introduction of the staphylococcus germ which causes small furuncles, or pimples.

Lubrication of the nose with simple baby mineral oil will help prevent recurrence of the pimples. Antibiotics and antibiotic ointment, when prescribed by the doctor, along with a gentle application of heat, can usually control these infections. Occasionally, a vaccine is injected to reduce their frequency and severity.

Boils and carbuncles of the neck seem to plague me. Could these be caused by a deficiency of vitamins or by poor diet?

A boil, or furuncle, is a small collection of pus. It is almost always caused by the staphylococcus germ. Often boils occur in clusters in the same area of the skin. A carbuncle is a far more serious infection. It affects the underlying layers of the skin and the muscle beneath it.

311

An inadequate diet and vitamin deficiency may devitalize the body and make a person more susceptible to such skin infections. However, in a person of your size, who undoubtedly eats a nourishing diet, the chances are greater that some local skin irritation is causing your problem. Some medical conditions such as diabetes, and other debilitating conditions, may predispose some people to infections of this type. The irritation of starched collars may abrade the skin and allow bacteria to be introduced. Lubricating the skin around the neck to prevent "collar rub" is one thing you might try.

Some doctors are enthusiastic about using a staphylococcus vaccine to immunize people against recurring and troublesome bouts of boils and carbuncles. Its value and effectiveness are not completely accepted by physicians everywhere. More important is rigid cleanliness and hygiene in the area of these recurrent infections.

Prompt treatment of tiny insignificant infections with wet dressings, and antibiotics if suggested by the doctor, can prevent complications of these superficial infections.

Only in the past few months have I noticed that the skin on my hands gets red and itchy. Can detergents and other soaps cause this?

Allergic reactions of the skin can most certainly be caused by an increased sensitivity to soaps, detergents and those with added "power-cleaning action chemicals." These are rather frequent reasons for dermatitis of an allergic nature. But then I have seen patients with bizarre allergies to perfume and hand lotions. Almost every other substance can be the causative culprit.

One study of this problem attributed itching, burning, redness and irritation of the hands to detergent powders that contained enzyme active chemicals.

It may be that the enzymes make the skin more susceptible to soaps and powders. If any woman has an unusual reaction she must, of course, discontinue the use of these enzyme soaps immediately.

Can a playful cat cause an infection of the skin with a scratch? How can we tell if I am allergic to it?

Skin scratches caused by a cat do occasionally become infected. It is rare, but does occur. Any deep scratch should be cleaned with soap and water. A mild antiseptic is an added precaution.

A virus can be introduced under the skin by a cat if it harbors it. A condition known as cat scratch fever sometimes occurs even after a scratch wound has healed. Fortunately, it is not dangerous but can be an annoying and debilitating condition.

It is wise to cut the cat's nails short and to keep them clean so that, even if the virus is present, the danger can be minimized.

There is only one way to tell if you are allergic to cat's fur or dander. If you developed any symptoms shortly after the cat arrived, a skin test can readily show special sensitivity. Then a process of desensitization can be tried, since few cat-lovers would dream of giving their cats away.

What changes occur in the skin as we grow older? Why are the hands such a telltale indication of age?

The process of aging is not understood completely. Why some people show their age while others do not may have some hereditary basis, but there are many variables in this picture. Those who live past one hundred are venerated for their age and are always asked to account for their longevity. Some insist that cigars, hard liquor, and carousing kept them going. Others feel that a regime of milk and total abstinence is the only answer. The skin, however, doesn't agree with either.

The most obvious change because of age is the color, the pigment, the texture, and the tone of the skin. It becomes thinner, less elastic, and the wrinkles show. The appearance of the skin, however, does not reflect the health of the heart, the brain, and other organs.

Are there any new forms of treatment for psoriasis?

The chronic disease psoriasis still eludes many of the scientific studies of skin specialists. What is known is that the sun is beneficial. Ointments and salves of all kinds are still used with only moderate success.

Skin specialists or dermatologists have been injecting small quantities of cortisone directly into the silvery, red patches that appear on the skin of the knees, the scalp and the elbows. Your own physician, of course, is in the best position to evaluate the possible use of cortisone. There are some reasons why it cannot be used by all people.

Is scabies a contagious skin disease?

Scabies is most certainly contagious and is highly communicable from one person to another. It is caused by a tiny insect or parasite, the sarcoptes scabiei. This small mite is frequently passed from one school child to another, and causes intense itching of the skin. Sulphur ointment is one of the most effective forms of treatment. Other drugs, too, are available. Sterilization of clothing and bed linen is essential if treatment is to be effective.

Can impetigo be passed on from one child to another at school?

Impetigo contagiosa is known to pass from child to child to adult with forest fire speed. To safeguard the health of children in schools, camps and nurseries, it is imperative that the person with impetigo be isolated and treated.

Rigid cleanliness and avoidance of family towels and utensils can halt the spread. Impetigo can be controlled more readily by high doses of antibiotics in addition to special doctor-directed applications to the skin.

Is ringworm of the skin caused by an actual worm?

The name ringworm is confusing because the condition is caused by a fungus. There are many varieties of ringworm that are called by different names depending on the part of the body that is affected. Ringworm of the scalp is known as tinea barbae. There is also a ringworm that involves the nails, the groin, and the skin in between the toes, commonly known as athlete's foot.

Ringworm must be considered as being contagious although it certainly is not nearly as easily contracted from other people as are the common diseases, such as measles and chicken pox.

Cleanliness and good personal and family hygiene are excellent precautions against passing it on from person to person. Common towels or slippers should be avoided, especially in gymnasiums where the fungus seems to be so prevalent. Ringworm responds to local application in addition to hygenic precautions. There now are a number of excellent medications which, taken by mouth, have remarkable effects on this distressing condition. Griseofulvin is a preparation which is used effectively but only under the doctor's constant supervision.

Ringworm of the scalp occurs rather frequently in children.

There is an excellent lamp which is used for diagnosis of tinea of the scalp. It seems that infected areas of the scalp light up in a special way when this lamp, called the Wood lamp, is used.

What causes shingles and what can be done to make them less painful?

There are few more painful and probably less understood conditions than that which is commonly called shingles. This is an inflammatory condition in which tiny blisters appear in regular formation on the trunk of the body. Almost always it follows the course of one of the nerves. Technically, shingles is called herpes zoster and sometimes zona because the condition girdles the body.

The cause of this distressing condition is an infectious virus which inflames the nerve endings. These blisters are not unlike those that accompany chicken pox. Almost always they come out after a few days of very tender skin sensations with a feeling of pins and needles.

Shingles may affect any part of the body and are seen on the face and even in the outer ear canal. Most often they occur on the skin of the chest wall, the abdomen, the thigh, and the back.

For some strange reason children are rarely affected with this condition. It is definitely a communicable disease and can be transmitted from person to person with direct contact. With advancing age shingles occur more frequently.

The prominent symptom is long lasting pain. Sometimes in patients who are undernourished or who are recovering from a severe illness, shingles may last for weeks and even months. Long after the blisters have disappeared and the skin surface seems to be normal, momentary sharp shooting sensations of pain may occur.

Most of the treatment is devoted to relieving the pain with pain-killing drugs. Rigid cleanliness prevents the tiny blisters from becoming contaminated and infected.

With the discovery of cortisone and ACTH there has been a radical change in the control of this disease. When these are used in the very early phase of shingles, the symptoms can be markedly relieved. When they are given in large doses in the stage before the blisters appear, many of the distressing effects can be modified. Antibiotic ointments are used to cover the blisters to prevent secondary infection.

Some physicians have felt there is great value in the use of an immune serum which is taken from the blood of a patient who has recently recovered from herpes zoster. There may be some advantage to this because it is said to help the body combat the disease.

What is infantile eczema? Can it be prevented? How is it treated?

This type of skin condition is known as atopic dermatitis. It occurs particularly in infants and almost always is considered to be an allergic reaction.

The word eczema is derived from the Greek meaning "to boil." This is exactly the appearance of the skin that is affected. The face is the most common site, but the under surface of the knees, armpits and buttocks may show the characteristic red, angry appearance.

Itching is frequently severe and distressing. It has been noticed that breastfed infants almost never develop infantile eczema. Cow's milk may therefore be the offender. Children with this condition frequently show other evidence of allergy.

The skin should be lubricated with the gentlest preparations, creams and lotions in order to avoid further irritation of the sensitive areas.

It takes a great deal of combined effort by the parents and the doctor to find the offending substance and to bring relief from the skin infection and to avoid its recurrence.

Can cold sores of the lips be caused by a poor diet or vitamin deficiency?

Cold sores have been attributed to many causes, some real and some fanciful. Technically they are known as herpes simplex and almost always are caused by a virus. They can develop at any season of the year, in any climate and in any geographic area.

Overexposure to the sun, stomach and intestinal upsets and allergy can be contributing causes. Emotional upheavals and stress can also be responsible.

Inadequate diet and vitamin deficiency are not directly the cause of cold sores. The only possible relationship could be that these conditions lower the body resistance and invite the virus that causes this condition.

Antibiotics and cortisones are used with discretion by physicians. They seem to be effective in speeding the healing process.

Each year I develop a terribly irritating reaction to poison oak and poison ivy. Sometimes I have been laid up for weeks. How does the poison get into the system? Is there any way to protect oneself against it?

I have often wondered why plants with such lovely sounding names as sumac, ivy, oak, buttercup and primrose can cause so much misery when they touch the skin and yet look so lovely to the eye. Nevertheless, they do contain a very irritating substance, urushiol, which produces all the unpleasant symptoms in highly sensitive people. The sap of a plant can be just as irritating to the skin as the leaf.

When I say sensitive people react to this ingredient, I do so because I'm aware that there are hundreds of people who can be in contact with these leaves and never have the slightest reaction. The secret perhaps lies in the fact that other people are allergic to the plant oils and react violently to the slightest contact with these plants.

To avoid the regular distress you describe, stay away from these plants, especially the three-leafed poison ivy.

Poisonous substances in the plants can be spread from one part of the body to another. They can be passed from one person to another by simple handshaking contact when the irritating urushiol is on the skin. Clothing and tools can become contaminated and pass on irritants from one user to another.

The specialist in allergy should be consulted by people who are markedly distressed by these irritating spring and summer plants. There are ways of effectively desensitizing most people.

When is it necessary to have all the skin tests done for an unknown allergy?

An allergic or highly sensitive person reacts to an offending substance by releasing histamine into the tissues and blood stream of the body. Almost any foreign substance can produce this histamine reaction. In general, allergens or offenders are classified in a number of ways. First, there are contactual materials like cosmetics, furs, feathers, woolens and metals. Next, there are those substances which we eat and these may include any and every conceivable food. To make matters a little more difficult, an allergic reaction can occur following a combination of foods. A person may not be sensitive to ham or to cheese but may be allergic to the combination. That is why it is so difficult to track down the real causes even with the most diligent effort.

Inhalants like pollen are most commonly responsible for the hay fever group. Drugs, vaccines, bacteria, insect bites, serum may all cause reactions that vary from mild to severe, depending on the degree of sensitivity of the person.

Allergic reactions vary. Some people may develop giant hives or urticaria. Others may develop local swelling and some may have a severe asthmatic attack.

The decision to skin test a person depends on the severity of the allergic response. Sometimes it takes the patience of a saint to track down the cause in an effort to free the victim of these distressing symptoms.

My skin itches a great deal and I get hives without any special reason. My doctor seems to think that "it is all nerves." What have the emotions got to do with skin problems?

It is an accepted fact that there is a very close relationship between the emotions and skin disorders. This does not mean that the skin does not also suffer from infections, inflammations, tumors and injuries. It becomes necessary, therefore, that all physical disease must be ruled out before a psychological basis for a skin condition is considered.

Itching and tickling sensations of the skin are all part of the body's pain system. Itching, therefore, becomes a symptom to be evaluated just as pain would be anywhere else in the body.

Highly nervous, anxious, tense and even depressed patients frequently complain of severe and distressing itching. This is an accepted fact, but before this diagnosis is made every effort should be made to uncover a physical reason for these unpleasant symptoms.

It is well known that, during severe emotional periods of anger or fear, marked sweating occurs. Psychological testing has shown how excessive perspiration on the forehead, the hands, and soles of the feet is directly related to the emotions.

Giant hives, with intense itching, can occur even in the absence of allergies, drugs, insect bites or other obvious causes.

When your physician says that "it is all nerves," he undoubtedly arrived at that conclusion by careful judgment. There are now a great many drugs which, by reducing anxiety and emotional tension, can relieve distressing skin symptoms such as yours. The local applications of creams with cortisone is also suggested in some instances.

Patients must learn not to take it as an insult when their physician comes to the conclusion that the emotions may be responsible for a symptom. It is not a sign of weakness or inadequacy.

Is there any harm in using a sun lamp for a half-hour a day? I have read that overexposure to sunlight can cause dangerous tumors of the skin. Does this hold for artificial sunlight too?

A sun lamp gives off ultraviolet rays which have the same effect as exposure to a hot midday sun. The lamps produce the typical redness and pigmentation of the skin if they are used without moderation. One half-hour under an ultraviolet one strikes me as being a very long time, even if the lamp is old and weak and if you have been slowly building up your time of exposure.

The reports of dangerous growths on the skin due to overexposure to sunlight may be true, but they do not deserve to induce terror in those people who enjoy the sunlight. A consultation with a skin doctor, or a dermatologist, can give you assurance and suggest a safe period of exposure to the sun and to the sun lamp.

Is sunburn really a burn? How can it be avoided?

Sunburn is a real burn even though acquiring it may be, for the moment, very pleasant. Anyone who has ever been incapacitated by such a burn attests to the pain and hardly remembers any fun attached to it.

Burns by fire, scalding liquids, sun lamps and sun injure the skin and underlyinng tissues with the same degrees of severity. The degree is a technical one and depends on the redness of the skin, the blistering, the leakage of serum and the toxic effects of all burns.

It is unfortunate that enthusiastic sun worshippers, in their anxiety to acquire a healthy-looking tan quickly, lose their sense of moderation when first they expose winter tenderized skin to the ultraviolet sunrays. Slow, gradual tanning allows the pigment to protect the skin from the concentrated rays of the sun.

A general rule of safety is to begin the tanning process with twenty to thirty minutes' exposure on the first day. There then should be a gradual increase of time, depending on one's past experience, skin coloration and sensitivity. The fair-skinned are much more susceptible to sun hazards than are swarthy, dark-skinned people.

When sun is reflected off the sand and water the intensity of the rays is magnified even through clouds. Sunburn creams and lotions offer excellent protection and may produce earlier bronzing. They, too, can be dangerous if careless overexposure occurs in the false belief that they are completely protective. The eyes are vulnerable to the ultraviolet rays of the sun and should be protected by good tinted glasses. I emphasize *good* because the poor ones offer little or no protection and may permit rays to damage the eyes.

If, despite all warnings, the late Sunday night anguish of a burn has occurred, clean the skin gently with a mild antiseptic soap and absorbent cotton. Do not rub the tender, painful skin with harsh gauze or rough towels. Four heaping tablespoons of bicarbonate, or baking soda, in a quart of cold tap water can be soothing and protective. Cold compresses offer temporary relief. Don't smother the burned skin with heavy greasy ointment. This is good advice for all burns. There are now some excellent anesthetic ointments that can be used with safety. Yet they and pain-killing drugs should be used on the advice of your doctor. Every family has its own special "tribal" remedies for sunburn which include compresses of white vinegar, herbs and tea. Many of them work well, but not as well as the preventive advice of sunning sanely.

Should blisters be opened if they form after a burn of the skin of the hands?

When a blister forms it should be left intact as long as possible. The skin that covers the blister, if unbroken, is an excellent protection against infection.

Sometimes a large blister is filled with fluid and seems ready to burst. The fluid should be freed in a particular way. Gently wash the edge of the blister and apply some mild antiseptic. Sterilize a needle over a flame, wait until it cools, and then carefully puncture the blister at the edge. Press out the fluid through the opening and cover the blister with a sterile or clean piece of gauze.

An excellent treatment for burns that may prevent blistering is to dip the hands immediately into ice cold water. Running cold water over the burns also can be effective in reducing the pain, the blistering and the swelling. Extensive burns should, of course, be treated by the physician.

The temptation to smother the area with greasy solutions must be avoided; they only interfere with subsequent treatment.

I am embarrassed by the appearance of my skin. I can't wear a bathing suit because of white patches over my body. My condition has been called vitiligo. Is there a cure?

Vitiligo is a condition in which there is a marked loss of pigmentation on large patches of skin. The edges are sharply defined from areas of normal pigmentation. The cause has never been definitely found. A heredity factor has been suspected. The skin depigmentation can occur in all races and has no known physical affect on general health. As in your case, the cosmetic affect is most distressing.

A drug has been tried with some success and some disadvantages. Oxpsoralen when taken by mouth seems to help return some of the pigment when the skin is later exposed to sunlight. The drug has some definite toxic side effects and, therefore, must only be used under the direction of the doctor who prescribed it.

We live in an area with insects, mosquitoes and wasps. How can they be discouraged from biting? What is the first aid treatment for severe bites?

The best way to discourage insects from biting is to avoid unnecessary exposure to them. When this is not possible some precautions can be taken. It is an accepted fact that mosquitoes are attracted to people who wear perfumes and fragrant after shave lotions. They also seem to be drawn to highly active people who perspire profusely. And a recent study shows that mosquitoes have a greater affinity for dark clothing. They favor black, dark hues and dark reds, rather than whites, yellows and green colors.

There are many insect repellents which, when applied to the skin, are very effective in preventing the distressing annoyance of insect bites. Some stings can be serious, especially to those who are highly sensitive to toxins. Severe reactions of hives, swelling, pain and itching and asthma demand immediate attention.

The Thayer Hospital in Waterville, Maine, issued the following valuable list of first aid suggestions for very severe insect bites:

1. An injection of adrenalin into the site of the sting and another injection in another part of the body. This site should be massaged to hasten the absorption. The amount of adrenalin should, of course, be controlled by a physician.

2. If adrenalin is not available a pill, Isuprel, kept beneath the tongue should be absorbed, not sucked or chewed. This pill can be repeated once.

3. Put a tourniquet above the site of the sting if it is on an arm or leg.

4. Apply an ice pack to the site of the sting.

5. Antihistamines and cortisone by mouth or injection, under the direction of a doctor, are very effective.

6. Go to a hospital or doctor's office if possible.

7. It is important to identify the insect for more effective treatment.

Vaccines and desensitization techniques can be used for individuals who are known to be particularly sensitive to the bite of insects.

When our daughter was born with a portwine birthmark that covered twenty percent of her face, my wife and I searched for someone who could remove the mark. We were told to try X-ray treatment, but we were frightened to do so. A prominent skin surgeon advised against skin grafting. Our daughter is thirteen now. She is becoming very self-conscious, even though she uses a special make-up to cover the birthmark.

Let me first explain that there are many types of birthmarks and moles that are classed medically as nevi. Sometimes an extensive strawberry mark or portwine stain covers a large part of the face and becomes a psychological oppression to the child and to the parents.

You have had the opinions of excellent physicians and surgeons who mutually agreed not to do extensive plastic surgery on her. Their judgment is based on years of surgical experience and their understanding of the urgency of your problem. If they felt that the surgery would be worthwhile they undoubtedly would have performed it.

There are many forms of treatment that are carefully chosen for each individual case. Surgery, X-ray, dry ice, skin grafting, tattooing, electrocoagulation and abrasion have all been used in some selected cases.

If none of these has been suggested to you, you must now devote yourself to giving your daughter the maximum psychological support so that she may grow into happy adult womanhood. You will be amazed how her young men and women friends completely disregard a birthmark if your child is secure, charming and lovely. Young adults with birth-marks make wonderful marriages and live happy normal lives, often with people who are particularly understanding and sensitive.

At this time it might be wise to have your daughter screened by a physician to find out if she needs any psychological testing to bring out the areas that need your help. With your understanding and the doctor's advice your daughter can be shown the way to grow into maturity without the feeling of an emotional handicap. This takes a great deal of energy on everybody's part, but the results are rewarding.

Can scars of chicken pox be safely removed?

Facial scars and blemishes due to chicken pox, acne and injuries can be removed by a number of ways. Usually the smaller ones can be eliminated by the dermabrasion method. It is simple and safely done with a high speed rotary abrasive brush after the skin has been anesthetized. This electric "sandpapering" removes the outer layers of skin. When healing follows, a smooth surface replaces the pitted marks. A crust appears and remains for about ten days. When it falls off there is left a healthy, normal skin.

Some surgical methods are chosen to fit more extensive needs of a patient.

I had tattoos made on my chest and arm when I was sent overseas. I would go to any length to get rid of them. Is there any operation for this?

I wish your letter could be reprinted in every one of the armed services magazines so that thousands of young men could think twice before they impulsively submit to tattooing. The consistency with which most adults regret their youthful impulse to be tattooed should be emphasized so that fewer young men will fall into the same trap.

Surgery, chemicals, and abrasive skin-peeling techniques have been tried in an effort to remove these telltale evidences of youthful misjudgment. Unfortunately, the results are not consistently good. Sometimes, the scars that are left may be even more disfiguring than the tattoos themselves.

Many highly trained plastic surgeons have been reporting successful methods for disguising tattoos. An opinion from one of these in your own city might be helpful. Do not, however, become involved with tempting, but unreliable, mail order advertisements about miracle methods of removing tattoos.

I had a war injury and am worried about the need to have a skin graft. Do these always take?

You are surrounded in your hospital by highly trained, skillful surgeons. You can be certain that with modern techniques for skin grafting, the chances are great that the graft will take and there will be no need for repeated operations.

Many readers have been interested in the different types of skin grafts. The grafts vary in thickness; some are called full-thickness grafts, others are thin-split grafts. The choice of graft depends on the area that must be recovered. Antibiotics and other treatments protect the graft against infection. The results are often spectacular and the cosmetic effect can be excellent.

Why do some people bruise so easily and develop ugly black and blue marks?

Black and blue marks under the skin are not nearly as pretty and attractive as their medical name, ecchymosis. They are all caused by leakage of blood from a broken vessel. The blood vessel may be a tiny one just underneath the skin, or it may lie more deeply and may bleed because of more severe injury.

People with fair skin, especially those with an extra layer of soft fat, seem to be blemished rather easily. The combination of fair skin, blonde hair and blue eyes seems to bruise more easily than others.

Only rarely is there an important medical reason. In some individuals the blood vessels and capillaries seem to be more fragile and break with the slightest touch. This capillary fragility need have no important blood disorder to produce it.

There are some types of anemia and, of course, hemophilia, the bleeder's disease of royalty, that are responsible for bleeding almost without provocation.

The resistance of some people to physical injury is as difficult to explain as is the resistance of others to emotional disturbances. There are psychological and bodily thresholds in all people that vary from time to time.

Chapter XV

Answering The Unexpected

Just when I think there isn't a question of medicine left in the world that I haven't heard, I get a letter from a worried woman with a cough who says it all started when her husband brought home some pigeons. Could it be her husband or the pigeons that she's allergic to? Naturally in my response to her query I explained that exposure to pigeons may indeed be responsible for lung infections and advised her to have a skin patch test to locate the source of her problem. But I couldn't resist adding that perhaps, for her health's sake, those pigeons should be encouraged to fly in one direction only.

It was weeks afterward that I received another letter from the same woman, thanking me for my advice and saying that her husband had taken up bowling. The pigeons had flown the coop and she no longer coughed continually. "And there's no smell in a bowling ball," she added.

I tell this story only to demonstrate how important a sense of humor can be when discussing one's medical problems. Humor is one of the most effective tools we doctors have for solidifying the relationship between ourselves and our patients. Properly employed, it can help dispel the formality of that super-sterilized atmosphere that can easily become a part of a physician's image and intimidate a patient into becoming over-respectful and non-communicative.

Humor can reduce anxieties; it can even speed recuperation. A patient who maintains a cheery outlook and who avoids thoughts of gloom and doom after an illness makes a far more comfortable quicker progress, too, than the patient who loses himself or herself in a welter of self-pity and distress.

Often patients unwittingly ask questions that bring a smile to my lips. A woman asked if one could live after the spleen is removed by surgery. "Why operate at all, if there was no chance to live?" I reminded her gently.

On the whole, the history of medicine is remarkably free from refreshing evidences of humor. In my travels, even today, I've observed that European medicine especially still exhibits all the pomposity it has had for centuries. Fortunately, American medicine is relinquishing stiffness and stuffiness for caring, warmth, empathy—and a touch of humor. It makes a difference.

That's why I am always delighted when some of my correspondents ask the unexpected, the naive, the incredible. And why I like to answer in kind—whenever possible. I close with one more irresistible example. A husband wrote me at length about his wife's allergies, adding that the one bright aspect to the situation was her allergy to mink. His joy didn't last long. It turned out she was not allergic to sable! I chuckled all day at that one.

Here are some examples of the surprise questions that tumble out of my mailbag from time to time.

My husband has become a pigeon fancier and flies them from our rooftop. It may be a coincidence, but from the day he bought them I have been coughing. Is it possible to be allergic to them?

The old axiom about birds, "for some people they sing," must be extended to "for some people they cause coughs."

Actually, there are many people who are allergic to the dander and the excretions of birds and frequently develop chronic bronchitis and asthma. Exposure to pigeons may be responsible for long-standing and severe irritations and infections of the lungs.

A strange yeast-like fungus, the cryptococcus, has been found in diseased pigeons in various parts of the world and in many areas of the United States. This fungus causes very serious effects in man. Not only the lungs but all other organs of the body can be affected if this fungus invades the human body.

If you have been able to trace a relationship between the time your husband began to fly pigeons and the onset of your cough, the chances are good that an allergy exists. A skin patch test can be performed to find out if you are allergic to the dirt, dust and excretions of pigeons. For your health's sake, the pigeons should be encouraged to fly in only one direction.

Can wax in the ears cause deafness?

The normal skin in the ear canal produces wax. The purpose is to lubricate the outer ear and to protect the delicate lining from dirt, debris and irritating foreign particles.

When there's a chronic infection in the middle or outer ear, wax doesn't form. Wax accumulates when there's a narrowing or unusual curve in the canal.

Wax only rarely can cause deafness. If you were to plug both your ears with cotton or even your fingers, you would immediately notice how difficult it is to block out ordinary sound or speech. Try it.

Deafness that interferes with normal hearing deserves immediate attention for the more important causes of deafness.

Do animals really hear better than man?

Animals may not hear better than man, but they do hear better the sounds of higher pitch.

The normal hearing range for most humans is about 20,000 to 30,000 cycles. This is the technical term for the measurement of pitch.

Animals can hear sounds with a pitch as high as 50,000 to 75,000 cycles.

Can ether be used as an antiseptic for open cuts, wounds or sores?

Ether has been used for its cleansing action rather than for its antiseptic value. There are many better antiseptic solutions valuable for this purpose. Any one of these can be purchased at the pharmacist.

I do not believe that ether should be a household cleansing agent. The fact that it is highly inflammable adds another unnecessary hazard to the home. There is no point in subjecting you and your family to a drug for which there are safer substitutes.

What is the immediate remedy for a bump on the head that is beginning to turn black and blue?

A black and blue mark on the head, or anywhere on the body, means that a blood vessel has been broken by the injury and that blood is seep-

327

ing into the soft tissues. The very first and immediate treatment should be pressure over the site of the injury. Then ice packs should be used in order to slow down the seepage of blood. This combination generally is excellent for injuries.

When the bleeding has stopped, as it does with pressure after a half hour or more, heat can later by applied to hasten the recovery of the hurt tissues. Heat helps to absorb the blood under the skin more rapidly and facilitates the return of the soft tissues to their nomal condition.

During the past ten years a new idea has been used successfully for the more rapid absorption of blood after an injury. A special type of enzyme is now taken in tablet form.

In a very complex way these enzymes help to reduce the swelling and make the black and blue marks technically known as ecchymoses disappear more rapidly.

What causes the embarrassing, growling noises of the stomach that always seem to happen in a quiet restaurant?

The only thing that can compensate for these rumbling noises is the loveliness of the technical name. It is known as borborygmus, and is the splashing, gurgling sound caused by air trapped in the stomach or the intestines.

Other places that seem to induce noisemaking are churches and quiet theaters. When this happens to me, I look intently and accusingly at the person next to me and pretend that this strange organ music is not related to me in any way.

Actually, air is always present in the intestinal tract. Doctors can listen for it with their stethoscopes. In some conditions, it has important meaning. Almost always borborygmus is unimportant, although if it persists, its cause should be sought. Many people are chronic air swallowers, especially those who eat rapidly and carry on excited conversations while eating.

I recently visited a relative who told me he had a hookworm. Can this be transmitted to me even with a short contact?

Hookworm, a parasitic infection, occurs mostly in warm, moist climates. It is usually introduced by way of the skin from contaminated soil. I doubt that a short contact and exposure to your relative means that you have had this worm transmitted to you. It is wise that your physician thoroughly examine the stool for parasites. Modern drugs can keep this condition under control when once it is known to exist.

I would be grateful if you would explain what trichinosis means. Is it contagious?

Trichinosis is a disease caused by a parasite, trichinella spiralis. Infection by this parasite, a round worm, can occur when raw pork is eaten or when it is inadequately cooked. The parasite is sometimes found in bear meat, too.

The larvae, when eaten, are taken into the blood stream and carried to many of the tissues and organs of the body. When they enter the muscles they cause inflammation followed by deposits of calcium which cause pain on motion.

Many other muscles of the body become involved and can cause many unpleasant, although not always dangerous, complications. The incubation period from the time the pork is eaten until the onset of symptoms is about seven to fourteen days.

The symptoms are so strange and diversified that doctors suspect it because of the indistinct pattern of the illness. Swelling of the eyelids and face along with intestinal symptoms in patients that give a story of eating pork suggests the diagnosis. Blood studies are helpful in confirming the suspicion.

Sometimes a small piece of tissue, a biopsy, is taken from a muscle and inspected for the parasite.

The disease is not contagious. It occurs in families because all the members may have eaten the same poorly-cooked fresh pork at the same time.

Do deep furrows on the tongue have any significance? Both my mother and I have them. She insists she developed this condition at my age of forty-seven.

The condition you describe is the one referred to as a "geographic tongue." This rather interesting description came into being because of its resemblance to a relief map.

There may be some hereditery link that caused this in two members of the same family. The chances are great that your mother and you had these furrows all your lives and that they were not deep enough to attract your attention.

There is no serious implication to this appearance of the tongue. Rarely does it ever indicate a dietary or vitamin deficiency. There is no treatment that will alter the appearance or the depths of the furrows.

What causes a "charley horse" and what can be done about it?

Many of us have been awakened at one time or another from a deep, comfortable sleep by a sudden painful cramp in the muscles of the leg. If you have, then you know how distressing, even terrifying these spasms can be. Although they may last only a few minutes, they cause great anxiety.

Painfully annoying, too, are the cramps that occur while you are awake. The charley horse, which plagues athletes, falls into this last category.

Cramps are caused by narrowing or spasm of the arteries that bring nourishing blood and oxygen to the muscles of the legs. The causes are many and varied. In the elderly, arteriosclerosis is one of the major causes that impair the normal flow of blood.

There are many simple causes of leg cramps, too. Bed sheets too tightly bound down, tight garters that restrict the circulation of blood, even improperly fitting shoes may cause leg cramps.

In most instances, night cramps are more uncomfortable than serious. However, if they persist, the exact cause should be determined and removed.

When a painful cramp wakes you, don't slap, kick or bruise that tender leg as somebody may suggest. It has troubles enough without that old wives' remedy.

Better, try to walk slowly, or gently massage the leg. The spasm of the blood vessels responsible for the cramps will soon disappear. Generally, if you relax, the spasm will.

If pain persists, warm moist towels applied to the leg bring comfort and relief. Recently, quinine prescribed in special doses by doctors and taken at bedtime seems to prevent these recurrent spasms.

Does a phobia mean that a person is afraid of everything?

Phobia comes from the Greek word *phobos* meaning fear. To be phobic is to be afraid or to have a severe aversion or dislike to something.

Almost always a person's fear is directed to one or more situations. Therefore, in front of the word phobia is another Greek derivative which describes the specific type of fear.

A morbid fear of high places is called acrophobia (*acro* means highest). The fear of dark places is called nyctophobia while a fear of strangers is called xenophobia.

Cancerphobia is used to describe people who suffer from an intense fear of developing cancer. Claustrophobia is a fear of closed, locked-in spaces.

Aerophobia is an intense fear of fresh air or drafts. So bizarre and extensive are the types of phobias that there is even one called astrophobia or fear of celestial space and outer world galaxies.

There are endless phobias and many of them exist in people without disturbing their capacity to function as normal productive human beings. Sometimes the phobia may become so severe and insistent that it actually changes the pattern of living of the individual.

Can severe rages, anger and bad temper cause physical ailments?

It is an accepted fact that the emotions play a vital role in all physical disorders. This is the basic law of psychosomatic medicine. The *psyche* (mind) and the *soma* (body) are a single unit that determines the total health of the total patient.

I can flatly say that in all the years I have practiced medicine I have never seen a single patient who did not have some emotional factor in his illness. Everyone is concerned about the nature of his sickness. Some are more distressed than others. Some hide their anxiety while others express it.

Anger, bad temper, fears and anxieties undoubtedly upset the normal functioning of the body.

Psychological problems are known to produce asthma, stomach ulcers and ulcerative colitis. Diseases of the colon particularly seem to be identified with aggression and frustration.

Constipation, diarrhea and abdominal strain are only a few of the complaints noted by people under tension. Headaches, especially of the migraine type, have similar identification with controlled or uncontrolled anger.

When people are made to realize that bad temper and anger are an expression of inner turmoil, perhaps they can be induced to seek some

331

psychological guidance in order to bring a greater stability to their lives.

What can cause hiccups to last for weeks? How can they be stopped?

Hiccups are also called singultus or hiccoughs. By any name they are most annoying and not nearly as amusing as they seem to be to people who are the observers.

A hiccup is caused by a sudden spasm of the muscles of the diaphragm, which divides and separates the chest from the abdomen. A complex series of nerves that run from the brain to the neck and down through the chest can be responsible for the spasm of the diaphragm.

The phrenic nerve, particularly, may be irritated by extremely hot or cold foods and may cause an occasional hiccup. When this condition lasts for a long time it is devitalizing. Conditions in the esophagus, stomach, intestines, pleurisy and alcoholism are a few of the causes. There are many emotional reasons for hiccups.

Everybody who has ever had an attack of hiccups has his own personal remedy to stop them. Drinking a pint of cold beer without a stop is not too unpleasant an idea on a sultry day.

For teetotalers a glass of plain cold water may do the same. Re-breathing into a paper bag and thus building up the carbon dioxide in the body can stop it.

Swallowing crushed ice or hard bread, holding the nose tightly squeezed, smelling snuff to sneeze and pressure on the eyeballs may all singly or individually stop the attack.

There are now a number of drugs used under a doctor's supervision that can control these spasms. Hypnosis in specially chosen cases has been effective when used by physicians, psychiatrists and psychologists, all specially trained in the use of this method.

I notice that I become very uncomfortable when I go to a high altitude. This happened in Mexico City, and twice while I was skiing. It seems that I'm the only one who's bothered.

It is difficult to understand why some people are affected more than others by "mountain sickness."

Mountain climbers, skiers and ordinary travelers who are suddenly transported to high altitudes may develop dizziness, rapid respiration, headache, a sense of weakness and an increased heart rate. Many people affected by altitude complain that, for a day or two, they are unable to sleep.

Here are a few suggestions from experts for your plight. When a trip to a high altitude is anticipated it is prudent to decrease the total food intake and increase the carbohydrate proportion. It is often helpful to carry hard candy as a dietary supplement.

A barbiturate, taken for one or two nights before and the first few nights after the traveler's arrival, will minimize the insomnia.

Skiers and travelers who have followed these suggestions, by also eliminating tobacco and alcohol, have markedly reduced the headache and nausea that may result from high altitudes.

It would be wise, of course, to find out if there are any special medical reasons for your discomfort.

Can the lines in the hands tell a person's future? I was frightened to death by a palm reader at a party.

It is sad that you have been caused so much misery by one who, unscientifically, takes the responsibility of guessing your future. I know that I will be bombarded by believers who will send me limitless case reports of great diagnoses of disease, speculations about the fate of the world, a person's longevity and the exact time to make crucial decisions. Put me down as a nonbeliever who accuses them of scientific fraud and often financial exploitation.

Whether or not you paid for that advice in money is not important. You paid a heavy price in emotional distress and that is far more expensive than an outlay of cash.

The science of dermatoglyphics is a highly complex one because every human being has his own set of fingerprints, with ridges and furrows that last throughout his lifetime.

Although some physical conditions show characteristic creases in the skin, none of these furrows can be used to tell fortunes, life expectancy or the possibility of disease. You have paid an emotional penalty for allowing yourself to be victimized.

I know someone who consults an astrologist and a palm reader before any important decision is made. What does this mean?

The first thing that impresses me is that this person is in such a state of conflict and confusion that she cannot even decide whether to consult an astrologist or a palm reader.

After years in the practice of medicine I have learned that arguments about politics, religion, astrology, palm reading, yoga, health foods, megavitamins and "magical" scientific forms of treatment usually wind up the way they started, with two people in disagreement.

Whatever support individuals get from palm reading and astrology must fulfill a personal need. So long as it does not harm their physical health you should not be too concerned.

Why do doctors examine the nails of a patient?

Fingernails that scar, split, break, discolor or have ridges can be important diagnostic signs. The color of the nails (unpolished, of course) is of significance in severe anemia.

Fragile, thin nails can sometimes be associated with vitamin deficiencies and inadequate diets.

Brittle nails can be due to special intestinal disturbances in some rare instances.

Marked thickening or clubbing of the fingernails and tips of the fingers are sometimes strangely connected with chronic lung conditions such as emphysema.

The nails tell an important story only to the doctor. Don't inspect your nails and interpret your findings based on these rare possibilities.

What is the cause of a black furry discoloration of the tongue?

Long-continued concentrated use of some antibiotics is known to cause such a discoloration. The dark furry patch usually lasts a short time and then disappears. The color of the tongue soon returns to normal.

It is believed the condition is due to a temporary overgrowth of a fungus. Fortunately, this is more of a nuisance than a medical problem.

A too vigorous effort to scrub the tongue clean can injure it.

My wife is a laxative bug. She is constantly giving some to me or one of the three children. She actually keeps a chart of our regularity. How can I break her of this habit?

This is indeed a new switch on the concept of breaking the laxative habit. It is difficult enough to break one's own but to break your wife's laxative habit may be a yeoman's job.

I can understand that the children fall into the trap of taking laxatives because of their mother's pressure. What are you deprived of if you were to say, "I just won't take it?"

We in the practice of medicine are always amazed by the number of people who believe there should be a state law and a Constitutional amendment that make it necessary for everyone to have a bowel movement every day. It is absolutely ridiculous to find this compulsive, unreasoning concentration on regularity.

Almost always it goes hand in hand with "special diets," expensive food supplements and wheat germ mash in everything except an ice cream soda. Your own doctor must show your wife the faults of becoming a laxative-centered family. When she sees the light, with simple education, all of you can be spared the dependence on laxatives that comes with their prolonged and unecessary use.

I am about to marry a young man who is twenty-eight years old. He, like his father, has had gray hair since he was twenty-one. My sister insists that graying hair in a young man means that there is a greater likelihood of early aging. Is there any validity to this idea?

The tendency toward premature graying of the hair has never been thoroughly understood or explained. Some people have studied the problem from the point of view of thyroid and other hormone deficiencies. Others have considered the psychological basis for this condition. The secret still persists. You may rest secure in the knowledge that there seems to be no relationship between graying of the hair in the young and good health and a normal life span.

The added distinction that graying of the hair gives to the personality is an additional reason for your good judgment in proceeding with the wedding.

There seems to be a possibility that my ancestry goes back to the American Indian. Is there any way of determining this medically?

No chemical tests, blood tests, or X-ray studies can throw light on the ancestry of anyone.

335

The only way to determine ancestry is by a diligent research into family history.

Is it possible to live after the spleen is removed by surgery? I know it is a very important organ but do not know exactly what it does.

The spleen is a very special organ that lies in the left upper portion of the abdomen. It plays a most important role during the development of the embryo by manufacturing both white cells and red blood cells.

After birth and throughout life it produces very important specialized white blood cells. It is also the burial ground for red blood cells that have worn out their usefulness and are being replaced by others.

Throughout life it answers emergency calls when the body needs extra blood or extra cells during illness. It is felt, too, that the spleen acts as a filtering agent to clean the blood of germs that may be circulating in the bloodstream.

The spleen is removed for certain kinds of anemia which threaten the life of the patient. Patients with hemophilia, the royal bleeding disease, are markedly benefited by the removal of the spleen in certain well-chosen cases. The decision to remove the spleen is only made after intensive study and consultation between the physician, the general surgeon and the blood specialist, or hematologist.

When once the spleen is removed its important function is taken over by other organs. The bone marrow, too, is an active blood-forming organ and takes over some of the properties of the removed spleen. One can live just as long as any other person if the spleen is removed.

How is trench mouth acquired? Is it a venereal disease?

Trench mouth is the common term used for a medical condition known as Vincent's angina. It is caused by a germ known as the fusiform bacillus which can be passed from one person to another by kissing or by the use of a common glass or eating utensil.

It is a rather disagreeable infection with inflammation of the gums which may extend to the tonsil area, the floor of the mouth and the linings of the cheeks. The fact that it is contagious when passed on from person to person by direct contact does not mean that it is a venereal disease such as syphilis or gonorrhea. A venereal disease such a syphilis or gonorrhea is one that is acquired as a result of sexual contact with one who is afflicted with the condition.

Trench mouth usually begins with a mild fever and a general feeling of being washed out and tired. The swelling and redness and pain in the gums is associated with bleeding on pressure and a foul odor to the breath. The glands of the neck may become enlarged and tender, especially when there is a secondary infection on top of the original condition.

Poor dental hygiene is probably one of the ways to invite this type of infection. Only occasionally are vitamin deficiencies and nutritional disturbances a cause. Treatment is directed to relieving the painful symptoms while antibiotics are used intensively to destroy the germ. Consultation with a dentist after the acute phase has subsided may uncover areas and pockets that may house the cause of its germ.

What is meant by thin blood?

Thin blood has no meaning either to doctors or to the advertising people who created this medically pointless term. It may be true that blood is thicker than water but it is also true that gold is thicker than blood. And gold in many forms is reaped in by people who sell expensive blood thickeners that have no medical value.

This does not mean that anemia of the blood is not present in some people. However, there is only one way to find out if a person has anemia, and that is by a complete blood study. This shows the number of red cells and the amount of hemoglobin. When a blood study is accompanied by a complete physical examination, the causes of anemia can usually be found.

Simple anemia, with an iron deficiency, can be controlled with iron replacement. Expensive tonics and fancy named supplements make medical suckers out of all who fall prey to such advertising.

A few years ago, I contracted serum hepatitis from a blood transfusion after surgery. Some friends still think that it is not safe to visit me because they think it's contagious.

The type of hepatitis you acquired through a blood transfusion is known as homologous serum hepatitis. Like other forms of hepatitis, or infections of the liver, the cause is definitely some type of virus.

Blood contaminated with this virus, when introduced into the bloodstream of a patient during transfusion, may set up an inflammation of the liver. For this reason, all blood now in use is under strict surveillance to be sure that donors are not obviously carriers of illness.

Rigid attention to sterilization of all instruments has materially re-

337

duced the danger of this complication to transfusion. New chemical methods are now being tried to detect the presence of a substance known as the "Australian antigen" to further reduce the complication of hepatitis.

Your friends do themselves and you an injustice by falsely believing that contact with you presents any hazard to them. The condition you had is certainly not contagious or transferable to them.

Is there really an illness called butterfly disease? Can it be the result of working with butterflies?

The term butterfly is a descriptive one, named because of its appearance over the bridge of the nose and the side of the face. The skin is red and, to some people, seems to resemble the shape of the head of a wolf. This is how the technical name lupus erythematosus was first used to describe a very serious skin condition that has no relation to the handling of butterflies.

The cause of this condition is still unknown. There have been many speculations that lupus is caused by intense exposure to sunlight, to drugs, allergy and tuberculosis.

The disease for some unexplained reason happens more frequently in women past the age of thirty. With it there may be involvement of the blood vessels, nervous system, heart and the kidneys.

Before the days of cortisone and ACTH, the results of treatment were not encouraging. Today with earlier recognition and more intensive treatment, the severe complications can sometimes be avoided.

What is a horseshoe kidney? Is it dangerous and can it affect a normal life?

This unusual condition occurs in about one in every five hundred people. In the absence of any infection, people who have this unusually shaped kidney are as healthy and live as long as those with two kidneys.

Is it a sign of illness or trouble if one sneezes when looking into the light? Does this mean that the person should stay out of the sunlight?

One of the gentlest and most remarkable mechanisms is involved in this perfectly normal process of sneezing while looking into the sunlight. It is called the naso-ocular reflex and is a perfectly normal mechanism of the body.

This reflex occurs to many people when they look into any strong light. It need not be the sun. Chronic sneezers know that there is nothing more frustrating than to come to the very edge of a sneeze, prepare for it with a covering handkerchief, only to find that the sneeze maliciously disappears.

When this happens and a sneeze is "almost there," look into any bright light and the chances are good that an explosive sneeze will follow.

The fact that this perfectly normal physiological experience happens does not mean that there is a need to avoid the sun. Remember it is a bright light, not the sun itself, that is responsible for the reflex.

Comedians make so many jokes about surgeons leaving sponges in the abdomens of patients that I honestly am concerned about an operation I am about to have.

Exploitation of a serious situation by comedy acts as a psychological release not only for the comedian but for the listener as well.

There is no reason why you should be anxious or fearful about this very rare situation in the operating room.

These accidents almost never occur because there is a "sponge count" at the end of all surgery. This means that every sponge given to the surgeon must be accounted for.

A surgical sponge is not a sea sponge, but rather a large pad of gauze to which is attached a metal ring for added safety and indentification.

Can alcohol fumes be dangerous to a young child who is given a sponge bath to reduce fever?

Yours is a very valid question that only recently has been given serious consideration. Doctors have suggested that heavy concentration of alcohol vapors may be toxic to a young infant. Tepid water as a sponge bath is almost as effective. In older children, this concern is of course minimized.

I like to sleep with the windows wide open. I find that I get a better night's sleep when it's cool. My husband insists that the windows be kept closed because night air is poisonous and dangerous. Can this really be a health hazard?

339

I have always believed that any marriage that lasts more than twenty minutes is a testimonial to the adaptability of a man and his wife. The conflict as to whether to eat Chinese food or steak, to watch television rather than go to a movie and to keep a window open or closed is somehow always resolved by the give and take of mature people.

Let me immediately tell you that night air is no more poisonous than day air because both of them are so completely polluted in every large city in America. The only time that night air is more dangerous than day air is if you live near a factory which is spewing its filthy smoke into your windows during the night shift. Air is air, depending not on the time of day but on the cleanliness and control of air pollution.

I never could quite understand the great need for some people to "freeze to death" at night. These same people are the very ones who bundle themselves up carefully during the day, wear scarves, hats, warm clothing, fleece-lined boots and thermal underwear.

When nighttime comes, some strange psychological disease overtakes them. After being so completely protected during the entire day, women get into delicate nightgowns and men get into ill-fitting, baggy, thin pajamas and go to bed. First, however, they convert their bedroom into a homemade refrigerator and then proceed to freeze themselves into unconsciousness.

I don't mean to get involved in your marital happiness. Why don't you do exactly as I do. Tell your husband to learn to freeze with the window wide open as I have learned to do. I lost that battle a long time ago.

Is it possible for the stomach and intestines to fall out of place?

A condition does exist in which the organs of digestion fall from their normal place in the upper abdomen. This condition is known as visceroptosis. In many cases, this displacement of the stomach and intestines may be due to the general body build. In other cases, there may be a general loosening of the attachments that hold these organs in their proper position.

The true diagnosis, rather than just the patient's suspicion of it, can be determined by X-ray examination. If this is substantiated, supportive belts, corsets and girdles may alleviate the painful symptoms, even though the basic condition is not cured.

In severe cases of visceroptosis, surgery may be the best way of repositioning the organs.

Should a hot water bottle or an ice bag be used for stomach pains?

I assume that, when you refer to the stomach, you mean the abdomen. The stomach is only one of the many organs that are housed in the body's abdominal cavity.

Because pain is one of the important symptoms, its character, severity and duration can only be judged by a physician. The location of the pain and the direction in which it shoots suggests to the doctor many possibilities.

It is for this reason that pain must not be suppressed with heat, ice bags and pain-killing drugs without the definite approval of a doctor.

The regular and easily recognizable pain of menstrual cramps can, of course, benefit from heat. A cyst of the ovary or an attack of appendicitis may definitely be harmed by heat. Freezing with ice is sometimes suggested by a doctor for appendicitis but only when the patient is under his constant observation.

Pain is so important in the diagnosis of abdominal disorders that doctors use pain-killers very sparingly so that this important symptom will not be masked or hidden.

The decision to use heat or cold is a responsibility that must not be taken by anyone who is not trained. It takes the most astute knowledge to know what disorders are present within the abdomen.

When food is swallowed, where does digestion first begin?

Saliva produced by three sets of salivary glands contains enzymes that start the process of digestion while food is chewed. Saliva moistens the food and makes it easier to be broken down by digestive juices.

The process of digestion continues in the stomach where hydrochloric acid and a new set of enzymes begin to break down starches, sugars and fats into substances that can then be absorbed and used by the bod,. The pancreas and the liver bile continue the work in the small intestine.

Is the black lung disease caused by pollution of the air?

The black lung disease is one of a group of lung conditions known as pneumoconioses. These conditions consist of abnormalities, inflammations and infections of the lungs due to constant inhalation of dust particles. People who are exposed to the fumes of iron for many years may develop siderosis. Anthracosis is caused by inhalation of coal dust that becomes deposited in the lungs.

The most dangerous is the coal miner's or black lung disease which can lead to many complications. Thousands of coal miners become chronic invalids because adequate protective devices are not used against deposits of coal dust in the lungs.

Those who live in the area of coal mines must, of course, suffer from the polluted air but certainly not to the same degree as those who are actually mining coal deep in the shafts.

It is shameful that so many people must spend their lives as invalids when modern technology can clear the air even in the most ghastly working environment.

___

Is sclerosis of the brain the same as multiple sclerosis?

Sclerosis of the brain or cerebral sclerosis refers to degenerative changes in the brain caused by blockage of the arteries that carry blood to the brain. The term is not really a good one because it can be vaguely used and serve only to confuse rather than to clarify.

Occasionally symptoms of cerebral sclerosis or atherosclerosis may be confused with those of multiple sclerosis. But they are two distinctly different diseases.

Multiple sclerosis is a disease whose cause is still unknown and one which affects the brain, the spinal cord, and the nerves that lead from it. Much is known and much information is being accumulated about this strange, slowly progressive disease which is characterized by periods of remissions or good health.

Cerebral sclerosis may be associated with changes in behavior or marked forgetfulness. These symptoms are rarely found in multiple sclerosis.

___

Is it safe to borrow someone else's lipstick? I have a friend who is constantly forgetting her own.

It is unwise to trade cosmetics in this way. I recall a bacterial study that revealed powder puffs contaminated with staphylococcus germs.

Many people may build up an immunity to their own personal mouth and skin germs and be free from infection. Yet the germs that are safe for them may cause infections in others.

Several cases of severe eye infections were recently traced to an infected mascara brush that had been passed around at a school play.

Cosmetics are very personal and should be kept that way.

Chapter XVI

New Horizons —The Best Is Yet To Come

The history of civilization is mirrored in the history of medicine. The art and practice of medicine and science is interwoven in every phase of man's accomplishment. And plainly, the history of a nation's economy, intellectual and artistic attainment has been dependent on the health of all of its people.

New and revolutionary ideas in science and medicine have, through the ages, opened new horizons for the benefit of man. Every generation brings with it newer achievements, newer forms of treatment and newer aids in diagnosis. Within our memory span is the discovery of the miracle of anti-biotics, the creation of cortisone and the eradication of what seemed to be an unconquerable disease, poliomyelitis or infantile paralysis.

These and many other brilliant achievements show the hope that lies within the framework of science. No period in modern mankind's history has had greater visionary horizons than those that exist today. Here are just some of the scientific dreams that have become or are becoming practical reality:

Greater understanding of the genes and the chromosomes may markedly reduce the catastrophes of birth defects.

Synthetic blood may soon be available for transfusions. This would eliminate severe reactions and the constant search for special types of blood.

Vaccines against syphilis, gonorrhea, herpes viruses, and the common cold are imminent.

Nuclear powered artificial hearts are being tested.

The possibility of a blood test for the early diagnosis of cancer is more than a fanciful idea.

Drugs to improve the memory of the aged are already being studied.

A technique by which peaceful sleep can be induced by electric stimulation to parts of the brain through the skull is being developed.

Studies to keep the body from rejecting transplants of the heart, the liver, and the kidneys are a practical reality.

An "insulin machine" which can be implanted in the bodies of patients with diabetes is possible. Whenever the blood sugar level rises, an exact amount of insulin will be poured into the blood.

Learning to teach chimpanzees how to talk may help brain-damaged and autistic children to learn and remember.

New techniques for surgery for deafness are increasing.

Prostaglandins can become the wonder chemicals for the control of asthma, high blood pressure, kidney disease, ulcers of the stomach, thrombo phlebitis, arthritis, glaucoma and, perhaps, even cancer.

There is possible treatment of loss of taste and smell, using copper and zinc.

There will be highly complicated intensive care units in hospitals.

Heart-lung machines that make possible all open heart surgery, are possible.

Kidney dialysis machines will be more common.

Radioactive isotopes are already in use for the scanning of the brain, the heart, the lungs, the kidneys, for diagnosis and treatment.

Artificial replacement of joints of the body, the hip, the fingers, the elbows, the shoulder, the knee and toes is now possible.

The early recognition of an RH baby and the prevention of birth abnormalities associated with it is a real potential.

Drugs for the control of severe mental illness, including schizophrenia and paranoia, are increasing.

Tranquilizing drugs, psychotropic drugs and psychic energizers are being improved.

Expansion of aerospace medicine and the use of the by-products of nuclear fission and nuclear fusion offer great possibilities.

Rehabilitation of the injured, the handicapped, those born with birth defects and the victims of stroke is improving.

The diseases of malnutrition can be prevented with the newer knowledge of total nutrition, vitamins and minerals.

New surgical techniques for the replacement of the larynx will give better speech to patients with cancer of the larynx.

Early diagnosis of cancer of the breast with mammography and thermography exists.

Electrocardiograms can be transmitted by telephone to a central computer.

Computers can be used for diagnosis and even outline of treatment.

Synthetic skin to be used for burns and for plastic surgery is possible.

A ten-minute operation in the eye surgeon's office may soon be safe for eye cataracts.

Blindness from glaucoma may soon be prevented by a drug inserted into the eyelid. The drug will control the tension within the eyeball responsible for glaucoma.

Teeth implants and metal implants into the gums will avoid the need for dentures.

The complete eradication of tooth decay with drugs and the laser beam is almost a reality.

Bones from cadavers may replace cancers of the long bones to prevent amputation.

Electric currents may be painlessly applied to the brain from the outside for the relief of intense pain, for the control of epilepsy, for the eradication of male impotence, for safe anesthesia and even to control appetite to lose weight.

There can be chemical antagonists to drug addiction and alcoholism.

Detoxification of alcohol by chemicals is the subject of experimentation.

There will be electrical devices making it possible for completely paralyzed paraplegics to walk up steps and to function independently.

Corneal transplants are being improved.

Anti-virus drugs are being developed.

Bypass operations for coronary heart disease are becoming more common.

Safety of anesthesia can be increased through the use of new drugs.

Complex systems in recovery rooms can offer better care of post-operative patients.

The prevention of blindness from glaucoma with highly sensitive instruments that detect it in its earliest possible phase.

New operations for the removal of cataracts make possible, in selected cases, hospitalization no longer than forty-eight hours.

Vaccines against meningitis and hepatitis will be added to the many vaccines that already exist.

The control of Parkinson's disease by surgery and with L-dopa will be improved.

There will be universal use of the pap test for the earliest detection of cancer.

Fiberoptic instruments will "see around corners" in the lungs, in the gall bladder and in the intestines.

Newer studies will result in the development of immunoglobulins and other forms of immunity.

There will be a one-dose cure for rabies.

Biofeedback techniques can control pain, sleep, overweight, excess tobacco and overabuse of alcohol.

The use of hypnosis will become an effective tool in the study of psychoneurosis and for the control of pain.

The discovery of new drugs will make it possible for thousands of mental patients to leave psychiatric hospitals and to be able to function in society.

Newer ways of controlling drug addiction and alcoholism will appear.

Yes, the best is yet to come!

An Afterword:
On Fear

You hold this book in your hands because you fear illness or disease, as all of us do. Yet, fear itself is an illness. Fear is a communicable disease, transmitted, not by bacteria or viruses, but by human to human. Sometimes, fear is transmitted unwittingly, sometimes in error and sometimes, purposely.

Fear is an all-pervasive disease that slowly insinuates itself into our lives, devitalizing them and destroying our physical and emotional fibers.

Fear, as an illness, is a circle whose circumference is everywhere and whose center is nowhere.

Fear is a powerful destructive force that can play havoc with careers, with social attainments, with relationships between husbands and wives, and between parents and children. It can alter productivity and sociability, whether at work or in the community.

The greatest potency of fear lies in its being hidden. Because it cannot be counted or contained, fear is not charted in disease statistics. Yet it ranks first as a demoralizer and as a threat to emotional and physical health.

For many years in the practice of medicine I have noted the increase in the number of patients who come to my office overwhelmed with fears disproportionate to the severity of their illnesses. Their fears have nothing to do with sex, age, occupation, social, financial or intellectual level, or ethnic, religious or geographic groupings.

They suffer from fear of all diseases—cancer, heart attacks, tuberculosis, arthritis, strokes—of growing old, of cataclysmic destruction by nuclear bombs, of economic upheaval. These fears constantly bombard our inner security and cheat us of tranquility.

Yet children are born into this world unafraid. But from the moment they enter this society, forces set in motion by the complicated emotional machinery of their parents exert fear-producing pressures on them. Later, these fears are magnified until they play an active part in the emotional growth and security through adolescence to adulthood.

351

This magnification occurs because fear is big business. Under the guise of medical education, fear has been exploited and has become a gigantic, lucrative, money-raising device. Jugglers of statistics, using ingenious advertising techniques, have used terror masquerading as health education to haunt all of us and devitalize our emotional energies.

Such man-made threats overwhelm us with persuasiveness. If we were to believe the statistics of death and destruction used in some fund-raising campaigns, our destiny would be a disaster. We could not shake off the threats that one out of five would be dying of cancer next year or that one out of twenty of us would be assigned to a mental institution. There we would be visited by our children, one a victim of cerebral palsy, another with multiple sclerosis, a third with leukemia or rheumatic heart disease, and the last would be at home unable to break his appointment with his psychotherapist. And this could occur only if we were fortunate enough to escape the ever-compounding effects of tobacco, alcohol, heart disease, arthritis, tuberculosis and strokes.

Now add to these the mortality statistics of Memorial Day, Fourth of July and Labor Day accidents, and there is practically no chance of survival. Anyone who is alive at the beginning of any month must indeed be the beneficiary of good fortune.

Such induced fear drives many people into the outstretched arms of every conceivable form of quackery within and without the boundaries of the law. All of us in the practice of medicine are confronted daily by evidence of the invasive forces of fear.

The utilization of fear is indeed big business. Fund-raising campaigns induce us to give generously to these health organizations. Many of these do serve an extremely useful purpose. Some do not. For, in addition to the money paid by the public, it pays a heavier price in destroyed inner tranquility. Fund-raisers know that fear and anxiety, when pushed to outer limits, pay off in greater contributions. Sympathetic understanding for the needs of others is a characteristic trait of the American people. They give generously. But often there is the unexpressed hope that by giving they are buying themselves an immunity to that special disease.

It is not unusual for patients to tell their doctors how carefully they inspect and examine themselves every day of their lives. This is part of the teaching by some of the intensive fund-raising campaigners. Patients literally look at their tongue in the morning for changes in color. They inspect their gums and mouths for their daily cancer checkup. Then comes the routine examination of the breasts for hidden cancers and tumors. After this, there is a careful inspection of the urine and stool for unusual color or bleeding. The more terrified ones count their pulse rate, take their temperature and some even take their own blood pressure. When the daily careful inspection is complete, many read the obituary columns to see how closely their age group compares to the recent dead.

Yet since the beginning of this century, the longevity rate has increased to where it is the highest in the history of mankind. The child born today has a life expectancy of almost seventy-five years, because of gigantic strides made in medicine, surgery, technology, chemistry and the bio-medical fields. It is sad to find so many people who are dying their lives in fear rather than living their lives in hope and in potential happiness.

Are there any rules to control the insidiousness of fear? There are. It is necessary to face fear frankly. The attitude that this too shall pass is a treacherous error. For time is no healer of fears. The cure for the disease of fear does not lie in any wonder drug. It starts with the recognition that it exists and that there is a need for psychological guidance and direction.

It is no shameless thing to seek psychotherapeutic help. It is no greater shame than seeking help for pneumonia or a broken leg.

The family doctor, the psychologist, and the psychoanalyst are bulwarks of support for the anxious ones. Some patients may need only redirection of their energies and a clearer understanding of their emotional conflicts. Speaking out their fears and confronting them minimizes their potency.

It is an arduous task to dig deeply into one's background and extract painful memories that for years have been covered by the facade of pretense. When these memories are recalled and inspected with the help of a trained specialist in the field of psychotherapy, a refocusing of the patterns of living evolves. When completely understood, fears can be converted into a positive, constructive force. Fear is a highly complicated alarm system which, when properly used, can protect our physical and emotional stability.

To surrender to fear is to forsake ourselves and abandon our hopes and dreams. Fortunately, the disease of fear, like all other diseases, is vulnerable and yields to the "miracle drugs" of hope, courage, faith, inner security, education and freedom from superstition.

Index

361